SMOKING AND WOMEN'S HEALTH

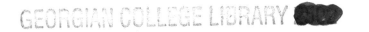

SMOKING AND WOMEN'S HEALTH

MERIDETH K. WESLEY AND
INGRID A. STERNBACH
EDITORS

Nova Science Publishers, Inc.
New York

Library of Congress Cataloging-in-Publication Data

Smoking and women's health / Merideth K. Wesley and Ingrid A. Sternbach (editors).
     p. ; cm.
  Includes bibliographical references and index.
  ISBN 978-1-60456-148-7 (hardcover)
  1. Smoking--Health aspects. 2. Women--Tobacco use. 3. Women--Health and hygiene. I. Wesley, Merideth K. II. Sternbach, Ingrid A.
  [DNLM: 1. Smoking--adverse effects. 2. Smoking--epidemiology. 3. Smoking Cessation--methods. 4. Tobacco Use Disorder. 5. Women's Health. QV 137 S6668 2008]
  RA1242.T6S58846 2008
  362.29'6082--dc22
                                2007049413

Published by Nova Science Publishers, Inc. ; New York

Contents

Preface

The Office of the US Surgeon General, in a detailed report entitled "Women and Smoking," made the following statement: "When calling attention to public health problems, we must not misuse the word 'epidemic.' But there is no better word to describe the 600-percent increase since 1950 in women's death rates for lung cancer, a disease primarily caused by cigarette smoking. Clearly, smoking-related disease among women is a full-blown epidemic." -- David Satcher, MD, PhD

Tobacco use accounts for nearly one third of all cancer deaths. Tens of thousands of women will die this year from lung cancer, which has greatly surpassed breast cancer as the leading cause of cancer death among women. More than 90% of these deaths will be due to smoking.

In addition to increasing the risk for lung cancer, smoking is a risk factor for cancers of the cervix, mouth, larynx (voice box), pharynx (throat), esophagus, kidney, bladder, pancreas, and stomach. It is also connected to some forms of leukemia. This new book presents the latest research in this field from around the world.

Short Communication A – Cancer of the head and neck is the fifth most frequent worldwide. One of the principal locations within this region is the oral cavity, with approximately 3% of all cancers occurring in this area with a rising in incidence. In some geographic areas, such as south-west Asia, oral cancer is the most frequent cancer in men and the third most frequent in women. Oral Squamous Cell Carcinoma [OSCC] represents more than 90% of all tumors of the oral cavity, the remainder are distributed between melanomas, non-squamous cell carcinomas, and adenocarcinomas of the minor salivary glands, sarcomas, malignant odontogenic tumors, lymphomas, leukemias, myelomas and metastasis.

Two distinct precancerous lesions are described in the oral cavity: leukoplakia and erythroplakia. Of these, the first is undoubtedly the most frequent. Its prevalence varies from one country to another; a recent study in Germany found a prevalence of 2.3% in males and 0.9% in females. As with oral cancer, its principal etiologic factor is smoking, and at a time when this habit is shifting towards a younger population and increasing in females, it is to be expected that the prevalence of leukoplakia will increase in young women. Attending to these established data in the western population, the authors wish to focus on the epidemiology of oral cancer and its presentation in the female population.

This paper proposes two objectives:

- On the one hand, to highlight the changes seen in the epidemiologic distribution of oral cancer with particular reference to its increase in young people, women and the principal etiological agent: smoking.
- On the other, to demonstrate that the most efficient measures that can be taken in order to diminish the morbidity and mortality associated with OSCC, are to increase the diagnosis of precancerous lesions, and to make aggressive efforts aimed at reducing alcohol, and above all tobacco consumption, especially among women (primary prevention), and at the early detection of malignant lesions (secondary prevention).

Short Communication B – By encouraging women to stop smoking or to avoid smoking in the first place, public health officials could prevent untold amounts of morbidity and mortality in a vulnerable population. For example, smoking is linked to several forms of cancer (oral and throat, esophageal, pancreas, kidney, bladder, uterine) and, in particular, lung cancer—the leading cause of cancer mortality among women. A total of 90 percent of women's deaths from lung cancer are believed to be caused by smoking. In addition to lung cancer, smoking is associated with other lung diseases, coronary heart disease, and stroke. Each year, cigarette smoking kills an estimated 178,000 women in the U.S. For much of the 20th century smoking was regarded as a lifestyle issue that affected men primarily. Recognition of smoking as a crucial women's health issue would help to reduce the toll that smoking-related morbidity and mortality take increasingly upon female smokers.

In the U.S., the gender gap for rates of smoking has narrowed since the 1960s to a level for women presently within a few percentage points of men's rates. During the mid-1960s, more than one-half of men and one-third of women smoked. Then, following the publication of the U.S. Surgeon General's Report on Tobacco and Health in 1964, the rates of cigarette smoking declined substantially among both men and women. However, between 1965 and 1990, the rate of decline was much greater among men than among women. Since the beginning of the 21st century, smoking frequency among both genders has continued to decline. Nevertheless, despite declines in smoking rates over the past four to five decades, nearly one-fifth to one-quarter of the U.S. population continues to smoke. As of 2003, the female-male differential in smoking rates was only about five percent (19 percent versus 24 percent, respectively). As a result of earlier and persisting high rates of smoking, mortality rates from lung cancer among American women increased by 600 percent from 1930 to 1997.

Women, in comparison with men, should be regarded as a special risk group to health impacts related to smoking. The risks of death for respiratory and vascular disease are higher for women who inhale while smoking than they are for men. Cigarette smoking has been linked to abnormal menstrual function, infertility, menopause at a younger age, and lower bone density after menopause with increased susceptibility to hip fracture.

Although evidence indicates that smoking endangers the health of mothers and their developing fetuses during pregnancy, the percentage of women who continue to smoke during pregnancy is cause for alarm. Although this percentage has tended to decline over time, it was, nonetheless, about 12 percent in 2001. The contribution of maternal smoking to low birth weight as well as miscarriages and prematurity has been documented extensively.

Among young women who smoke, those who are rearing children are more likely to be current smokers than those women who are not raising children.

Chapter 1 – Cigarette smoking among female college students continues to be a daunting problem. During this developmental period, choices made often have long term consequences for the health and well being of women. The factors affecting young women's decisions to smoke are in some ways distinctive from those influencing young men's. Clarifying these factors is important because it may provide information valuable to the development of more effective prevention methods.

This chapter summarizes several empirical investigations examining psychological issues affecting young women's decisions to smoke. The role of affect and appetite regulation, young women's ambitions, and the interpersonal context in which smoking occurs, are considered in this research aimed at describing the issues shaping young women's smoking choices. Female students showed higher levels of empathy, which may play a role in their greater vulnerability to depression and use of tobacco to regulate emotional states. Although it was hypothesized that appetite regulation would play a prominent role in women's decisions to smoke, the data failed to support this expectation. In these undergraduate samples, no gender differences in career ambitions emerged. The majority of the females expected to remain employed outside the home after having children, although several hoped to reduce their involvement in work during their children's early years. Most women expected an egalitarian division of household responsibilities in their future families. Interestingly, the majority of the males studied did not anticipate having an employed spouse after starting a family, and few expected to contribute equally to household chores. In general, young women perceived maternal employment more positively than their male counterparts did. Young women endorsed the benefits of maternal employment for children more strongly than males. Males also were more likely to perceive maternal employment as posing hazards to the development of children. These gender differences were mitigated somewhat by the respondent's maternal employment history (evaluations of maternal employment were generally more positive among children whose own mothers had worked outside the home), but still emerged among those from all family backgrounds. There was no evidence that women undergraduates use substances, including tobacco, more than men in order to manage the pressures associated with educational, career, and family ambitions. Women were also similar to men in their reactions to social situations prompting cigarette smoking. Both men and women reported greater tobacco use in interpersonal campus contexts involving alcohol use. Finally, both men and women reported similar responses to contexts involving smoking restrictions. The implications of these findings for prevention program planning are explored.

Chapter 2 – Every year nearly one million women die from tobacco-induced diseases worldwide. The majority of tobacco-related deaths are due to cardiovascular diseases followed by lung cancer. Although smoking related cancer deaths are decreasing among men, they are increasing among women – 90 % of female lung cancer deaths are attributable to smoking. Moreover, smoking contributes to osteoporosis, breast cancer, and pregnancy complications. Because prevalence of smoking has not decreased as successfully among women as men, the authors can expect that smoking-related illnesses will continue to increase among women. Health burden is further enhanced by the fact that the current female smokers are more likely to have other co-morbidities (high nicotine dependence, depression, physical inactivity, low education) contributing to more severe and chronic conditions. Smoking cessation is the most rapid way to decrease tobacco related morbidity and mortality. Although majority of tobacco users would like to quit, less than 10% succeed in a given year. Weight concerns, stress, depression, lack of social support, and low education level are some of the factors contributing to poorer outcome in cessation treatments for women than men. Women report also greater physical and emotional dependence on tobacco than men do. Successful treatment for tobacco dependence among women should include both pharmacological and non-pharmacological components. Pharmacological tobacco dependence treatments have been actively developed during the past decade. They include wide selection of nicotine replacement therapies, bupropion, and varenicline. Non-pharmacological treatment includes behavioral interventions such as relapse prevention or cognitive-behavioral counseling and should always be added to pharmacotherapy. Hindrances to success come from findings that nicotine replacement therapy alone may not be as effective for women as for men, and that none of the pharmacological treatments are recommended for pregnant or breastfeeding women. Cognitive-behavioral therapies addressing negative affectivity and weight concerns have been found promising. Similarly, exercise has been tested as a novel and particularly suitable treatment for female smokers. In order to reduce the health burden of tobacco among women worldwide a lot more work needs to be done both in prevention and cessation. First, we need to find ways to reduce the initiation and development of dependence of tobacco use among young women. Second, we need continue to develop treatments that offer social support as well as address weight concerns and negative affect. Third, we need to identify and remove barriers preventing women from utilizing treatments.

Chapter 3 – Smoking is a critical hazard for women in their reproductive years, particularly when they are pregnant. It is a well-established fact that smoking is very detrimental to health, and for pregnant woman smoking is detrimental also to the health of the fetus, the newborn and the infant. Smoking in early gestation and through pregnancy is associated with adverse outcomes, and some of these effects can be avoided by reducing smoking or quitting entirely. Research on the health consequences of smoking has obtained results indicating that smoking is associated, among other things, with early pregnancy loss and complications of labor and delivery, preterm delivery, stillbirth, high rates of sudden infant death syndrome (SIDS), and low birth weight, in addition to intrauterine growth retardation.

Research over the years has clearly established both short- and long-term benefits for women who do not smoke during pregnancy. Therefore, it is an important task of health professionals to influence people's smoking behavior and to disburse information about the negative effects of smoking on health. However, achieving changes in smoking behavior in pregnant women is not an easy task. Of women who quit smoking spontaneously, i.e., persons who stopped smoking before entering prenatal care, many went into relapse and resumed smoking sometime before obstetrical delivery. Similar patterns of resumption are noted with both sudden cessation and gradual reduction in smoking. Persons with a more positive attitude toward smoking cessation more often intend to quit smoking. Therefore, smokers' intent to quit smoking should receive additional support.

An increasing number of health care professionals recognize the problem of smoking during pregnancy and workers in health education have developed several smoking cessation programs for pregnant women with the expectation that these educational projects would produce positive results in terms of behavior change. Subsequent evaluations of the programs, however, suggest that behavioral change often is temporary. When it comes to health and preventive programs, the difficulty of improving future health status is a well-established fact. The likelihood of persuading mothers to quit is not always promising, especially with regard to heavy smokers. Apparent expectations to quit are not always followed by behavioral change.

Chapter 4 – Research studies have consistently shown a relationship between smoking cessation and weight gain. Unfortunately, concern about postcessation weight gain prevents many individuals from attempting to quit smoking and may contribute to treatment attrition and relapse. Postcessation weight gain is currently of particular concern given the rising prevalence of overweight and obesity in the United States. Effective interventions that target both smoking cessation and postcessation weight gain are needed to address the public health concerns associated with smoking and obesity, in addition to the weight concerns that prevent many individuals from successfully quitting smoking. This chapter provides a qualitative review of the research on combined smoking cessation and behavioral weight control interventions. Fourteen studies that included dietary or physical activity components in combination with a smoking cessation intervention met the inclusion criteria for the present review. Overall, findings suggest that adjunctive weight management interventions provide little or no long-term weight control benefits, although such interventions do not generally have a negative impact on cessation outcomes. Future directions for research are discussed.

Chapter 5 – There is some growing empirical evidence suggesting significantly lower success rates of Nicotine Replacement Therapies (NRTs) in women than in men despite a generally lower self-reported nicotine dependence in women, fewer number of cigarettes smoked per day and lower nicotine exposure. Nevertheless, some more recent reviews question the significance of such findings suggesting that the observed trends may be of little clinical significance. At the same time several lines of basic nicotine research provide converging evidence that men and women respond to nicotine treatment differently in a variety of domains: physiological, affective and cognitive. Moreover, such response differences may be further accentuated by underlying genetic differences in a particular type of dopamine receptor. Overall these findings seem to add empirical support to conclusions that gender differences observed in smoking cessation trials are real and may be clinically important. Yet, experimental nicotine studies have often been plagued by methodological shortcoming related to nicotine dose used, types of cognitive and affective tasks, types of nicotine replacement, duration of nicotine deprivation, lack of control for the stages of the menstrual cycle and use of oral contraceptives in women. Therefore, evaluation of available evidence and interpretation of emerging findings becomes increasingly challenging when one considers the above confounding factors. The present review is thus aimed at a systematic critical scrutiny of extant research on gender differences in response to nicotine and suggests most promising avenues for future investigations in this area.

Chapter 6 – Background: Studies on the effects of gender and smoking on cardiovascular and peptic ulcer disease have been reported in Western countries, but data from Asian countries are limited and inconsistent.

Methods: The authors examined the effects of gender and smoking on cardiovascular and peptic ulcer disease using the longitudinal data of the Adult Health Study collected during biennial health examinations from 1 July 1958 to 30 June 1998. The examinations included medical history, chest x-ray, ultrasonography, and fluoroscopy or endoscopy. Smoking histories were obtained from 5 questionnaires self-administered during different time periods. The authors estimated the relative risks for being female and for "ever" versus "never" smoking after adjusting for significant effects of age, city, birth cohort, calendar time, alcohol intake, and radiation dose. They also examined the interaction between gender and smoking.

Results: Eight hundred and fifty four strokes, 215 aortic aneurysms, 1093 gastric ulcers, and 437 duodenal ulcers were detected between 1958 to 1998: and, from 1978 to 1998, 125 myocardial infarction were detected. The incidence of myocardial infarction, stroke, and gastric and duodenal ulcer was significantly higher in men than in women, but the authors found no gender difference for aortic aneurysm incidence after adjustment for smoking status. The authors detected positive associations of smoking with myocardial infarction (RR for ever smoked to never smoked, 1.96), stroke (RR, 1.26), aortic aneurysm (RR, 1.80), gastric ulcer (RR, 2.06), and duodenal ulcer (RR, 1.32). The interaction between gender and smoking status was not significant for any of the diseases.

Conclusions: Male gender and smoking were significant risk factors for cardiovascular and peptic ulcer disease in a Japanese population.

Chapter 7 – The current study used latent class analysis to describe longitudinal patterns of regular cigarette use among a sample of 1,214 high school girls from a low-income township in Cape Town, South Africa. It also sought to test whether participation in a comprehensive leisure, life skills and sexuality education program was related to these patterns. There was support for the presence of three patterns of regular cigarette use: non-smokers, initiators, and consistent smokers. Intervention participants were more likely to be non-smokers than were control group students. In addition, girls with the highest risk in a number of domains (academics, peer norms, use of other substances) were more likely to be consistent smokers and less likely to be non-smokers, as compared to girls with less risk. These results suggest that smoking prevention efforts need to begin prior to or early in high school and that there may be concrete markers that allow for the targeting of intervention to those most at risk of early smoking initiation.

Chapter 8 – Cigarette smoking among women is unfortunately still very frequent despite its negative consequences. In addition to its economic and medical implications, smoking might affect women's mental health, inducing cases of dependence, depression and anxiety disorders, and even suicidal behavior.

In this paper the authors will describe the epidemiology of smoking among women, present several psychiatric complications frequently reported in smokers, and will elaborate on the link between smoking and suicide. Smoking has been related to increased risk of suicidal behavior in the general population, in a cohort of nurses, among male soldiers and in psychiatric patients. They also report the results of their study on the link between smoking and suicide risk, in patients with schizophrenia.

It is unclear, however, whether the abovementioned connection results from a causal effect of smoking or whether it derives from the confounding effect of low mental well-being, impulsivity or of mental disorders, clustering with other substance abuse. The link may result from the effect of smoking on brain serotonin levels or from lower monoamine oxidase activity found in smokers. The link between suicide, psychopathology and smoking is important due to its potential ramifications and due to the frequent use of nicotine in today's culture. Further studies in males and in females are crucial to clarify the role of smoking in mental health.

Chapter 9 – Many studies have tried to evaluate the effects of smoking on women's oral health and women's oral microcirculation. Oral side effects of tobacco are: sticky tar deposits or brown staining on the teeth; 'smoker's palate' - red inflammation on the roof of the mouth; delayed healing of the gums; increased severity of gum disease; bad breath or halitosis; black hairy tongue; oral lesions; gum recession - with chewing tobacco at the site of the tobacco "wad", the gums react by receding along the tooth root, exposing the root; oral cancer, aesthetics: tobacco stains and discolours teeth, dentures and restorations.

A significant relationship between women's smoking and the presence of capillary tortuosity emerged too.

A pathological situation was characterized by architectural confusion or by the presence of clear morphological anomalies.

Smoking causes an abnormal pattern formation of chorioallantois membrane blood vessels in chicks, which alters the composition of the extracellular matrix in the chorioallantois membrane mesoderm.

According to these studies, nicotine has no direct effect on vascular caliber, but it may interact with certain intravenous substances (norepinephrine, acetylcholine, adenosine phosphate), consequently determining vascular constriction.

The microcirculation variations observed in correspondence with oral microcirculation can compromise the phlogistic defense response. In particular, it can compromise one of the first phases of phlogosis: vasodilatation and the resulting vasopermeabilization, with consequent impossibility on the part of defense mechanisms to react. Such events would make smoker women more sensitive towards exogenous noxae, since they cannot respond effectively. This could explain why smoking represents a risk factor, especially for women's oral health.

Chapter 10 – Mortality rates from diseases related to environmental tobacco smoke exposure (ETS) are constantly increasing. The potential impact of ETS on the development of cardiovascular diseases has recently been under debate, but has so far remained uncertain among children. In order to address this issue the authors examined plasma and urinary levels of 8-epi-prostaglandin-$F_{2\alpha}$ (8-epi-$PGF_{2\alpha}$) as a measure of in-vivo oxidation injury in 158 children (71 boys, 87 girls, aged 3-15 years). Children were grouped according to smoking habits of their parents: one or both parents smoking, < 20, > 20, or > 40 cigarettes smoked a day, and compared to a non-smoking control group.

Plasma and urinary 8-epi-$PGF_{2\alpha}$ levels were elevated in children of smoking parents. An increased number of smoked cigarettes correlated with higher 8-epi-$PGF_{2\alpha}$ levels and smoking by mother had a trendwise more pronounced influence compared to smoking by father. These data clearly demonstrate a significant in-vivo oxidation injury in children of smoking parents and indicates that development and progression of later vascular disease may already be triggered in childhood by ETS. Considering that worldwide nearly half of the children are exposed to ETS these data clearly underline the importance of the implementation of preventive strategies.

In: Smoking and Women's Health
Editors: M.K.Wesley and I.A. Sternbach, pp.1-11

ISBN 978-1-60456-148-7
© 2008 Nova Science Publishers, Inc.

Short Communication A

Smoking and Women's Oral Health. A Review Focus on Oral Cancer and Precancer

C. López-Carriches, M.I. Moreno-López[1] and M.I. Leco-Berrocal

Universidad Europea de Madrid, Policlínica Universitaria,
Pza Francisco Morano s/n. 28005 Madrid, Spain

Introduction

Cancer of the head and neck is the fifth most frequent worldwide. One of the principal locations within this region is the oral cavity, with approximately 3% of all cancers occurring in this area [1] with a rising in incidence [2]. In some geographic areas, such as south-west Asia, oral cancer is the most frequent cancer in men and the third most frequent in women. Oral Squamous Cell Carcinoma [OSCC] represents more than 90% of all tumors of the oral cavity, the remainder are distributed between melanomas, non-squamous cell carcinomas, and adenocarcinomas of the minor salivary glands, sarcomas, malignant odontogenic tumors, lymphomas, leukemias, myelomas and metastasis [1].

Two distinct precancerous lesions are described in the oral cavity: leukoplakia and erythroplakia [3]. Of these, the first is undoubtedly the most frequent. Its prevalence varies from one country to another; a recent study in Germany found a prevalence of 2.3% in males and 0.9% in females [4]. As with oral cancer, its principal etiologic factor is smoking, and at a time when this habit is shifting towards a younger population and increasing in females, it is to be expected that the prevalence of leukoplakia will increase in young women. Attending to these established data in the western population, we wish to focus on the epidemiology of oral cancer and its presentation in the female population.

This paper proposes two objectives:

1 carmen.lopez@uem.es.

- On the one hand, to highlight the changes seen in the epidemiologic distribution of oral cancer [5] with particular reference to its increase in young people, women and the principal etiological agent: smoking.
- On the other, to demonstrate that the most efficient measures that can be taken in order to diminish the morbidity and mortality associated with OSCC, are to increase the diagnosis of precancerous lesions, and to make aggressive efforts aimed at reducing alcohol, and above all tobacco consumption, especially among women (primary prevention), and at the early detection of malignant lesions (secondary prevention).

Epidemiology

Oral Squamous Cell Carcinoma [OSCC] is found fundamentally in males in the sixth or seventh decade of life. The most frequent sites are the lateral borders and ventral surface of the tongue, and floor of the mouth. Epidemiologically, oral cancer and oropharyngeal cancer are usually grouped together due to their close anatomical relationship and their similar risk factors [6].

Of the risk factors involved in oral cancer, it has been demonstrated that smoking has a direct carcinogenic effect on the epithelium of the oral cavity. In 1950 The M:F ratio for occurrence of oral cancer in the United States was 6:1; however the increase in smoking in women in recent decades has led to a higher incidence in women, the M:F ratio becoming 2:1 [7]. It is thought that this continued difference is due to the inequality in exposure to risk factors between the two sexes, including smoking.

Alcohol consumption was for a long time thought to be a cofactor together with smoking, the association of smoking with alcohol increasing the risk by between 6 and 15 times, nevertheless, diverse epidemiological studies have also demonstrated it to be an independent factor [8].

Regarding age at presentation, Silverman et al. [7] found that 90% of oral cancers occur after the age of 45, the average age at diagnosis being beyond 60 years. However, there has been an increase in the number of adults between the ages of 20 and 30 who develop cancer, especially on the tongue [9]. In recent years this change in the epidemiologic distribution of these tumors has become apparent, and an increase in incidence and mortality has been found, especially in patients under 45 and in women both in Europe and the US [10,11,12].

For this reason, research has more recently focussed mainly on other factors besides the customary ones. One of the most important of these new factors implicated in the development of oral cancer in young patients and women is HPV infection, especially genotype 16, considered to be involved in the production of both malignant and premalignant lesions in the oral mucosa [13].

Nevertheless, the reason for an increasing incidence of oral cancer, particularly amongst younger persons is unclear. It has been hypothesized either to be a result of an increase in exposure to known risk factors amongst certain groups in the community, or to be due to new etiological agents as commented above. Prior to conducting large, expensive, population-based studies, it seems appropriate to conduct initial smaller-scale surveys to assess evidence for each of these two hypotheses. Some of these surveys of young persons with oral cancer suggest that most are exposed to the traditional risk factors of smoking tobacco, drinking alcohol and a low consumption of fruit and vegetables [14].

Together with an increase in the incidence of oral cancer in women, a worrying change in the evolution of mortality has also been observed.

The level of mortality of oral cancer within the mortality for all tumors is very different in men than in women. This, as previously mentioned, was until a few years ago due to the different exposure to risk factors between the two sexes. The mortality rate for oropharyngeal cancer in the European Union in 2000 was 5.6 in men, with large variations from one country to another, finding a maximum of 21.2 in Hungary. In contrast, in women the European average was 1.1%, the country with the highest mortality again being Hungary with 3.3% [15].

When we study the evolution of this mortality over a number of years, we can see from the data obtained regarding these tumors that changes are taking place in the relationship between women, smoking and mortality. In the European Union, the mortality of smoking-related tumors such as lung, bladder and the oral cavity has reduced in males since 1955, but has increased in females. The data corresponding to tumors of the oral cavity and oropharynx are shown in figure 1. This difference in evolution clearly demonstrates the need for action to prevent smoking in women [16].

It is true that within the European Union large differences exist as previously indicated. Studies on the evolution of mortality indicate how the accession of the latest 10 new members has increased the average mortality rate in the Union. It is argued that this increased mortality could be reduced if all current knowledge regarding prevention, diagnosis and treatment were applied in these central and eastern European countries [16].

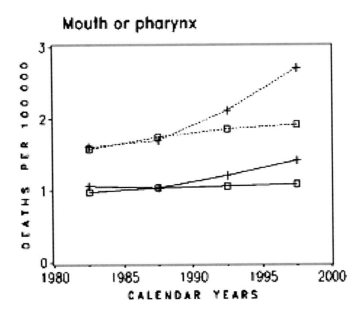

Figure 1.Trends in directly age-standardized [world population] death certification rates per 100,000 females [oropharyngeal cancer] in accession and the European Union [EU] from 1980 to 2000. Solid lines, all ages; dashed lines, 35–64 years; +, accession countries; squares, EU. [16].

In the particular case of oral cancer, the tendency towards an increase in mortality in women is highlighted, principally among the new-member countries from east and central Europe. This tendency is interpreted terms of exposure patterns to tobacco and alcohol, and should imply urgent action to control these factors, in addition to improving the diagnosis and treatment of these tumors [17, 18].

Smoking as a Risk Factor in Oral Cancer

Different case-control studies have found that tobacco and / or alcohol use are the biggest risk factors for OSCC in adults at any age. Smoking and / or alcohol consumption are present in more than 80% of patients with OSCC [19]. With regard to other risk factors, various case-control studies have found that patients with oral cancer have a diet low in fruit and vegetables [20], and that the intake of fruit and vegetables is a protective factor in both smokers and drinkers [21].

Although oral squamous cell carcinoma of the oral cavity is clearly associated with tobacco and alcohol use [22], a minority of patients do not consume these substances, and as commented earlier, the number of these patients appears to be increasing, which therefore implies the presence of other etiologic agents [5]. In cases of oral cancer in non-smokers or non-drinkers, nutritional deficiencies and human papilloma virus infection are the principal factors, as well precancerous conditions such as intraoral lichen planus, although the malignant potential is very small [23,24]. In contrast to cases associated with tobacco and alcohol consumption, cases that present in non-smokers or non-drinkers are more frequent in women at a proportion of 3:1. [25]. It has not been demonstrated a relationship with chronic trauma from broken teeth or maladjusted dentures, although these are frequent findings in patients with oral cancer [26]. Exposure to the sun is clearly related with cancer of the lip, a lower incidence has been recorded in relation to a decline in working in the open air, reducing the number of workers in the countryside and at sea [27].

Smoking habits vary according to gender. When analyzing the differences in smoking between men and women in different countries, three patterns are observed. The proportion of smokers is similar in both sexes in Scandinavian countries [Denmark and Sweden], United Kingdom, Ireland and Holland. Differences between sexes are significant, but with a tendency to converge, in central European countries such as Belgium, France, Luxembourg, former West Germany and Austria. On the other hand, in countries in southern Europe [Spain, Italy, Greece and Portugal] and in former East Germany, there are large but decreasing differences between the rates of smokers in both sexes. This convergence in smoking patterns is not so much due to a decrease in the number of male smokers, but rather to an increase in the number of female smokers [28].

This tendency towards higher tobacco consumption in women was clearly expressed in the framework report of the World Symposium on Tobacco in Prague in 1997. William Ryan, Director General of the multinational tobacco company Rothmans International, expressed his optimism about the sector's promising future in these terms [29]: "The fact is that the worldwide profits for the tobacco industry are continuing to grow steadily and substantially, to such a point that the tobacco sector is an object of envy among multinationals of other sectors. The worldwide sales volume continues to grow and it is expected to maintain this tendency, especially considering the positive tendencies of tobacco consumption in women..." – obviously the director's interpretation of 'positive tendencies' is in complete contrast to our own in this context, but it serves to show how our current data are also reflected in business results and in marketing strategies.

Within this increase in smoking in women one fact expressed on many occasions must be taken into account: the role played by tobacco in controlling weight. [The fact is that data exists which can support this idea] [28].

Women worry more about their weight than men, for young women physical appearance is very important and they often perceive themselves to be overweight. However, fear of being overweight is more common than actual excess weight, and evidence suggests that fear of weight-gain can maintain women smoking, and that considerations about how to control weight influence young women in the decision to start smoking. Advice on how to control weight should form part of smoking treatment programs directed towards young women [30], and any preventative measure for adolescent female smokers should take into account and deal with the question of weight gain [31].

Smoking prevalence is lower among women than men in most countries, yet about 200 million women in the world smoke, and in addition, millions more chew tobacco. Of female smokers worldwide, approximately 22% live in developed countries and 9% in developing countries, but because developing countries represent a higher proportion of the world population, there are numerically more women smokers in developing countries. Unless effective, comprehensive and sustained initiatives are implemented to reduce smoking uptake among young women and increase cessation rates among all women, the prevalence of female smoking in developed and developing countries is likely to rise to 20% by 2025. This would mean that by 2025 there could be 532 million women smokers. Even if prevalence levels do not rise, the number of women who smoke will increase because the population of women in the world is predicted to rise from the current 3.1 billion to 4.2 billion by 2025. Thus, while the epidemic of tobacco use among men is in slow decline, the epidemic among women will not reach its peak until well into the 21st century. This will have enormous consequences not only for women's health and economic well-being but also for that of their families. The health effects of smoking for women are more serious than for men. In addition to the general health problems common to both genders, women face additional hazards during pregnancy, and female-specific cancers such as cancer of the cervix. In Asia, although there are currently lower levels of tobacco use among women, smoking among girls is already on the rise in some areas. The spending power of girls and women is increasing so that cigarettes are becoming more affordable. The social and cultural constraints that previously prevented many women from smoking are weakening, and women-specific health education and quitting programs are rare. Furthermore, evidence suggests that women find it harder to quit smoking. The tobacco companies are targeting women by marketing light, mild, and menthol cigarettes, and introducing advertising directed at women. The greatest challenge and opportunity in primary preventative health in Asia and in other developing areas is to avert the predicted rise in smoking among women [32].

Although it has been demonstrated that in developed countries the cost of smoking exceeds the income generated by the industry, the data in relation to this topic are limited

[33]. There is a connection between the duration of the habit, the number of cigarettes smoked and an increased risk of oral cancer, and also between the time elapsed between quitting smoking and the reduction of this risk.

Smoking and Oral Cancer among Women in Spain

Smoking

Figure 2 shows the evolution in the number of male and female smokers in Spain. From this discrete information on tobacco smoking, collected from Health Surveys conducted in Spain during the last century and in 2001 and 2006, the prevalence of daily cigarette smokers has been reconstructed for the period 1945-2006.

In males, the prevalence of smokers in 1945 was 42.4%, increasing to 59.1% in 1975 and stabilizing until 1985, then reducing to 48.9% in 1995, and continuing to reduce to 32.6% in 2006. In women, the prevalence of smokers was below 5% until the 1970s, from which point it began increasing continuously. In 1995 the prevalence had reached 22.5%, maintaining sustained growth until 2001 with 24.6%, experiencing a small reduction in 2006 to 22.1% of female smokers. This analysis allows us to appreciate the different dynamic of the smoking epidemic between males and females in Spain [34].

It has previously been established how, at least in Spain, the narrowing of the gap between genders is due fundamentally to an increase in the number of female smokers.

Between 1982 and 1998 the proportion of habitual smokers among males between 15 and 64 years of age in the Catalan region reduced from 58.3% to 39.3%, while in women it increased from 20% to 30.7%. These changes began at the beginning of the seventies when Spanish women took up smoking in large numbers, and since then the number of female smokers has increased rapidly.

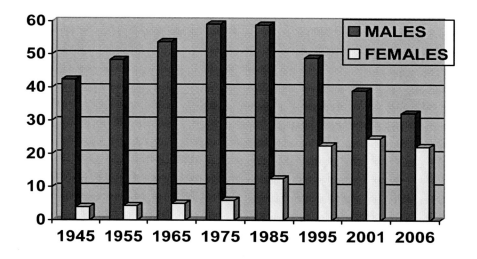

Figure 2. Percentage of smokers [adult habitual smokers]. Males and Females. Spain 1945-2006.

Even so, since 2001 there has been a decrease of 18% in male smokers, and 9% in women. If we look at the numbers of people who have never smoked, we see an increase in men from 2001 to 2006 [from 33.0% to 35.5%], but in women this decreases from 63.2% to 62.8%. However, if we consider the population aged between 16 and 24, there is a 31.15% of female smokers against 25.53% of male smokers, that is, there is still a serious problem of new smokers among the young female population

At this point we should highlight that at the beginning of 2006 important progress was made against smoking in Spain on the part of the Government, with the implementation of a very restrictive law. This law, amongst other measures, has prohibited smoking in offices and public places, and has encouraged the giving up of this habit in a significant section of the smoking population.

Oral Cancer

Although the increase in smoking among women has taken place relatively recently, we can already find data related to oral cancer that is attributable to this evolution.

In the first place, we can study the mortality of all tumours and oral tumors. In the case of mortality for all tumors [figure 3] we observe how from a peak in 1998 the number of deaths from cancer in Spain has tended to decrease in both men and women [35].

In contrast, mortality of oropharyngeal cancer has not followed the same pattern. In males there has been a decrease since 1998 as in all cancers, while in females it has remained stable with figures similar to those of 1991; data which is in accordance with that of other EU countries.

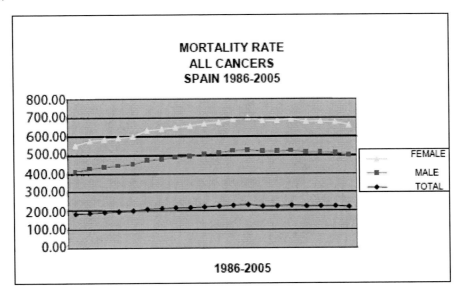

Figure 3.

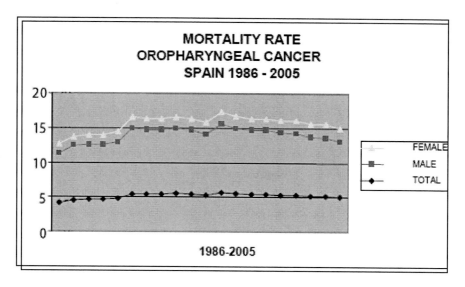

Figure 4.

Regarding the incidence of oral cancer in Spain, this is between 5.7 and 12.9 cases per 100,000 in males / year, and 0.6 to 2.1 cases per 100,000 females / year [36] with rising trends [37].

In a study carried out by Borrás [38], on trends in incidence of smoking-related cancers between men and women in the tumor registry in Tarragona, it was observed that the incidence increased by 3% in males and by 4.5% in females. By location, the annual increase was 4.3% in the oral cavity for men, and 7% for women at the same site. Similar results were found in an study in the south of Spain in Andalusia [39].

The lowest incidence for a cancer in a European country in any determinate age group would represent the minimum possible achievable at any given moment. This is assuming that the lower incidence is due to a lower prevalence of risk factors and not to genetic predisposition, which contributes little to the variations between countries [except for those cancers related to climate and skin type]. The excess of cancer cases compared with the minimum data would presumably be caused by a higher prevalence of risk factors and other indicators such as lifestyle, diet and other occupational and / or environmental factors.

In Spain there was a high incidence of oral cancer among men compared with other countries of the EU (at the time when the EU consisted of 15 members). This is associated with the traditional use of dark tobacco and its interaction with alcohol. Dark tobacco was the most common type in the first years of tobacco consumption in Spain, while Virginia tobacco is currently the most prevalent, and most women have smoked Virginia tobacco since the beginning. In public health terms, these findings are very important when defining and establishing smoking-related oral cancer prevention and control programs [38]. All indications are that preventative measures should be increased at school level, especially in females where a significant increase in cases of oral cancer has been observed [40].

Final Recommendations

Oral cancer has predominantly been found among males, and is now an emerging disease among the female population of western countries. This increase is due to various factors, principally the increase in smoking in females, especially young women. In order to reduce the number of new tumors, it is essential to implement primary prevention programs directed towards reducing the risk factors of this disease as well as secondary prevention through the early diagnosis of a disease that presents with easily visible lesions.

References

[1]   Jemal A, Siegel R, Ward E, Murray T, Xu J, Thun MJ. Cancer statistics, 2007. *CA Cancer J. Clin.* 2007;57[1]:43-66.

[2]   Shiboski CH, Shiboski SC, Silverman S. Trends in oral cancer rates in the United States, 1973-1996. *Community Dent. Oral Epidemiol.* 2000;28[4]:249-56.

[3]   Kramer IR, Lucas RB, Pindborg JJ, Sobin LH. Definition of leukoplakia and related lesions: an aid to studies on oral precancer. *Oral Surg. Oral Med. Oral Pathol.* 1978; 46[4]:518-39.

[4]   Reichart PA. Identification of risk groups for oral precancer and cancer and preventive measures. *Clin. Oral Investig.* 2001;5[4]:207-13.

[5]   Llewellyn CD, Johnson NW, Warnakulasuriya KA, Risk factors for oral cancer in newly diagnosed patients aged 45 years and younger: a case-control study in Southern England. *J. Oral Pathol. Med. 2004; 33[9]:525-32*

[6]   Moreno-López LA Esparza-Gómez G. Oral cancer vs oropharyngeal cancer vs head and neck cancer. *Oral Oncol.* 1998;34[6]:576-7].

[7]   Silverman S. Demographics and occurrence of oral and pharyngeal cancers, the outcomes, the trends, the challenge. *JADA* 2001;132:7-11.

[8]   Moreno-López LA, Esparza-Gómez G, Gónzalez-Navarro a, et al. Risk of oral cancer associated with tobacco smoking, alcohol consumption and oral higiene: A case – control study in Madrid, Spain. *Oral Oncology 2000; 36[2]:170-4]].*

[9]   Riera P, Martínez B. Morbidity and mortality for oral and pharyngeal cancer in Chile. *Rev. Med. Chile* 2005;133:555-63.

[10]   Annertz K, Anderson H, Biorklund A, et al. Incidence and survival of squamous cell carcinoma of the tongue in Scandinavia, with special reference to young adults. *Int. J. Cancer 2002; 101:95-9*

[11]   Schantz SP, Yu GP, Head and Neck cancer incidence trends in young Americans, 1973-1997, with special analysis for tongue cancer. *Arch. Otoryngol. Head Neck Surg.* 2002; 128: 268-74.

[12]   Zavras AI, Laskaris C, Kittas C, Laskaris G. Leukoplakia and intraoral malignancies: female cases increases in Greece. *J. Eur. Acad. Dermatol. Venereol* .2003;17[1]:25-7.

[13]   Luo CW, Roan CH, Liu CJ. Human papillomaviruses in oral squamous cell carcinoma and pre-cancerous lesions detected by PCR-bases gene-chip array. *Int. J. Oral. Maxillofac. Surg.* 2007; 36[2]:153-8.].

[14] Mackenzie J, Ah-See K, Thakker N, Sloan P, Maran AG, Birch J, Macfarlane GJ. Increasing incidence of oral cancer amongst young persons: what is the aetiology? *Oral Oncol. 2000 Jul;36[4]:387-9].*

[15] Levi F, Lucchini F, Negri E, Boyle P, La Vecchia C. Mortality from major cancer sites in the European Union, 1955-1998. *Annals of Oncology 2003;14:490-5].*

[16] Levi F, Lucchini F, Negri E, Zatonski W, Boyle P, La Vecchia C. Trends in cancer mortality in the European Union and accession countries, 1980-2000. *Annals of Oncology 2004;15:1425-31.*

[17] La Vecchia C, Lucchini F, Negri E, Levi F. Trends in oral cancer mortality in Europe. *Oral Oncology 2004;40[4]:433-9.]*

[18] Tarvainen L, Suuronen R, Lindqvist C, Malila N. Is the incidence of oral and pharyngeal cancer increasing in Finland? An epidemiological study of 17,383 cases in 1953-1999. *Oral Dis* 2004;10[3]:167-72.

[19] Mclaughlin JK, Gridley G, Block G et al. Dietary factors in oral and pharyngeal cancer. *JNCI 1988; 80:1237-43].*

[20] Oral and oropharyngeal cancer in Spain: influence of dietary patterns. *Eur. J. Cancer Prev. 2003;12[1]:49-56].*

[21] Lissowska J, Pilarska A, Pilarska P, Samolczyk-Wanyura D et al. Smoking, alcohol, diet, dentition and sexual practices in the epidemiology of oral cancer in Poland. *Eur. J. Cancer Prev.* 2003;12[1]:25-33.

[22] Eisen D. The clinical features, malignant potential, and systemic associations of oral lichen planus: A study of 723 patients. *J. Am. Acad. Dermatol* 2002; 46[2]:207-14].

[23] Hsue SS, Wang WC, Chen CH, Lin CC, Chen YK, Lin LM. Malignant transformation in 1458 patients with potentially malignant oral mucosal disorders: a follow-up study based in a Taiwanese hospital. *J. Oral Pathol. Med* .2007;36[1]:25-9.

[24] Wiseman SM, Swede H, Stoler DL, Anderson GR, Rigual NR, Hicks WL et al. Squamous Cell Carcinoma of the Head and Neck in Nonsmokers and Nondrinkers. An Analysis of Clinicopathologid Characteristics and Treatment Outcomes. *An Surg. Oncol.* 2003;10[5]: 551-7.

[25] Gorsky M, Silverman S. Denture wearing and oral cancer. *J. Prosthet. Dent.* 1984;52:164-70.

[26] Lissowska J, Pilarska A, Pilarska P, Samolczyk-Wantyra D, Piekarczyk J, Bardin-Mikollajczak A, Zatonski W, Herrero R, Muñoz N, Francezchi S. Smoking, alcohol, diet, dentition and sexual practices in the epidemiology of oral cancer in Poland. *Eur. J. Cancer Prev.* 2003;12[1]: 25-33.]

[27] Joossens L, Sasco A, Salvador T, Villalba JR. Las Mujeres y el tabaco en la Unión Europea. *Rev. Esp. Salud Publica* 1999;73:34-9.

[28] Joosens L. La igualdad se va con el humo. Las mujeres y el tabaco en la Unión Europea. Bruselas: European Network for Smoking Prevention; 1999.]:

[29] Rieder A, Schoberberger R, Kunze M. Helping women to stop smoking. *Int. J. Smoking Cessation* 1993; 2: 34-39.].

[30] Crisp AH, Stavrakaki C, Halek C, Williams E, Segwick P, Kiossis I. Smoking and pursuit of thinness in schoolgirls in London and Ottawa. *Postgrad. Med. J.* 1998; 74: 473-479.].

[31]   Mackay J,Amos A. Respirology 2003; 8:123–130.

[32]   Sturgis EM. A review of social and behavioral efforts at oral cancer preventions in India. Head Neck 2004.26:937-44.

[33]   Borrás JM, Fernández E, Schiaffino A, Villalbí JR, García M, Saltó E. Prevalencia del consumo de tabaco en España entre 1945 y 1995: Reconstrucción a partir de las Encuestas Nacionales de Salud. Med Clinica 2003;120[1]:14-6.

[34]   Encuesta Nacional de Salud de España. Online Resource: http://www.ine.es/jaxi /menu.do?type=pcaxisandpath=/t15/p419andfile=inebaseandL=0. Access June, 30th, 2007.

[35]   Cáncer en España. Madrid: Ministerio de Sanidad y consumo. Online Resource: http://www.isciii.es/htdocs/centros/epidemiologia/epi_cancer.jsp. Access July, 10th, 2007.

[36]   Nieto A, Ramos MR. Rising Trends in oral cancer mortality in Spain, 1975-94. *J. Oral Pathol. Med.* 2002;31[3]:147-52.

[37]   Borrás J, Borras JM, Galcerán J, Sánchez V, Moreno V and González JR. Trend in smoking-related cancer incidence in Tarragona, Spain, 1980-96. *Cancer Causes and Control* 2001;12:903-8.

[38]   Ruiz Ramos M, Nieto A. Mortality trends from oral cnacer in Andalusia, Spain, 1975-1998. *Public Health* 2001;115[5]:338-44.

[39]   Blanchaert RH. Oral and oral pharyngeal cancer: an update on incidence and epidemiology, identification, advances in treatment and outcomes. *Compend Contin. Educ. Dent.* 2002;23[12 Suppl]:25-9.

In: Smoking and Women's Health
Editors: M.K. Wesley and I.A. Sternbach, pp. 13-22

ISBN 978-1-60456-148-7
© 2008 Nova Science Publishers, Inc.

Short Communication B

Smoking and Tobacco Use Among Asian-American and Pacific Islander (AAPI) Women

Robert Friis, Claire Garrido-Ortega, Sarah Long,
Paula Griego and Veronica Acosta-Deprez
Department of Health Science
California State University, Long Beach, USA

Introduction—Women and Smoking

By encouraging women to stop smoking or to avoid smoking in the first place, public health officials could prevent untold amounts of morbidity and mortality in a vulnerable population. For example, smoking is linked to several forms of cancer (oral and throat, esophageal, pancreas, kidney, bladder, uterine) and, in particular, lung cancer—the leading cause of cancer mortality among women. A total of 90 percent of women's deaths from lung cancer are believed to be caused by smoking.[1] In addition to lung cancer, smoking is associated with other lung diseases, coronary heart disease, and stroke. Each year, cigarette smoking kills an estimated 178,000 women in the U.S.[2] For much of the 20th century smoking was regarded as a lifestyle issue that affected men primarily. Recognition of smoking as a crucial women's health issue would help to reduce the toll that smoking-related morbidity and mortality take increasingly upon female smokers.

In the U.S., the gender gap for rates of smoking has narrowed since the 1960s to a level for women presently within a few percentage points of men's rates.[3] During the mid-1960s, more than one-half of men and one-third of women smoked. Then, following the publication of the U.S. Surgeon General's Report on Tobacco and Health in 1964, the rates of cigarette smoking declined substantially among both men and women.[4] However, between 1965 and 1990, the rate of decline was much greater among men than among women. Since the beginning of the 21st century, smoking frequency among both genders has continued to decline. Nevertheless, despite declines in smoking rates over the past four to five decades, nearly one-fifth to one-quarter of the U.S. population continues to smoke. As of 2003, the female-male differential in smoking rates was only about five percent (19 percent versus 24 percent, respectively). As a result of earlier and persisting high rates of smoking, mortality rates from lung cancer among American women increased by 600 percent from 1930 to 1997.[5]

Women, in comparison with men, should be regarded as a special risk group to health impacts related to smoking. The risks of death for respiratory and vascular disease are higher for women who inhale while smoking than they are for men.[6] Cigarette smoking has been linked to abnormal menstrual function, infertility, menopause at a younger age, and lower bone density after menopause with increased susceptibility to hip fracture.[1]

Although evidence indicates that smoking endangers the health of mothers and their developing fetuses during pregnancy, the percentage of women who continue to smoke during pregnancy is cause for alarm. Although this percentage has tended to decline over time, it was, nonetheless, about 12 percent in 2001.[7] The contribution of maternal smoking to low birth weight as well as miscarriages and prematurity has been documented extensively. [1] Among young women who smoke, those who are rearing children are more likely to be current smokers than those women who are not raising children.[8]

Characteristics of Asian Americans and Pacific Islanders (AAPIs)

The AAPI group is highly diverse and contributes more than four percent of the U.S. population.[9] AAPIs constitute one of the fastest growing racial/ethnic groups in the U.S., representing a diverse population of more than 50 distinct subgroups defined by ethnicity and language.[10] Since 1980, the AAPI population in the U.S. has grown approximately ten times faster during each decade than the overall population.

The U.S. Census Bureau states that the term "Asian" denotes "...people having origins in any of the original peoples of the Far East, Southeast Asia, or the Indian subcontinent (for example, Cambodia, China, India, Japan, Korea, Malaysia, Pakistan, the Philippine Islands, Thailand, and Vietnam."[11] For the 2000 census, the U.S. Office of Management and Budget subdivided the category of Asian-Pacific Islander into "Asians" and "Native Hawaiians and other Pacific Islanders."[12] However, this classification is not sufficient to characterize the vast geographic span and cultural differences among the AAPI group.

Although heart disease is the top killer among the general population of the U.S., cancer is the leading cause of death among AAPIs, both women and men.[12] In addition, mortality statistics reflect great disparities in cancer death rates across Asian-American sub-populations. For example, data for the years 1997 to 2001 demonstrated that South-Asian females in California had age-adjusted cancer death rates of 57.8 per 100,000 in comparison with Korean-American males who had rates of 203.4 per 100,000.[9,13] Cigarette smoking is a well-known risk factor for cancer mortality, although other lifestyle and environmental factors are implicated in the high cancer rates found among AAPIs.

Prevalence of Tobacco Use Among AAPIs

In many Asian countries, the prevalence of cigarette use tends to be high among the general population and much higher among men than women. In Asian countries such as China, Indonesia, Thailand, and Korea, the male to female smoking ratio averages about ten to one.[14] This discrepancy contrasts with developed countries including those in Europe and North America, where smoking rates tend to more equalized among genders.

The high frequency of smoking in Asia has affected not only Asian-American immigrants but also their offspring who are born in the U. S.[15] Mirroring the gender differences found in Asian countries, Asian women in the U.S. smoke less frequently than Asian men, 4.8 percent versus 17.8 percent, respectively.[16] These smoking rates exclude Native Hawaiian or other Pacific Islanders. Excluding Asians of multiple races, AAPI women also are less likely to be classified as "ever-smokers" than AAPI men.[17]

Nationally, smoking prevalence among AAPI women 18 years of age and older (including Native Hawaiians and Pacific Islanders) is 9.1 percent and varies according to Asian subgroup, ranging from 3.0 percent among Asian Indians to 6.9 percent among Filipino Americans.[18] Among Asian-American female teenagers, the national smoking prevalence is as high as 8.9 percent among Filipino Americans and 8.0 percent among Vietnamese Americans.

Because national data on smoking prevalence among adult members of some Asian subgroups is not readily available, prevalence studies tend to regard the AAPI population as a composite. This approach is inappropriate given the variation in smoking rates among AAPI subgroups that have been observed in several small studies. For example, smoking rates as high as 70 percent have been observed among Laotians and Cambodians and more than 40 percent among Native Hawaiians and Chuukese.[19]

Data from the 2001 California Health Interview Survey indicated that among California residents, the female smoking prevalence rates varied from 1.1 percent among Vietnamese Americans to 21.4 percent among Pacific Islanders. The rates for Japanese, Filipinos, and Koreans were 12.7 percent, 9.3 percent, and 9.2 percent, respectively.

Factors that Influence Tobacco Use among AAPI Women

The prevalence of smoking may be underestimated in some groups of AAPI women due to cultural proscriptions against women's smoking, which is highly stigmatized in some Asian communities. Asian-American women and girls may secret themselves in private areas of the household where they feel that it is safe to smoke without being observed; although they are active smokers, they tend to deny this fact when interviewed. The remainder of this paper will cover variables that influence AAPI women's use of tobacco. The factors include the following:

- Acculturation
- Socioeconomic status and educational level
- Advertising and the media

- Awareness of smoking-related health risks

Acculturation

The process of acculturation takes place when an individual or group selectively accepts some aspect of a dominant culture, though does not entirely give up its own.[20] For AAPIs, acculturation has both positive and negative impacts on tobacco use, depending on gender and age. Greater acculturation is associated with increased smoking rates among Asian American male youth and with decreased rates among male adults.

In contrast with men, more acculturated Asian-American women tend to have higher smoking rates than their less acculturated counterparts. Asian-American women are more likely to smoke if they are more proficient in English when compared with women who are less proficient, though the opposite relationship between smoking and English language proficiency has been observed among Asian-American men.[21] When the relationship between acculturation and smoking was studied among AAPI subgroups, more acculturated Chinese-American women, Filipino-American women, Korean-American women had higher rates of smoking than less acculturated women.[15] In addition, acculturation did not appear to have an effect on Japanese-American women; little information regarding smoking has been reported among other Asian subgroups.

Socioeconomic Status and Education

The associations between smoking prevalence and poverty status as well as with level of education have been documented extensively.[22] Within the general U.S. population, women who have lower incomes and lower levels of education are more likely to smoke than those who have higher incomes and education levels. In 1990, approximately 40 percent of Cambodian Americans were living below the poverty line.[23] In this low income group, smoking rates tend to be high overall, although smoking frequency is much lower among Cambodian-American women than among Cambodian-American men.[24]

Advertising and the Media

During the early 20th century, smoking in the U.S. was predominantly a male habit, reinforced by gifts of free cigarettes to American soldiers as part of their rations during World War I. In many parts of the world, smoking has become more frequent among women and has been linked to substantial increases in diseases attributed to smoking.[6] Smoking prevalence appears to increase with increased worldwide economic development.

One influence associated with the feminization of smoking has been the advent of tobacco marketing themes that tie together social desirability, independence, and weight control.[25] These themes seem to cross generations and tend to influence women from almost all ethnic and racial groups, including AAPI women. Cultural constraints that dissuaded AAPI women from smoking in their country of origin are more relaxed in the U.S.; as a result, AAPI women may be more likely to smoke in the U.S. than in their countries of origin.

Today, women continue to be targeted by tobacco companies.[25] These advertising efforts are being directed increasingly toward APPI women and young females.[26] Adding to the influence of advertising campaigns is the reported higher density of billboards and posters that promote tobacco use in many Asian neighborhoods in comparison with white neighborhoods.[27] The tobacco industry is known to support AAPI organizations and cultural events in order to gain a positive foothold in the community.

Awareness of Smoking-Related Health Risks

Prior studies have established that smoking status is linked to how the risks of smoking are perceived. Some studies suggest that Asian-American women may smoke less frequently than Asian-American men because they are more aware of the adverse health effects of smoking.[28] The concept of individualism is not valued as highly as the needs of the family within Asian-American cultures. The role of the female (a wife, mother, or sister) in Asian-American families may prove useful in increasing the awareness of health risks associated with smoking. Risk perception of smoking, however, may differ among specific Asian-American subgroups. The awareness levels of tobacco use as a health consequence was considerably higher among Korean Americans when compared to Vietnamese Americans.[28] Results for focus groups conducted with Cambodian-American women suggested that participants had only limited information regarding smoking-associated health risks.[24]

Smokeless Tobacco as a Substitute for Cigarette Smoking

The use of smokeless tobacco is generally low among women in the general population of the U.S. During 2004, only 0.3 percent of women were current users of smokeless tobacco.[2] Although smoking among women is often culturally unacceptable in Asian countries, the use of chew tobacco by women is sanctioned in form of chewing betel quid. Throughout Asia and the Asian Pacific region, it is common for women to chew betel quid (a mixture of betel leaf, areca nut, and slaked lime) mixed with tobacco.[29] Consumption of betel quid is associated with an oral precancerous disease such as submucous fibrosis. As little information exists regarding the extent to which immigrant AAPI women transfer this practice to the U.S., further studies need to be conducted on the prevalence of use of chew tobacco by AAPI women. In focus groups conducted by the senior author, older Cambodian American women disclosed that they engaged in practice of chewing betel quid combined with tobacco.[24]

Secondhand Cigarette Smoke

Exposure to secondhand cigarette smoke is also called passive smoking, referring to non-smokers' involuntary inhalation of tobacco smoke from smokers.[30] The U.S. Surgeon General has identified exposure to secondhand smoke as a significant health risk.[31] Even though the frequency of smoking is lower among AAPI women than among men, male family members who smoke expose women, (perhaps unwittingly) as well as developing fetuses and children to secondhand smoke. Exposure to secondhand smoke, which occurs at home, during leisure, while traveling to work, and during work, is particularly a health issue for women in many Asian countries where most men are smokers. Adults who are exposed to secondhand smoke experience increased risk of cancer as well as possible increased risk from coronary heart disease, respiratory problems, and impaired lung function.[30]

Barriers to Quitting

An important issue for future research is identifying and overcoming cultural barriers to smoking cessation; few studies have addressed cultural barriers among AAPI women that AAPI women experience when they attempt to quit.[32] Smoking cessation programs targeted to minority groups are less available to minority women, who appear to be less receptive to smoking cessation efforts than non-minority women. In addition, language barriers may be an issue in designing successful cessation programs as over 30 percent of AAPIs do not have anyone over the age of 14 in their homes who are proficient English speakers.[23] In order to be successful in their efforts to curtail smoking among women, smoking cessation planners need to tailor smoking cessation programs to specific AAPI subgroups by making the programs available in the women's preferred language. It may be inappropriate to attempt to apply "off the shelf" cessation programs designed for English speakers to non-English speaking AAPI women.

Implications for Practice and Prevention

Research suggests that quitting smoking is the most important behavioral change a woman can adopt to reduce her risk of morbidity and early mortality from smoking-related causes. Certainly, this assertion applies to AAPI women who tend to be a neglected population from the standpoint of research into the most culturally appropriate means for achieving smoking cessation. Minority women are at greater risk for the impact of morbidity and mortality for smoking-related conditions than women in the general population. The increased risk may stem from lack of awareness of the health consequences of tobacco use and reduced access to health care providers. Although AAPI women have a lower self-reported prevalence of smoking than AAPI men and members of the general U.S. population, they are vulnerable to the effects of exposure to secondhand cigarette smoke even if they do not smoke. Smoking prevalence rates are believed to be increasing among AAPI women as they become more acculturated to the U.S. society and as young AAPI females smoke more frequently.

According to the United States Department of Health and Human Service's Office on Women's Health, not only is there a dearth of information about the dimensions of smoking cessation among AAPI women, virtually no research on smoking cessation programs has targeted this population.[33] Consequently, research into interventions to curb tobacco use—vital to the health of AAPI women—needs to be developed. One focus of future studies should be on the frequency of use of alternatives to cigarette smoking such as chew tobacco. Researchers need to gain insight into why the use of chew tobacco is acceptable to some subgroups of AAPI women and how to increase awareness of the health risks associated with chew tobacco. Such research may lead to the identification of culturally appropriate methods for prevention and cessation of chew tobacco use.

Another need for research is the development of culturally appropriate smoking cessation programs for AAPI women. Descriptive epidemiologic studies would be helpful in confirming the prevalence and correlates of cigarette smoking among AAPI women. Because of language, cultural, and other barriers, "off-the-shelf" cessation programs may not be welcomed by AAPI women. Cessation programs that are likely to gain acceptance by this group should use culturally appropriate role models and be delivered in the woman's preferred language.

Further, researchers need to acquire information on preferred methods for delivery of a cessation program—whether AAPI women desire self-help literature, group or individual counseling, self-help telephone "quit-lines," or a combination of approaches. If the option of group counseling is chosen, some older less acculturated AAPI women may prefer groups that are composed of women only, whereas younger, more acculturated women may feel comfortable in mixed gender groups.

Finally, community involvement can lead to reduction of tobacco use among AAPI women. A united community is able to reject the placement of tobacco advertisements and win the political support of government officials for cessation efforts. Political support may, in turn, lead to the placement of government funded cessation programs in local health and social agencies. The community can support AAPI women in their efforts to adopt household rules that restrict indoor smoking in order to reduce family members' exposure to secondhand smoke.

Members of some immigrant and minority communities distrust government agencies that seek to conduct research within communities. The community itself can be empowered to conduct research on the most effective methods of smoking cessation through partnerships with academic and other organizations. Research activities by a community based organization would be less likely to be rejected by those minority community members who are distrustful of the government. Much can be done to reach AAPI women, a neglected and vulnerable minority from the standpoint of tobacco research.

Acknowledgements

This paper was supported by grants from the following sources:

Pilot CARA Award 12BT-2201, Cambodian Research Initiative from the Tobacco-Related Disease Research Program, University of California, Los Angeles.

CARA Award 16AT-1300, Determinants of Smoking Prevalence among Cambodian Americans funded by the Tobacco-Related Disease Research Program, University of California, Los Angeles.

Summer Fellowship Award from California State University, Long Beach.

References

[1]   Centers for Disease Control and Prevention. 2001 Surgeon General's Report—Women and Smoking: Health Consequence of Tobacco Use Among Women. Available: www.cdc.gov /tobacco/data_statistics/sgr/sgr_2001/highlight. Accessed: August 2, 2007.

[2]   Centers for Disease Control and Prevention. Smoking and Tobacco Use. Fact Sheet: Women and Tobacco, 2006. Available: www.cdc.gov/tobacco/data_statistics /Factsheets/women_tobacco.htm Accessed: July 11, 2007.

[3]   American Lung Association. Women and Smoking Fact Sheet, March 2006. Available: http://www.lungusa.org/site/pp.asp?c=dvLUK9O0E&b=33572   Accessed: May 29, 2007.

[4]   National Center for Health Statistics. *Health, United States, 2005. With Chartbook on Trends in the Health of Americans* Hyattsville, Maryland: 2005.

[5]   Patel JD, Bach PB, Kris MG. Lung cancer in US women: A contemporary epidemic. *JAMA*. 2004; 291:1763-1768.

[6]   Marang-van de Mheen PJ, Smith GD, Hart CL, Hole DJ. Are women more sensitive to smoking than men? Findings from the Renfrew and Paisley study. *International Journal of Epidemiology*. 2001; 30: 787-792.

[7]   Centers for Disease Control and Prevention. 2001 Surgeon General's Report – Women and Smoking: Tobacco Use and Reproductive Outcomes.   Available: http://www.cdc.gov /tobacco /data_statistics/sgr/sgr_2001/highlight_outcomes.htm Accessed: August 1, 2007.

[8]   Steueve A and O'Donnell L. Continued smoking and smoking cessation among urban young adult women: Findings from the research for health longitudinal study. *American Journal of Public Health*. 2007;97(8): 1408-1411.

[9]   Leistikow B, Chen M, Tsodikov A. Tobacco smoke overload and ethnic, state, gender, and temporal cancer mortality disparities in Asian-Americans and Pacific Islander-Americans. *Preventive Medicine*. 2006; 42: 430-434.

[10]   Lew R and Tanjasiri SP. Slowing the epidemic of tobacco use among Asian Americans and Pacific Islanders. *American Journal of Public Health*. 2003; 93(5): 764-767.

[11]   US Bureau of the Census.   The Asian Population: 2000.   Available: http://www.census.gov/prod/2002pubs/c2kbr01-16.pdf Accessed: August 28, 2007.

[12] Chen M, Jr. Cancer health disparities among Asian Americans: What we know and what we need to do. *Cancer.* 2005; 104(S12): 2895 – 2902.

[13] Kwong S, Chen M Jr., Snipes K, Bal D, Wright W. Asian subgroups and cancer incidence and mortality rates in California. *Cancer.* 2005; 104(12 Suppl):2975-2981.

[14] Mackay J, Amos A. Women and tobacco in *Invited Review Series: Tobacco and lung health. Respirology.* 2003;8:123-130.

[15] Kim SS, Ziedonis D, Chen KW. Tobacco use and dependence in Asian Americans: A review of the literature. *Nicotine & Tobacco Research.* 2007; 9(2):169-184.

[16] Centers for Disease Control and Prevention. Cigarette smoking among adults –United States, 2004. *MMWR.* 2005;54(44):1121-1124.

[17] Gomez SL, Kelsey JL, Glaser SL, Lee MM, Sidney S. Immigration and acculturation in relation to health and health-related risk factors among specific Asian subgroups in a health maintenance organization. *American Journal of Public Health.* 2004; 94(11): 1977-1984

[18] Centers for Disease Control and Prevention. Prevalence of cigarette use among 14 racial/ethnic populations – United States, 1999-2001. *MMWR.* 2004;53(03);49-52.

[19] Lew, R. A national effort to reduce tobacco use among Asian Americans and Pacific Islanders. *Cancer Supplement.* 1998;83(8):1818-1820.

[20] Ma G, Tan Y, Toubbeh J, Su X, Shive S, Lan Y. Acculturation and smoking behavior in Asian-American populations. *Health Education Research.* 2004; 19(6):615-625.

[21] Tang H, Shimizu R, Chen M Jr.. English language proficiency and smoking prevalence among California's Asian Americans. *Cancer Supplement.* 2005;104(12): 2982-2988.

[22] Centers for Disease Control and Prevention. 2001 Surgeon General's Report—Women and Smoking: Patterns of Tobacco Use Among Women and Girls. Available: http://www.cdc.gov/tobacco/data_statistics/sgr/sgr_2001/highlight_tobaccouse.htm# Accessed: August 29, 2007.

[23] Ro M. Moving forward: Addressing the health of Asian American and Pacific Islander women. *American Journal of Public Health.* 2002; 92(4): 516-519.

[24] Friis RH, Forouzesh M, Chhim HS, Monga S, Sze D. Sociocultural determinants of tobacco use among Cambodian Americans. Health Education Research. 2006;21(3):355-365.

[25] Kaufman N, Nichter M. *The marketing of tobacco to women: Global perspectives* in Samet J, Yoon SY. (2001) *Women and the Tobacco Epidemic Challenges for the 21st Century.*

[26] Asian Pacific Partners for Empowerment and Leadership. *Tobacco use in Asian American and Pacific Islander communities.* Available: http://www.aapcho. com/links/AAPItobacco3-02.pdf Accessed: August 28, 2007.

[27] Elder JP, Edwards C, Conway TL. *Independent evaluation of Proposition 99-funded efforts to prevent and control tobacco use in California.* Sacramento: California Department of Health, 1993.

[28] Ma GX, Fang CY, Tan Y, Feeley RM. Perceptions of risks of smoking among Asian Americans. *Preventive Medicine.* 2003;37:349-355.

[29] Gupta PC, Ray CS. Epidemiology of betel quid usage. *Annals Academy of Medicine.* 2004; 33(S4): 31-36.

[30] Samet J, Yang G. *Passive smoking, women and children* in Samet J, Yoon SY. 2001. *Women and the Tobacco Epidemic Challenges for the 21ˢᵗ Century.*

[31] *The Health Consequences of Involuntary Exposure to Tobacco Smoke: A Report of the Surgeon General, U.S. Department of Health and Human Services: 6 Major Conclusions of the Surgeon General Report.* Available: http://www. surgeongeneral.gov/library/secondhandsmoke/factsheets/factsheet6.html   Accessed: August 22, 2007.

[32] King TK, Borrelli B, Black C, Pinto BM, Marcus BH. Minority women and tobacco: Implications for smoking cessation interventions. *Ann Behav Med.* 1997;19(3):301-313.

[33] Office of Women's Health. *Surgeon General's Report on Women and Smoking Asian or Pacific Islander Women and Smoking.* U.S. Department of Health and Human Services. 1991; p 2.   Available: http://www.4women. gov/owh/pub/factsheets /smoking_asian.htm Accessed: August 29, 2007.

In: Smoking and Women's Health   ISBN 978-1-60456-148-7
Editors: M.K. Wesley and I.A. Sternbach, pp.23-67   © 2008 Nova Science Publishers, Inc.

Chapter 1

Factors Affecting Women Undergraduates' Smoking

Catherine Chambliss, Amy C. Hartl, Megan K. Austin, Joanne Brosh, Kimberly Bean, John Paul Venuti, Dana Piraino, Jenna Filipkowski, Shelby Cochran, Noelle Bisinger and Jessica Kim

Ursinus College, Collegeville, PA, USA

Abstract

Cigarette smoking among female college students continues to be a daunting problem. During this developmental period, choices made often have long term consequences for the health and well being of women. The factors affecting young women's decisions to smoke are in some ways distinctive from those influencing young men's. Clarifying these factors is important because it may provide information valuable to the development of more effective prevention methods.

This chapter summarizes several empirical investigations examining psychological issues affecting young women's decisions to smoke. The role of affect and appetite regulation, young women's ambitions, and the interpersonal context in which smoking occurs, are considered in this research aimed at describing the issues shaping young women's smoking choices. Female students showed higher levels of empathy, which may play a role in their greater vulnerability to depression and use of tobacco to regulate emotional states. Although it was hypothesized that appetite regulation would play a prominent role in women's decisions to smoke, the data failed to support this expectation. In these undergraduate samples, no gender differences in career ambitions emerged. The majority of the females expected to remain employed outside the home after having children, although several hoped to reduce their involvement in work during their children's early years. Most women expected an egalitarian division of household responsibilities in their future families. Interestingly, the majority of the males studied did not anticipate having an employed spouse after starting a family, and few expected to contribute equally to household chores. In general, young women perceived maternal employment more positively than their male counterparts did. Young women endorsed the benefits of maternal employment for children more strongly than males. Males also were more likely to perceive maternal employment as posing hazards to the development of children. These gender differences were mitigated somewhat by the respondent's maternal employment history (evaluations of maternal employment were generally more positive among children whose own mothers had worked outside the home), but still emerged among those from all family backgrounds. There was no evidence that women undergraduates use substances, including tobacco, more than men in order to manage the pressures associated with educational, career, and family ambitions. Women were also similar to men in their reactions to social situations prompting cigarette smoking. Both men and women reported greater tobacco use in interpersonal campus contexts involving alcohol use. Finally, both men and women reported similar responses to contexts involving smoking restrictions. The implications of these findings for prevention program planning are explored.

Introduction

Cigarette smoking among female college students continues to be a pressing concern. Some studies have found use of cigarettes to be growing more rapidly among adolescent girls than boys (Fiore, 1992). During this developmental period, choices made often have long term consequences for the health and well being of both women and their families (due to the effects of secondhand smoke and smoking during pregnancy). Young women have even more reasons to refrain from smoking than their male counterparts. The health hazards of smoking cigarettes seem to be more pronounced for women. Most importantly, cigarette smoking shortens the lives of women more so than men. The average age of those experiencing lung cancer related fatalities attributable to smoking among women is 55, compared to the 65 years' average age for male smokers who contract lung cancer. Since women's average life expectancy exceeds that of men, and they would therefore normally be expected to die at a later age, this earlier age of smoking related fatality means that smoking exacts an even greater comparative toll on women. Research on the social hazards of smoking has been somewhat more equivocal, but some studies suggest that the stigma associated with smoking may be directed more harshly against females (Dermer and Jacobsen, 1986).

Forty years after the 1960s women's revolution, many young women should take pride in what their gender has accomplished. From the early grades on up, girls outperform boys academically, are less likely to be placed in special education classes or find themselves in detention, watch less television, and are more likely to participate in the arts (Kingsbury, 2007). The percentage of women age 25-64 who held a college degree in 1970 tripled by 2004, rising from 11% to 33%. Women have shown that they have the ambition and initiative to become educated and are now more likely than men to enroll in college (U.S. Dept of Labor, 2005). Today, women are highly credentialed, comprising 49% of law school graduates and 36% of business school graduates (Thomson and Graham, 2005). Women now earn more than half of all bachelors degrees and masters degrees, according to the National Center for Education Statistics (2005).

However, college women face pressing health concerns, including several under their own control. More than one third of undergraduates were found to be obese or overweight and two thirds of female undergraduates were found to be deficient in calcium, iron, or folate

(Kliff, 2007). Although almost 47 million Americans have quit cigarette smoking as of 2005, many young women on US campuses continue to start this dangerous practice each year.

Why Young Women should not Smoke

Cigarette smoking is arguably the single most preventable cause of death in the United States. However, roughly 21% of women and 24% of men still engage in this behavior, despite abundant evidence establishing cigarette smoking as harmful to health. Cigarettes are considered to be responsible for more deaths than AIDS, alcohol, drug abuse, automobile accidents, and fires combined (Garfinkel, 1997). Medical care costs associated with smoking-related illnesses have been estimated by the Center for Disease Control and Prevention to be more than 50 billion dollars annually in the U.S. In addition, the value of lost earnings and loss of productivity due to smoking-related health complications is estimated to be at least another 47 billion dollars a year (TTURC, 2001). Adult smokers have been found to be less socially connected and more depressed (Glassman, Helzer, Covey, Cottler, Stettner, Tipp, and Johnson, 1988; Anda, Williamson, Escobedo, Mast, Giovino, and Remington, 1990; Glassman et al., 1990; Hemenway, Solnick, and Colditz, 1993; Stein, Newcomb, and Bentler, 1996), possibly utilizing cigarettes as a form of self-medication (Gilbert, 1979; Clausen, 1987).

Despite countless programs disseminating this information, smoking prevalence among adolescents actually increased during the 1990s, from 20% in 1991 to 36% in 1997. Among adolescents who smoke, approximately half are expected to become regular adult tobacco users.

Smoking among young women risks their health, but increasingly it entails additional social burdens as well. Older adults are becoming more condemning of smokers, and overt discrimination against those who smoke is increasing. Negative stereotypes about smokers are pervasive, which can compromise young female smokers' educational, career, and personal prospects. Stigma directed against female and male students who smoke has been documented in high school, college, law school, and medical school settings (Chambliss, 2004). Within the business world, studies have found that potential customers find smoke exposure offensive. As a result, many workplaces have instituted smoking bans for their employees. Anti-smoking statutes increasingly curb this behavior in public settings.

Extensive empirical evidence suggests that smokers are perceived more negatively on a variety of dimensions than are their nonsmoking counterparts. A study of workers found that business managers who smoked were rated more negatively than their nonsmoking peers on several variables, including honesty, leadership, interpersonal ability, and delegation (Chaudhary, 1997). Bleda and Sandman (1977) found that nonsmokers did not discriminate between courteous and discourteous smokers, but they did discriminate between smoking and nonsmoking confederates. They rated the nonsmoker significantly more positively than the two smokers, viewing both smokers as being less considerate than the nonsmoker. Dermer and Jacobsen (1986) also documented public bias against smokers. In their study, college students were given a picture of a person either holding or not holding a cigarette and asked to rate this person on a series of characteristics including consideration, impulsiveness, sociability, maturity, health, intelligence, and sexiness. Four of the six smokers portrayed in this experiment were perceived more negatively. Interestingly, participants' own smoking status had no effect on their perceptions of smoking. The male smoker was rated as the most masculine out of all of the cases, suggesting that smoking is generally conceptualized as unfeminine. Consistent with this notion is the finding that out of all of the hypothetical cases, females were rated most negatively, and thus were the most socially disadvantaged by their smoking status. This documented differential bias against smokers provides a powerful reason for young women in particular to weigh the risks of cigarette smoking very carefully. In addition to compromising their health, smoking will likely reduce their perceived femininity and social attractiveness.

Bleda and Bleda (1978) showed that the majority of people opt to avoid exposure to smoke when given the chance. They observed the behavior of participants when a confederate, smoking or not smoking, sat 12 inches from them in a shopping mall. Most of the participants who sat beside the confederate left the bench when the confederate started to smoke. Polivy, Hachete, and Bycio (1979) examined college students' perceptions of smokers, through the presentation of photographs, and found that nonsmokers rated other nonsmokers most positively along all of the dimensions they used, and rated smokers most negatively. Additional studies have confirmed that smokers and nonsmokers are perceived as having different personality charactersitics. Srebro, Hodges, Authier, and Chambliss (1999) found that smokers are perceived as less mature than nonsmokers. Hines, et al.(1998) found that nonsmokers perceive smokers as less healthy, less desirable as a date, less attractive while smoking, less sexy, less feminine, less conventional, and less self-confident. In addition, they also found that nonsmokers believed that smokers were less sensible. Both smokers and nonsmokers seem to harbor negative attitudes toward smokers. Smokers perceived other smokers as less secure, intelligent, physically fit, energized, confident, and alert than their nonsmoking counterparts (Srebro et al., 1999).

Approximately half of college student smokers reported having been asked to not smoke at least once within the past year in various locations (Campbell, Svenson, and Jarvis, 1993). Nonsmoker college students also believed that smoking would lead to negative consequences, such as appearing less attractive or feeling sick (Grube, Mcbree, and Morgan, 1986). In addition, college students also have described smokers to be less desirable to be in a close relationship with, such as being a roommate, a date, or a future spouse (Hines, Fretz, and Nollen, 1998).

Anderson, Shah, and Julliard (2002) examined the perceptions of and attitudes toward cigarette smoking by junior high school students. They also wanted to examine those who helped to formulate students' impressions of smokers and what kind of familial influence shaped these impressions. The research was conducted by administering a survey addressing these issues to students who visited the nurse's office. The researchers found that only 2% of the sample reported that they were smokers and more than half of the entire sample credited their parents with teaching them not to smoke. However, it is interesting to note that the majority of these parents were smokers themselves. Overall, subjects had negative views of smoking; specifically, 90% of the students recognized the habit as harmful to their health. It is important to note that the context used in this research may have reduced the accuracy of self reporting due to demand characteristics, resulting in an underestimate of actual student smoking.

Douglas, Allen, Arian, Crawford, Headen, Spigner, Tassler, and Ureda (2001) also examined younger adolescents' perceptions of smokers. Specifically, they wanted to identify the actual images that teenagers have of smoking, smokers, and nonsmokers. Adolescents, whether smokers or nonsmokers, felt that not only the physical characteristics of smoking were negative (smell, taste, etc.) but also that the smokers themselves had negative qualities. Although the general perceptions of smokers were negative, the degree to which the teenagers condemned smokers based on their habit varied across the dimensions being examined. Smokers' pride was seen as more acceptable and justified by African American adolescents than those with other ethnicities. The link between smoking and drug use was seen as stronger for African American and Hispanic adolescents, while drinking and smoking were more associated with white and Native American groups.

Campbell, Bartlett, Liberati, Tornetta, and Chambliss (2000) found evidence of discrimination against both male and female cigarette smokers among undergraduates. Their data indicated that nonsmokers viewed fellow nonsmokers as generally appearing intelligent (91%) while only 50.7% of the nonsmokers perceived smokers as being intelligent. Seventy eight percent of nonsmokers perceived other nonsmokers as sophisticated while only 37.4% of nonsmokers observed smokers as sophisticated. Ninety one percent of nonsmokers thought that other nonsmokers were considerate while 65.6% of nonsmokers viewed smokers as considerate. Nonsmokers also perceived smokers as less fit than nonsmokers (92.6% versus 64.2%). Almost all (96%) of nonsmokers saw other nonsmokers as being mature, while only 67% of them perceived smokers as being mature. Clearly, cigarette smoking risks tarnishing a student's image in the eyes of many. When viewed as a group, male and female smokers are evaluated more negatively than students who refrain from smoking.

Gender Similarities in Stigma Linked to Cigarette Smoking

It is important to consider ways in which the social hazards associated with smoking differentially affect women and men. Some studies have suggested that male smokers are viewed differently than female smokers. For example, Brosh, Austin, and Chambliss (2003) found that male smokers were seen as more hostile, artistic, and independent than their female counterparts.

Baker, Katona, Shull, Brosh, and Chambliss (2004) extended previous research on the stigma associated with smoking cigarettes. Their study assessed the generality of previous findings by including both an adolescent and adult sample; secondly, it explored whether smoking cessation reverses the negative social stigma associated with smoking; finally, it examined whether a smoker's gender influences the magnitude of social stigma directed against the smoker. The subjects in the Baker et al. (2004) study were presented with four hypothetical situations – that of male smoker, a female smoker, nonsmoker, and former smoker – and asked to rate these cases along many descriptive dimensions.

The sample chosen for the Baker, et al. study included both high school and college students. This was done in order to explore developmental differences. Because college students may have more crystallized, reasoned ideals, their attitudes may be different from those of their younger peers. The high school sample selected was drawn from a suburban, middle socio-economic population, similar in background to the college students sampled

This research also assessed attitudes and perceptions of former smokers. This is important because the former smoker hypothetical case provides interesting clues about whether the stigma associated with smoking is eliminated after the smoking behavior ceases. Other research has found that perceptions of smoking behavior vary as a function of the respondents' own smoking habits

Respondents in the Baker et al. study were 215 college students from a small liberal arts college from a suburban area in the Northeast United States and 110 high school students attending a public school in the same area. The sample included 172 female and 153 male students. College students, with a mean age of 19.32, were enrolled in introductory and upper level psychology courses, and high school students, with a mean age of 16.94, were enrolled in health education classes were administered the anonymous survey during class meetings.

The survey consisted of 200 items pertaining to current and previous personal smoking habits, motivations for smoking and not smoking, and perceptions of smokers and nonsmokers, as well as those who quit. Additionally, a personality inventory and self-esteem scale were included.

Perceptions of male smokers, female smokers, nonsmokers, and smokers who had quit were assessed through eight five-point Likert-format items (1=extremely low, 2=somewhat low, 3=neutral, 4=somewhat high, 5=extremely high). Participants were asked to describe their impression of an average student in each of these four categories along the following dimensions: intelligence, hostility, judgment, artistic creativity, independence, conscientiousness, ambition, and consideration.

Directionally adjusted items were totaled to create summary character ratings each of the four hypothetical cases (male smoker, female smoker, nonsmoker, and former smoker). High scores indicate high levels of socially valued qualities. In order to determine if differences exist among perceptions of current male and female smokers, nonsmokers, and former smokers, paired sample t-tests were performed on character ratings of the four hypothetical target cases representing these groups. Significant differences were found among all the targets, with $p < .001$, except the male and female smokers.

Nonsmokers were rated most favorably. Table 1 summarizes the character ratings of the four targets, and Table 2 reveals the results of the within-subject t-tests. Further analysis revealed similar results regardless of the participants' gender, smoking status, and developmental level (high school versus college).

Table 1. Mean ratings of generalized perceptions of hypothetical targets among high school and college students

Perceptions Mean Standard Deviation

Nonsmoker	26.93	5.01
Former Smoker	25.73	3.96
Male smoker	20.16	4.26
Female smoker	19.89	4.22

Table 2. Within-subject t-test results of comparisons of character ratings of four hypothetical cases among high school and college students

Perceptions t df p

	t	df	p
Nonsmoker vs. Male smoker	16.07	315	.001
Nonsmoker vs. Female smoker	16.85	320	.001
Nonsmoker vs. Former smoker	5.06	318	.001
Former smoker vs. Male smoker	16.25	313	.001
Former smoker vs. Female smoker	17.18	320	.001
Male smoker vs. Female Smoker	1.60	317	ns

Multivariate ANOVA (gender x participant smoking status x developmental period) performed on the 4 hypothetical cases revealed no significant developmental period main effects. In addition, neither smoking status by gender nor smoking status by developmental period effects were obtained. Scores on three of the four hypothetical cases were found to be significantly different for smokers and nonsmokers. Specifically, smokers viewed the hypothetical male smoker significantly more favorably than nonsmokers did (smokers: x=22.20, sd=3.04, n=76; nonsmokers: x=19.51, sd=4.39, n=222; F=10.16, df=1/298, p<.05). Smokers also viewed the hypothetical female smoker significantly more favorably than the nonsmokers did (smokers: x=21.96, sd=3.25, n=76; nonsmokers: x=19.31, sd=4.25, n=222; F=14.18, df=1/298, p<.01). However, nonsmokers viewed the hypothetical nonsmoker more favorably than the smokers did (nonsmokers: n=27.79, sd=4.82, n=222; smokers: x=24.96, sd=4.99, n=76; F=8.60, df=1/298, p<.01).

Only two hypothetical cases, the nonsmoker and former smoker, significantly differentiated between male and female respondents. One significant two-way interaction emerged on summary ratings of the hypothetical nonsmoker. Female high school students rated the nonsmoker case higher than the other three participant groups on this item (F=7.54, df=1/298, p<.01) (Table 3). This indicates that the stigma associated with smoking cigarettes is most strongly evident among female high school students. More effectively tapping the norms of this group may have the potential to exert a strong influence on adolescent smoking choices.

In addition to the hypothetical cases, impressions of the prevalence of smoking and expectations of typical behavior towards smokers were assessed through MANOVA. Specifically, respondents were asked whether they thought the majority of students within their respective schools were smokers and also if they thought smokers were discriminated against by other students, teachers, and employers. This analysis revealed no significant interactions among sex, developmental period, and smoking status on any of the dimensions examined.

Within subject t-test comparisons revealed that nonsmokers were viewed more positively than both current and former smokers on the individual personality traits. Former smokers were evaluated less negatively than current smokers on most characteristics.

Table 3. Significant two-way interaction results based on a MANOVA (sex x developmental period) for the nonsmoker hypothetical case

	High School	College
Male	x = 43.10 sd = 5.69 n = 40	x = 42.17 sd = 4.10 n = 24
Female	x = 45.86 sd = 5.72 n=59	x = 42.41 sd = 4.55 n = 81

Table 4.

	Male Smoker		Nonsmoker				
	x	SD	x	SD	t	df	p
Intelligence	2.71	0.81	3.87	0.85	16.53	323	.001
Poor Judgment	3.16	0.87	2.55	1.07	6.94	322	.001
Conscientiousness	2.60	0.88	3.79	0.87	15.25	322	.001
Considerate	2.56	0.86	3.74	0.88	15.13	323	.001
Ambitious	2.59	0.86	3.82	0.89	15.86	323	.001
Artistic Creativity	3.02	0.84	3.38	0.76	5.53	323	.001
Hostility	3.22	0.83	2.81	1.01	4.90	323	.001
Independence	3.10	0.97	3.64	0.91	7.00	322	.001

Table 5.

	Female Smoker		Nonsmoker				
	x	SD	x	SD	t	df	p
Intelligence	2.61	0.84	3.87	0.85	17.88	329	0.001
Poor Judgment	3.22	0.89	2.55	1.07	7.32	326	0.001
Conscientiousness	2.61	0.84	3.79	0.87	15.74	326	0.001
Considerate	2.57	0.84	3.74	0.88	1.01	329	0.001
Ambitious	2.56	0.82	3.82	0.89	1.11	329	0.001
Artistic Creativity	2.85	0.80	3.39	0.77	0.41	327	0.001
Hostility	3.03	0.85	2.82	1.01	0.37	328	0.013
Independence	2.92	0.95	3.65	0.91	0.57	328	0.001

Table 6. Mean ratings and paired-samples t-test results for ratings of the nonsmoker and former smoker hypothetical cases along the individual personality dimensions

	Former Smoker		Nonsmoker				
	x	SD	x	SD	t	df	p
Intelligence	3.71	0.75	3.87	0.85	3.43	323	0.001
Poor Judgment	2.82	1.05	2.55	1.07	1.51	323	ns
Conscientiousness	3.63	0.76	3.79	0.87	2.59	323	0.010
Considerate	3.54	0.79	3.74	0.88	3.97	322	0.001
Ambitious	3.66	0.80	3.82	0.89	2.36	322	0.019
Artistic Creativity	3.15	0.61	3.38	0.76	5.26	323	0.001
Hostility	3.01	0.83	2.81	1.01	4.69	323	0.001
Independence	3.53	0.80	3.64	0.91	2.33	323	0.020

Baker, et al. (2004) found variable patterns of tobacco use across the adolescent and young adult populations they sampled, suggesting that rates of cigarette use rise with age. Specifically, 17.4% of high school students and 28.3% of college students surveyed engaged in smoking behavior classified as habitual and regular. Among these segments, only trivial sex differences were observed. Of the female students surveyed, 22.4% were regular smokers. Of the male students surveyed, 23.0% were regular smokers.

This study supported the notion that smokers are increasingly stigmatized in our society, but found few significant gender differences in stigma. Both high school and college students evaluated current smokers far more harshly on a number of personality dimensions, including intelligence, creativity, and independence. Participants' evaluations of former smokers fell between those of current smokers and nonsmokers, suggesting that cessation alleviates some, but not all, of the stigma associated with this behavior.

It is interesting to note that there was one personality characteristic that appeared to be exempt from the salutary effects of smoking cessation, at least for females. On the hostility character item there was no significant difference between ratings of former smokers and current female smokers. This finding seems to be primarily due to the female smoker's being seen as less hostile than her male peer. Since a female smoker is initially seen as less hostile (presumably because women are generally perceived to be less aggressive), there is less opportunity for her smoking cessation to have a measurable impact on her perceived hostility. This result is consistent with the notion that a strong gender stereotype competes with the smoker stereotype for women. Although smokers are generally seen as more hostile than nonsmokers (Srebro et al., 1999), according to the present finding, this is far less true for females than male smokers. In society, there is a general and often overriding perception that women are more docile and passive. Perhaps this stereotype affected the subjects' reasoning and their perceptions of female smokers. Other evidence from the Baker et al. (2004) study suggested that stereotyped thinking about gender might have pervaded the subjects' judgment; for example, male smokers were seen as significantly more creative and independent than their female counterparts.

In summary, Baker, et al. (2004) found few gender differences in the stigma associated with smoking. Male and female current smokers were viewed similarly by students.

Why do Young Women Smoke?

The factors affecting young women's decisions to smoke are in some ways distinctive from those influencing young men's. The role of the interpersonal context in which smoking occurs, affect and appetite regulation, and young women's ambitions have been considered in research aimed at describing the issues shaping young women's smoking choices. Clarifying these factors is important because it may provide information valuable to the development of more effective prevention methods.

There has been much speculation about the causes of the smoking increase seen among young women college students. The relatively recent upsurge of smoking among female undergraduates has made it imperative to examine what motivates young women to engage in this behavior. Relatively little research on the social and personal factors prompting college students to smoke has been done; most extant research focuses on the influences on adolescent and older adult smokers.

To discern the relationship between specific subjective determinants and smoking behavior, a comprehensive assessment of many possible factors is needed. One of the few empirical investigations that have attempted to examine motivational factors comprehensively was conducted by Campbell, et al. (2000). Three hundred and twenty-four college students completed a survey assessing smoking motivations. Respondents were asked to rate "When you smoke a cigarette, how does it make you feel?" on 16 Likert-format items (1=Never, 2=Rarely, 3=Often, and 4=Very Frequently), assessing four hypothesized subjective effects sought by smokers. Subjective smoking determinants of current smokers were assessed along the following dimensions: relaxation effects, image effects, competence effects, and stimulant effects.

To measure the motivational role of relaxation effects, scores were grouped and averaged for the following feeling items: high levels of relaxation, contentment, and trust, and low levels of anxiety and jitteriness. In order to assess the importance of image effects, scores were averaged and grouped for the following feeling items: high levels of attractiveness, sophistication, and maturity. In order to assess the importance of competence effects, scores were grouped and averaged for the following feeling items: high levels of alertness, competence, security, intelligence, and adequacy. In order to assess the importance of stimulant effects, scores were grouped and averaged for the following feeling items: high levels of physical fitness, and energy, and low levels of hunger.

Smokers reported using cigarettes in order to attain relaxation effects, image effects, and competence effects more so than stimulant effects. The rank-order of these factors, in descending order were: relaxation effects, image effects, competence effects, and stimulant effects (Campbell, et al., 2000).

A 2003 paper exploring motivations for smoking was authored by Austin, Brosh, and Chambliss. This study explored the experiential factors underlying smoking by administering a questionnaire consisting of the Rosenberg Self Concept scale and items assessing smoking habits and motivations to college and high school students. Directionally adjusted items were totaled to create summary scores for the 4 hypothesized motivational factors underlying smoking. Paired sample t-tests indicated the presence of significant differences between all possible factor combinations (p<.05). The rank-order of these factors, in descending order, were: relaxation effects, competence effects, stimulant effects, and image effects. A median split was used to divide participants into high and low self-esteem groups. 2 X 2 X 2 ANOVA (smoking status; developmental period; sex) revealed that female high school student smokers reported the greatest desire for more self-respect and expressed feelings of uselessness more than any other group (Respect: F=6.58, df=1/259, p<.01; Uselessness: F=4.44, df=1/261, p<.05).

Examination of nonsmoker motivations revealed significant differences between the primary reason cited, health concerns, and all other reasons (p<.001). Men's and women's use of cigarettes differed across the developmental periods examined. Of the female students surveyed, 12% of high school students and 30% of college students were regular smokers. Among the males, a quarter of high school students and a third of college students were regular smokers. This finding of slightly greater smoking among the males is consistent with the research linking this behavior to masculinity mentioned earlier in this chapter.

Table 7. Significant three-way interaction results based on a MANOVA (sex x developmental period x smoking status) on responses to the "I wish I could have more respect for myself" self-esteem item

Sex Developmental Period		Smoking Status	mean SD n
Male			
	High School	Smoker	1.64 1.03 11
		Nonsmoker	2.27 0.98 33
	College	Smoker	2.55 0.89 20
		Nonsmoker	2.13 0.98 46
Female			
	High School	Smoker	2.75 1.04 8
		Nonsmoker	2.46 1.08 56
	College	Smoker	2.22 0.97 27
		Nonsmoker	2.52 1.08 58

Table 8. Significant three-way interaction results based on a MANOVA (sex x developmental period x smoking status) on responses to the "I certainly feel useless at times" self-esteem item

Sex Developmental Period		Smoking Status	mean SD n
Male			
	High School	Smoker	1.64 1.03 11
		Nonsmoker	1.82 0.81 33
	College	Smoker	2.10 1.02 20
		Nonsmoker	2.04 0.94 46
Female			
	High School	Smoker	2.75 1.04 8
		Nonsmoker	2.04 0.93 57
	College	Smoker	1.93 0.87 27
		Nonsmoker	2.29 0.81 59

Situational and Stereotype Factors

Despite the fact that both adolescents and adults rate smokers more negatively than nonsmokers, some young women still see becoming a smoker as an appealing means of enhancing their self presentation. Jones and Carroll (1998) found evidence that smoking in a social context may be viewed quite positively by female undergraduates. They presented 40 female college students with video presentations of females engaging in stereotypical female behaviors while either smoking or not smoking a cigarette. The researchers believed that because the women would be able to see the context of the female's behavior rather than just a one-dimensional portrayal of her, the subjects would be more prone to rate a female smoker favorably along a variety of dimensions, such as being liberated and independent. The subjects were divided into two groups; one group saw a female talk on the phone for 10 minutes, light up a cigarette, and then proceed to read a book for 50 seconds, while the second group saw the same scene with the cigarette scene omitted. The female was portrayed as attractive, expressive, and engaging. After being presented with one of these two scenes, subjects were given a "Health Habits" questionnaire which assessed perceptions of the smokers and nonsmokers presented in the video.

The researchers concluded that the females viewing these scenarios, regardless of their own smoking status, rated the smoking female more positively than the nonsmoking female along most of the dimensions presented. In this study subjects received large amounts of dynamic information about the person they were supposed to rate, because subjects observed the target's social interactions with others, as well as her physical appearance, gestures, and attitudes. As a result, ratings were based on a wider variety of factors than subjects in other experiments. This may have contributed to findings which were discrepant with those of other experiments detailing the social hazards of smoking cigarettes. In addition, this sample consisted exclusively of female young adults, who may hold different views and beliefs about smoking.

Several studies have found that women and men react similarly to many social situations prompting cigarette smoking. For example, both men and women college students reported greater tobacco use in interpersonal campus contexts involving alcohol use. Campbell, et al. (2000) found that men and women responded similarly to contexts involving smoking restrictions. However, females seem to be more susceptible to such influences as smoking peers (Chassin, et al., 1996), smoke more in response to stress, and smoke more in social and emotional situations than do males (Zuckerman, 1994). Van Roosmalen and McDaniel (1992) found that men are more likely to recognize the benefits of quitting than women, which may account for their greater success at cessation. Women also voiced more concerns about job pressures linked to quitting.

Situational determinants of cigarette smoking behavior among adolescents were investigated by Lucas and Lloyd (1999), using qualitative research techniques. After quantitative survey research of 4,773 British respondents ages eleven to sixteen revealed a significant gender difference regarding current smoking behavior, 33 focus groups were formed. Due to the higher smoking prevalence among females, each focus group consisted of two to six girls who belonged to friendship groups prior to the study. Focus groups were classified by smoking status along the following dimensions: homogeneous non-smokers, homogeneous experimental smokers, and homogeneous regular smokers. Homogeneous non-smoking groups were composed of members who had never smoked a cigarette. Homogeneous experimental smoking groups were composed of members who tried smoking cigarettes, but no longer smoked cigarettes at the time of the study. Homogeneous regular smoking groups were comprised of members who were current regular smokers. Due to the requirement of homogeneous group composition, only 13 of the original 33 focus groups were examined.

The ten homogeneous non-smoking focus groups discussed situational determinants which they associate with smoking behavior. In a social context, members of homogeneous non-smoking groups asserted that smoking would alter group identity. Group members described other non-smokers as quiet, sensible, homebodies. When asked what they would do if a member of the group started smoking, respondents stated that their friends were autonomous, and therefore smoking was one's own decision. However, when discussing previous close friends who smoked, respondents recalled initial friendship maintenance, followed by persuasion to revert back to a non-smoking status. "Gone bad" or "badness" were the descriptors most frequently cited by respondents in reference to adolescent females who currently engage in smoking behavior. If a hypothetical non-smoker experimented with cigarette smoking and subsequently decided to quit, respondents concluded that she would remain a member of the group.

The two homogeneous experimental smoking focus groups regarded situational determinants along the following three dimensions: instigation, sense of place, and reassurance by smokers. Instigators were most frequently described as older acquaintances rather than close friends. A sense of place was cited as a designated location where the smoking ritual took place. Adolescents would go out and meet, with the purpose of smoking in mind. A sense of daring and fearlessness were cited most frequently, depicting the subjective experience associated with this location. Similar to the perceptions of the homogeneous non-smoking groups, homogeneous experimental smoking groups described smoking initiation in a persuasive context. Additionally, members of the homogeneous experimental smoking groups noted that individuals unable to produce persuasive counter arguments were more likely to smoke as a result of persuasion.

The one homogeneous regular smoking focus group described their subjective smoking experiences along the following three categorical dimensions: initiation, experimental smoking, and regular smoking. The initiation phase closely paralleled the perceived descriptions of peer influence given by respondents belonging to homogeneous non-smoking groups. A strong sense of place was expressed, similar to the homogeneous experimental smoking groups; however the role of an instigator was less pronounced. Additionally, when describing the experimental smoking phase, a desire to stay active and an unwillingness to make counter assertions regarding smoking claims was also evident. Regular smoking was characterized by the growing realization that they were addicted. When this occurred, respondents reported viewing themselves as a "smoker."

The possible role of parental and peer influence was assessed longitudinally by Brook, Whiteman, Czeisler, Shapiro, and Cohen (1997), over a period of 17 years, from 1975 to 1992. Participants ranged from one to ten years of age during wave one in 1975 and 18 to 28 years of age during wave four in 1992. A four-wave longitudinal analysis was conducted on 746 of the original 976 participants.

Due to the emergence of significant differences between those who completed all four waves of the study and those who dropped out, results were alternatively analyzed. A cross-sectional sample was obtained by dividing the sample by older and younger aged cohorts (older cohort= five years of age or older at wave one, younger cohort= younger than five years of age at wave one). A mutual parent-child attachment was positively correlated with nonsmoking status in both the younger and older cohort. Parent smoker status and child smoker status were positively correlated for the younger cohort. Deviant behavior, as well as usage of marijuana and cigarettes by peers, was positively correlated with child smoker status in the younger cohort.

In contrast, possessing friends who achieve good grades was negatively correlated with child smoker status in both the younger and older cohort. Regression analyses revealed the distinct role of parental and peer smoking influences during various developmental stages. At wave two, parental smoking behavior was the primary influence reported for smoking initiation. At wave three, peer smoking behavior was the primary influence reported for smoking initiation. Due to the significant difference between participants who completed all four waves of the study and those who dropped out, the findings were cross-sectional, not longitudinal, in scope.

Flay, Hu, Siddiqui, Day, Hedeker, Petraitis, Richardson, and Sussman (1994) examined the role of parental and peer smoking influence during smoking initiation and escalation. Respondents participated in the Television, School, and Family Project and as a part of this completed a smoking prevention program questionnaire. The first assessment, conducted in 1986, consisted of 6,695 seventh grade respondents. Fifteen months later, 4,896 respondents were re-administered the questionnaire as eighth grade students. Respondents who reported smoking more than one cigarette during the first assessment were excluded from the study, as well as those who reported disruptive family structure (single parent, orphan). Due to these restrictions, final analysis consisted of a 1,974 respondents, 1,402 respondents analyzed for initiation and 572 for examination of the escalation, respectively.

The structural model indicated that friends' smoking behavior directly affected smoking initiation of the respondent. Additionally, smoking intentions and negative outcome items indirectly affected respondent's smoking initiation, as smoking friends were associated with increased intent to smoke and decreased reporting of negative outcome. Parental smoking indirectly affected respondents' smoking initiation; as perceived parental approval increased, the likelihood of reported negative outcome decreased. Escalation was affected by parental and peer influences indirectly. Peer smoking was associated with increased levels of perceived peer acceptance of smoking, decreased levels of refusal self-efficacy, and a decline in reported negative outcomes. Parental smoking was associated with increased levels of perceived parental acceptance of smoking and a decline in reported negative outcomes.

Several features of the campus environment may promote young women's experimentation with smoking. The increased freedom of college, frequent unsupervised parties featuring alcohol, cigarettes, and other substances, and pressure to appear open and sophisticated can foster the decision to initiate smoking. Although most academic contexts on campuses are now ordinarily smoke-free, restrictions preventing smoking during classes may actually exert a counterproductive influence on some young women in the early stages of nicotine addiction. While policies forbidding smoking in public areas might seem to be of unequivocal benefit to novice smokers, because they increase the time they are engaging in non-smoking behaviors, forced abstention often has paradoxical effects on appetitive behaviors. The Campbell, et al. study discussed previously also explored the impact of campus smoking restrictions on student smoking, to assess whether young women's addiction to nicotine was accidentally being fostered by brief limits on access that enhanced the appetitive features of cigarettes. Since the pleasure associated with smoking is greater following a period of brief nicotine withdrawal, smoke-free classes of an hour or two might unfortunately serve to make smoking more reinforcing for women. Most of the smokers Campbell, et al. sampled acknowledged that try to conceal their habit from parents, faculty, staff, and others, although none confined their smoking to contexts including other smokers. Interestingly, less than a third of the smokers said they avoid situations because smoking is prohibited within them. It is encouraging to note that few of these college smokers reported craving cigarettes while in smoking restricted settings. In fact, most experienced reduced interest in smoking while in these situations.

On the other hand, the majority reported that they smoke wherever and whenever it is permitted. Although most of the smokers sampled by Campbell, et al. did not smoke within 30 minutes of waking (characteristic of those with nicotine addiction), almost all felt they were already addicted to nicotine. Roughly half of these college student smokers reported that they favor smoking restrictions, suggesting that some may find restrictions a helpful tool for self management at this point in the development of their habit.

The Campbell, et al. findings partially supported the notion that campus restriction might inadvertently enhance the appeal of smoking behavior; most smokers reported finding smoking more satisfying after a period of restriction (although only 43% found smoking more relaxing after abstinence). However, most did not feel constrained while in a smoke-free situation nor liberated upon less such situations. The Campbell, et al. findings suggest that while smoking restrictions may temporarily elevate the attractiveness of cigarettes and elicit increased smoking, they do not necessarily foster preoccupation with cigarettes, even among students who see themselves as already addicted to nicotine.

Social Image Factors

Several studies have obtained evidence supporting the notion that smoking behavior serves as a means of relating to peers within both adolescent and adult populations (Sarason, Mankowski, Peterson, and Dinh, 1992; Gillard and Bruchon-Schweitzer, 2001). Married, sensation seeking male adults, single, female respondents with poor self-refusal efficacy, and female adolescents all reported using cigarettes as a means of achieving greater social acceptance.

In one of the few studies explicitly examining concerns about image, Campbell, et al. (2000) found that these self presentation issues were second only to desire for relaxation as a motivation for smoking. The importance of image concerns found in this sample of young adult smokers was not paralleled by research using older samples of adults. This may suggest that self presentation figures into the decision to smoke more among college students than their older counterparts. It is also possible that college students are more willing to acknowledge the role of such factors in shaping their decision to smoke.

Direct assessment of the role of image concerns is difficult because it is not highly socially acceptable to acknowledge that one's smoking is motivated by the desire to enhance one's image. It seems plausible that few smokers would feel comfortable candidly acknowledging that they smoke "to look cool." However, reluctance to report this motivation does not necessarily mean it is not actually a causal factor. One way of indirectly estimating the influence of image factors is to consider the findings from research on various social situational determinants of smoking. Presumably those who are more likely to smoke in social contexts are at least partially doing so to enhance their self presentation.

During adolescence, it is typical to smoke for social purposes (Stein, Newcomb, and Bentler, 1996), and peer smoking behavior has been implicated as an influential contributor to smoking (Moore, 1998). Several empirical investigations have explicitly examined the psychological issues affecting young women's decisions to smoke. Both male and female adolescents who experimented with cigarette smoking often reported that they did so because they associated smoking with toughness, sociability, precociousness, and extraversion (Imperto and Mitchell, 1986; Hundleby, 1987) and wanted to project an image associated with these characteristics. In contrast, college student smokers perceived smoking to be relaxing (Hodges et al., 1999) as did older adult regular smokers (Chassin, Presson, and Sherman, 1990; Clausen, 1987; Gilbert, 1979), and as a means of relieving stress (Gilbert, 1979; Clausen, 1987; Chassin et al., 1990).

Female college students may start smoking if they believe they will be perceived positively in terms of sophistication, attractiveness, and/or social successfulness by their peers (Barton, et al., 1982; Burton, et al., 1989; Moore, 1998). A study by Hodges, et al. (1999) found that smoking for image purposes figured prominently into reasons why college students smoke, as did the research by Campbell, et al. (2000). It is interesting to note that students who frequently engage in high-risk behaviors also have a greater tendency to be smokers (Emmons, et al., 1998). Public engagement in dangerous behaviors is often used by young adults to demonstrate courage among peers and establish oneself as a leader. Smoking may thereby function as a tool for image enhancement in some social groups.

Advertising and Film Factors

Cigarette advertisements have been found to make a potentially enormous contribution to early smoking initiation (Reid, 1985; Potts, Gillies, and Herbert, 1986; Department of Health and Human Services, 1994; Zinser, Kloosterman, and Williams, 1994; Moore, 1998). Adolescents' environments have been found to be saturated with pro-smoking messages, especially in magazines (Schooler, Feighery, and Flora, 1996). Magazine advertisements for tobacco products frequently portray exciting, adventurous scenes depicting smokers as glamorous and appealing (Zinser, Kloosterman, and Williams, 1991; Hines et al., 1998; Moore, 1998). A study by Zinser, et al. (1991) discovered that both college student smokers and nonsmokers rated cigarette advertisements as more adventurous in comparison with advertisements for other products. Magazine ad content analyses validated the notion that advertisements were developed by the smoking industry to depict smokers as attractive, athletic, and lively (Altman, Slater, Albright, and Maccoby, 1987; Altman, Levine, Coeytaux, Slade, and Jaffe, 1996). It is important to note that because adolescence is a time of preoccupation with social image, young people often fall prey to the underlying suggestion that smoking will enhance their allure (Zinser, et al., 1991).

In addition to the pervasive influence of cigarette advertisements, film portrayals of cigarette smoking have been shown to increase smoking behavior among the young (Kaufman, 2003; Dalton, Sargent, Beach, Titus-Ernstoff, Gibson, Aherns, Tickle, and Heatherton, 2003). The influence of film images has been found to be especially pronounced among children of nonsmoking parents.

Rebellion Factors

Although interactions among various sociodemographic characteristics and environmental factors are presumed to influence women's decision to smoke, personality and developmental factors also come into play. As cigarette smoking has become less mainstream (the majority of adults no longer smoke, and smoking is increasingly rare among the power elite), its appeal as a form of adolescent rebellion has increased. Becoming a smoker in a family of nonsmokers may be seen as a manifestation of autonomy, rather than poor judgment; of courage rather than carelessness. The recent increase in smoking among college students noted by Wechsler, Rigotii, Gledhill-Hoyt, and Lee (1998) is especially intriguing because it runs counter to evidence showing that cigarette use is concentrated among the less academically successful. For example, Hu, Zihua, and Keeler (1998) used data from the 1990 California Youth Tobacco Survey to explore the correlation between school performance, smoking, and efforts to quit among teenagers. They hypothesized that a student's school performance would be related to their smoking status. It was assumed that the better a student performs in school, the less likely he or she is to become a smoker, and vice versa. School performance is seen as a broad indicator variable that reflects traits such as general educational commitment, motivation, competence in learning and value judgment, and academic success. The final sample of respondents included 5028 teenagers between the ages of 12 to 17. The teenagers were divided into 3 categories, that included current smokers, former smokers, and nonsmokers. Individuals who had smoked in the past 30 days were considered to be current smokers. A former smoker was a person who had smoked any time before, but not during the previous 30 days. Nonsmokers were persons who had never smoked before. School performance was self-reported as much better than average, better than average, average, and below average.

Results indicated that 72.9% of the teenagers were non-smokers, 17.2% were former smokers, and 9.9% were current smokers. The older the teenager was (16 or 17 years old), the more likely they were to smoke. No difference was found between boys and girls in smoking status. Although Black teenagers were less likely to be current smokers, those who did smoke were less likely to have made an effort to quit. Current or former smokers tended to perform below average in school.

Among the teenagers who were current smokers, 344 out of 496 (16.9%) had reported an effort to quit smoking. However, it seemed as though their efforts were largely unsuccessful; roughly one quarter had attempted to quit once, 31.4% had attempted to quit 2 or 3 times, and 25% had attempted to quit 4 or more times. Overall, 83% of the current smokers had tried to quit and failed.

Hu, et al. found that students who performed below average were more often current smokers and less likely to have stopped smoking. Poor educational attainment generally has been found not only to be the most powerful demographic predictor of smoking behavior (Chassin, et al., 1996) but is usually inversely related to smoking (Chassin, et al., 1996; Wechsler, et al., 1998).

Previous research has implicated socioeconomic status as an important predictor of smoking, both among adolescents and older adults (Hu, Lin, and Keeler, 1998; Green, et al., 1990; Stronks, et al., 1997; Emmons, et al., 1998). Clearly, rates of smoking tend to be higher among the less economically advantaged. Final level of educational attainment is also a powerful predictor of smoking behavior; smoking has consistently been found to be more common among the less educated (Chassin, et al., 1996). Other studies have shown a link between parental smoking behavior and children's choices regarding tobacco (Schooler, et al., 1996). Parental influence also plays a major role in the decision by youth to smoke cigarettes. Brook, et al. (1997) noted that the greater the parent-child attachment, the less likely the child will be to engage in cigarette smoking. Therefore, a child with a strong attachment is generally more likely to smoke if a parent is a current smoker.

Although some other studies have shown no direct relationship between smoking and school performance, it is possible that smoking may have an indirect effect on teenagers' academic behavior. Smoking seems to be associated with involvement in delinquent and drug abuse behaviors. These behaviors may, in turn, have a negative effect on school performance, and thereby account for the link between poor school performance and cigarette use.

Unlike some previous research, a study by Bartlett, Brackin, Chubb, Covatta, Ferguson, Hinckley, Hodges, Liberati, Tornetta, and Chambliss (1999) failed to observe a negative relationship between socioeconomic status and smoking behavior in college students, and in fact found smoking to be more common among students from higher income families. This finding was not explained by higher rates of parental smoking in the wealthier families (the majority of parents in all families were nonsmokers).

Smoking among some college students may represent a form of rebellion against affluent nonsmoking parents. This possibility received partial support from the finding that within the higher income family group, relatively few of the mothers smoked. In comparison, within low income families, nearly a third of the mothers smoked. However, the fathers in the higher income families were about as likely to smoke as their lower income counterparts. If for some college students smoking represents a way of asserting autonomy by engaging in behavior at odds with parental values, the offspring of wealthier nonsmoking mothers may quite unexpectedly be at higher risk.

Early smoking initiation has been linked to a history of conduct problems (Breslau and Peterson, 1996). Those high in sensation seeking seem especially prone to smoke. Young women who are drawn to risk and thrill-seeking may actually be more inclined to try cigarettes today, since smoking has so strongly been linked to dangerous health problems.

For daring young women, smoking may seem like a challenge, enhancing the excitement associated with this habit. In addition, the stimulation provided by nicotine may be experienced as especially reinforcing for such women.

Table 9.

Family income over $80,000, father's smoking status	
	Percent
No	69.7
Yes	30.3

Table 10.

Family income over $80,000, mother's smoking status	
	Percent
No	82.4
Yes	17.6

Table 11.

Family income under $80,000, father's smoking status	
	Percent
No	73.3
Yes	26.7

Table 12.

Family income under $80,000, mother's smoking status	
	Percent
No	73.3
Yes	29.7

Self Esteem Factors

A longitudinal study assessing adolescent self-esteem revealed that low levels of self-esteem present before smoking initiation may serve as a potential risk factor for future smoking behavior (Brynin, 1999). To assess the possible relationship between smoking and self-esteem, Kawabata, Cross, Nishioka, and Shimai (1999) conducted a three-year cohort study, surveying 2,090 fourth through ninth grade Japanese students. The 22-item questionnaire they used consisted of the following three self-esteem measures: the Harter Perceived Competence Scale, the Pope Self-esteem Scale, and the Rosenberg Self Concept Scale.

Between-group t-tests revealed a significant difference between ever smokers (current and previous smokers) and those who never smoked cigarettes. Female respondents and junior high school males classified as ever smokers were more likely to report lower levels of cognitive self-esteem than those who never smoked cigarettes. Additionally, significant differences regarding global self-esteem levels emerged between ever smokers and those who never smoked cigarettes. Female junior high school respondents who smoked were more likely to report lower levels of global self-esteem than those who never smoked cigarettes. However, measures of physical competence revealed that male respondents and female junior high school respondents who smoked were more likely to report higher levels of physical competence than those who never smoked cigarettes. Additionally, measures of social competence revealed that male junior high school respondents who smoked were more likely to report higher levels of social competence than those who never smoked cigarettes.

An examination of well-being and health-risk behaviors, conducted by Bergman and Scott (2001) revealed a relationship between low levels of reported self-efficacy and cigarette smoking, as well as unhappiness and cigarette smoking. Data in this study were derived from the 1994-1997 Youth Surveys of the British Household Panel Study, consisting of 1274 respondents, ranging from 11 to 15 years of age.

Stress Associated with Evolving Career and Family Ambitions

Various aspects of work and family life have been influenced by social changes in the past several decades, including the striking increase in the number of employed women in the United States over the past fifty years. While 43% of all women were employed either part-time or full-time in the 1970s, this percentage increased to 60% in 2003 (Barnett, 2004). Maternal employment has also increased dramatically, especially among women with young children (Greenberger and Goldberg, 1989). In 1968, only 21 percent of mothers who had a child less than a year old were employed, whereas in 2002 this percentage rose to nearly 60 (Hill, Waldfogel, Brooks-Gunn, and Han, 2005). The percentage of employed mothers with children under the age of 18 has also risen, from 36% in 1966 to over 70% in 2006 (Hoffman, 1998; United States Department of Labor, 2007). Since the majority of mothers now participate in the work force and dual-paycheck families account for over fifty percent of families, it is highly unlikely that the American society will return to the previous norm of the single-paycheck family (United States Department of Labor, 2007).

Some researchers attribute this trend to various economic changes. Although working-class women have always worked outside the home, economic changes in the 1970s made employment for more middle-class women essential (Scott and Tilly, 1975; Rubin, 1994). The number of dual-paycheck families increased as many women, especially those in the middle-class, entered the workforce in the 1970s due to inflation, wage stagnation, and the recession of 1973 (Rubin, 1994). Other researchers suggest that women's participation in the workforce was due to non-economic factors (Cherlin and Walters, 1981; Mason and Lu, 1988). One such factor was the Women's Liberation Movement, which encouraged women to reject the traditional housewife role and instead become educated and join the outside workforce. Research shows that women with higher levels of education are more likely to return to work after the birth of their child, and return sooner than mothers with lower levels of education. An increase in divorce and the prevalence of single motherhood are other factors which required women to return to the work force or become employed to support themselves and often their children (Hock, Gnezda, and McBride, 1984).

Increasingly, college women expect to shoulder the dual responsibilities of motherhood and career. This places pressure on them to prepare simultaneously for professional and personal success as undergraduates. Ambivalence about the feasibility of achieving all their ambitions may contribute to increasing levels of stress among many college women today, which may increase experimentation with cigarette smoking.

Cochran, Filipkowski, Cooper, Egresitz, King, Mack, Piraino, Sills, Bisinger and Chambliss (2007) investigated career and family ambitions among undergraduates in order to assess possible sources of stress for women students. Chi square analyses assessing the relationship between preschool maternal employment groups and children's career aspirations (professional, white collar, blue collar, no aspirations) showed that both males' and females' professional aspirations as young adults were positively associated with the extent of their mother's involvement in the workplace during their early years. Children whose mothers worked full-time were most likely to plan to have professional jobs (41%), while those whose mothers were not employed were least likely to have such plans (29%). Children of mothers who were not employed during their early years were roughly three times as likely to report no career aspirations as children whose mothers were employed (28% versus 10%; chi square=69.57(6), p<.001). Interestingly, no significant sex differences in young adults' career aspirations were found.

Cochran, et al. (2007) explored female and male college students' perceptions of the specific costs and benefits to children associated with maternal employment as a function of their mothers' work status during their preschool years. A sample of 1614 college students completed the Beliefs About the Consequences of Maternal Employment for Children (BACMEC) scale (Greenberger, et al., 1988). Two 2(sex) x 3(fulltime, part-time, non-employment) multivariate analyses of variance (MANOVA) were conducted to determine the relationship between gender and maternal employment during the preschool years and the students' perceptions of maternal employment. A gender main effect was found on both the summary measure assessing perceived benefits and the summary measure assessing perceived costs. Females' scores were higher on the benefits summary measure than males' scores (females: x=52.51, S.D.=8.92, n=445 versus males: x=47.85, S.D.=8.07, n=346; F=63.54, df=1/785, p<.01). Females' scores were lower on the costs summary measure than males' scores (females: x=31.64, S.D.=10.25, n=445 versus males: x=34.55, S.D.=9.38, n=346; F=19.69, df=1/785, p<.01). Responses to the statements describing the benefits associated with maternal employment suggest that the majority of students tend to agree that maternal employment has potential merit for children. In particular, maternal employment was widely linked to the development of independence and cooperation skills in children. The disparity between the attitudes of men and women is of considerable potential importance, since typically couples will need to reach a joint decision about maternal employment after their children are born.

Females' scores were higher on the Perceived Benefits Summary Scale (PBSS) and lower on the Perceived Costs Summary Scale (PCSS) than the males' scores. The maternal employment results were consistent with previous research showing that students with non-employed mothers perceived greater costs associated with maternal employment than students with part-time or fulltime employed mothers. Students whose mothers worked fulltime perceived there as being greater benefits associated with maternal employment than students whose mothers were not employed or employed part-time. For example, those with fulltime employed mothers were most likely to see working mothers as providing good role models for leading busy lives and as helping their children appreciate the value of money

On three of the PBSS items students whose mothers worked part-time scored the highest of the three groups. They more strongly believed that children whose mothers work are more independent and able to do things for themselves, pitch in and do tasks around the house, and develop more regard for women's intelligence and competence.

MANOVA also showed an interaction effect for gender and maternal employment. Females whose mothers had been employed part-time perceived maternal employment more positively than males whose mothers had been employed part-time.

This study also assessed how students anticipate they will share responsibilities with their future spouse. College students answered survey questions concerning expectations of future self and spouse in performance of household chores, contribution to the family income, and employment status. Independent samples t-tests comparing males' and females' responses were performed on data from all three maternal employment groups (fulltime, part-time, non-employed). Males and females of fulltime working mothers displayed the most preference for working throughout their child's development. However, males from all three maternal employment groups preferred that their spouses not work when their child is an infant, while females expect their husbands to be employed at this time. When the child reaches school age (6-12 years), most males and females expect themselves and their spouses to work fulltime. Both men and women anticipate that wives will contribute most to household chores, while husbands will contribute most to household income.

Across diverse maternal employment backgrounds, both males and females expect that females will contribute most to the completion of household chores, while males will contribute most to household income. Interestingly, expectations of spouses (for both household chores and contribution of income) are always less than what both the males and females actually plan to contribute. This suggests the possibility that some pleasant surprises await these future couples; their own sense of obligation exceeds the expectation of others.

In these undergraduate samples, no gender differences in career ambitions emerged. The majority of the females expected to remain employed outside the home after having children, although several hoped to reduce their involvement in work during their children's early years. Most women expected an egalitarian division of household responsibilities in their future families. Interestingly, the majority of the males studied did not anticipate having an employed spouse after starting a family, and few expected to contribute equally to household chores. In general, young women perceived maternal employment more positively than their male counterparts did. Young women endorsed the benefits of maternal employment for children more strongly than males. Males also were more likely to perceive maternal employment as posing hazards to the development of children. These gender differences were mitigated somewhat by the respondent's maternal employment history (evaluations of maternal employment were generally more positive among children whose own mothers had worked outside the home), but still emerged among those from all family backgrounds. These findings suggest that young women may encounter some resistance from their future husbands as they endeavor to fulfill their dual ambitions (career and motherhood). However, there was no evidence that women undergraduates use substances, including tobacco, more so than men in order to manage the pressures associated with their evolving educational, career, and family ambitions.

Psychopharmacologic Factors

Some individuals smoke in order to experience various physiological effects associated with cigarettes. Few notable differences in physiological response to smoking have been found between genders (Stein, et al., 1996). In order to clarify understanding of psychopharmacologic motivations for smoking, it is useful to consider the various desired physiological effects separately.

Relaxation Effects

Due to their harried lives, many women seek respite through cigarette smoking. As the demands upon the adolescent population become increasing more stressful, teenagers frequently cite smoking as a means of achieving relaxation effects. Although cigarette withdrawal periods are potentially stress-inducing events, as noted by Parrott (1999), smokers reported pursuit of relaxation effects as a powerful motivator for their behavior. Pursuit of relaxation effects was among the top two motivational factors reported by smokers (Sarason et al., 1992; Gillard and Bruchon-Schweitzer, 2001; Campbell, Bartlett, Liberati, Tornetta, and Chambliss, 2000; Jenks, 1994). Reported use of cigarette smoking as a means of relaxation was mediated by gender and frequency of smoking behavior. Female respondents and current smokers were significantly more likely to cite relaxation as a motive for smoking than males and former smokers (Sarason et al., 1992). Additionally, differential levels of relaxation motivation existed between heavy and light smokers, as heavy smokers regarded the perceived stress-reducing properties of cigarettes as a powerful motivator. Use of cigarettes to regulate negative affect may also be associated with relaxation. Gillard and Bruchon-Schweitzer (2001) discovered that high reported levels of anxiety among females were associated with endorsement of relaxation as a reason for smoking.

Several researchers have examined the relationship between current smoking status and reported use of smoking as a means of reducing distress, with somewhat contradictory results. Parrott (1999) demonstrated the positive relationship between smoking and stress. Paradoxically, although many smokers believe that smoking relaxes them, in actuality it results in increased levels of stress, especially for those who smoke regularly. Regular smokers report increased levels of stress and irritability when refraining from smoking (Office of the U.S. Surgeon General, 1988; Hughes, Higgins, and Hatsukami, 1990; Parrott, Garnham, Wesnes, and Pincock,, 1996; Parrott, 1999). Therefore, the source of positive affect experienced while smoking may result from the reversal of abstinence affect, rather than from any actual net improvement in mood. There is evidence in both adult and adolescent populations that self-reported stress levels differ by smoking status. Adult smokers tend to report levels of stress comparable to nonsmokers after engaging in smoking behavior. However, smokers report significantly higher levels of stress following even a brief period of abstinence (Parrott and Garnham, 1998; Parrott, 1999). Nonsmoking adolescents reported the lowest levels of self-reported stress in comparison to occasional and regular smokers (Lloyd and Lucas, 1997; Parrott, 1999). Regular smokers reported the highest levels of subjective stress. Although the design of these studies precluded an assessment of causal direction, learning to recognize the positive correlation between stress and smoking behavior may influence smokers to choose alternative behaviors to effectively relieve stress more effectively.

A study conducted by Wills, Sandy, and Yaeger (2002), further explored the relationship between stress and cigarette smoking. Wills, et al. (2002) examined the relationship between smoking and stress in the context of Parrott's model and the etiological model. Parrott believed that smoking behavior resulted in an increased level of stress. In contrast, the etiologic model proposed that stress is a risk factor for smoking behavior. A long-term repeated measures design was used to assess smoking status and stress level over time. Both smoking status and negative affect increased over the four-year period. Negative life events did not vary systematically over time. A latent growth model revealed the following positive paths for female respondents: level of negative affect, change in negative affect over time, and change in smoking status over time. The path from level of negative affect to change in smoking status was significant. However, no significant path was determined from smoking status to change in negative affect over time.

Stimulant and Cognitive Enhancement Effects

The stimulant effects of nicotine parallel those of other stimulants used by young people to enhance cognitive and academic performance, including caffeine and Ritalin. Gillard and Bruchon-Schweitzer (2001) found that while many women use cigarettes to ameliorate depression, male smokers often seek the stimulant effects of cigarettes, desiring a heightened sense of arousal . Although use of cigarette smoking as a stimulant was consistently ranked as the least important factor, evidence of tobacco's effectiveness as an appetite suppressant and metabolic stimulant has been well documented (Brannon and Feist, 1992).

Although there is accumulating evidence that nicotine is associated with cognitive enhancement, at least in some populations (Torrey, 1999), most young smokers do not report this as a prime motivation for smoking. For example, Bartlett, et al.(1999) were surprised to find that very few college students smoke in order to experience stimulant effects. These smokers report that they rarely experience the appetite suppression effects commonly associated with nicotine, infrequently feel energized by smoking, and almost never feel physically fit while smoking. This reality stands in sharp contrast to the lively, invigorating image of the smoking experience ubiquitously depicted in advertisements. Apparently these stimulant effects are less pronounced than commonly assumed, or misattributive processes may operate which prevent college smokers from recognizing the association between their intake of nicotine and these physiological effects. The energizing effects of smoking are evidently short-lived; smokers did not report enjoying stimulant effects on a regular basis. Similarly, cognitive enhancement was not commonly reported; the majority of smokers almost never experienced heightened intellectual ability while smoking.

Appetite Regulation

Several studies have suggested that many women smoke as a way of curbing appetite in order to maintain a desirable body weight. Many girls and women seem to use tobacco as a means of weight control, exploiting its metabolic enhancement and appetite suppressant effects (Tomeo, Field, Berkey, Colditz, and Frazier, 1999). Smoking for weight control seems to be especially common among young women (Charlton, 1984). Cawley, Markowitz, and Tauras (2005) examined the role of body weight in smoking initiation by adolescents. They estimated discrete-time hazard models of the decision to initiate smoking using data from the Children of the National Longitudinal Survey of Youth, 1979 Cohort. Cawley, et al. found clear gender differences. Leaner girls were less likely to initiate smoking, while current weight was uncorrelated with initiation among boys. Among girls, smoking initiation was unrelated to cigarette prices. For boys, rising prices seemed to deter smoking.

Although several researchers have hypothesized that appetite regulation plays a central role in girls' and women's decisions to smoke, the empirical findings have been inconsistent. Contrary to expectation, Bartlett, Brackin, Chubb, Covatta, Ferguson, Hinckley, Hodges, Liberati, Tornetta, and Chambliss (1999) found that female smokers were not more likely to report appetite suppression effects in conjunction with smoking. Furthermore, in a study examining college students' subjective experience of cigarette smoking, appetite reduction was rarely reported among either male or female smokers (Hodges, Srebro, Authier and Chambliss, 1999). In this and a related study (Srebro, Hodges, Authier and Chambliss, 1999), the main motivation for college student smoking was a desire to relax, followed closely by concerns about image. Cognitive enhancement and weight control were rarely cited as reasons for smoking by students of either sex. Similarly, Brynin (1999) found that respondents classified their smoking behavior as a means of seeking pleasure and relaxation more frequently than the use of cigarettes as a means of weight control. The ranked reasons explaining the smoking behavior of others, in descending order, were: relaxation, psychological addiction, physical addiction, pleasant activity, and weight control. Respondents were significantly more likely to perceive others' cigarette smoking as a means of relaxation than anything else.

Although findings establishing the importance of appetite regulation as a motivator for smoking have been contested, Van Roosmalen and McDaniel (1992) found that when compared with males, females are less likely to perceive the benefits of quitting and are more concerned about weight gain related to quitting. This may make it especially difficult to reduce the rate of smoking among the young female population.

Affect Management

Wills, et al.(2002) found a relationship between smoking and levels of negative affect. Research indicates that many individuals smoke as a means of self-medication to reduce symptoms of depression and to increase pleasurable relaxation (Gilbert, 1979; Clausen, 1987; Stein, Newcomb, and Bentler, 1996), and manage stress or mood (Chassin, Presson, and Sherman., 1990; Stein, et al., 1996). Stein, Newcomb, and Bentler (1996) performed a longitudinal study of 133 men and 328 females, who were recruited in junior high school, and assessed personality traits associated with the smoking adolescent population and those who continued to smoke into young adulthood. The researchers found that early adolescent smoking was positively correlated with cheerfulness, more socialization with peers, and extraversion. As the group was reevaluated across time on these variables the researchers discovered a displacement of the positive qualities associated with smoking. Four years after the study began, cigarette use and depression were positively correlated; cigarette use was negatively correlated with good social relations and minimally correlated with extraversion. These correlations were consistent and substantial as the study progressed over thirteen years. Stein and her colleagues concluded that early smokers initiate smoking for social reasons (peer identification) and that those who continue to smoke into adulthood did so for emotional reasons (relief from stress).

Gillard and Bruchon-Schweitzer (2001) investigated smoking behavior among 150 adults who currently smoke. A 42-item survey was devised after interviewing 35 adult smokers and performing thematic analysis of previous surveys created over the past thirty years. Each item represented one theme related to personal smoking motivations. Varimax rotation yielded the following four factors: dependence, social integration, regulation of negative affect, and hedonism. The dependence factor was characterized by the uncontrollable urge to smoke, automatic smoking behavior, and a reported need for nicotine. The social integration factor was characterized by impression management, social acceptance, and use of cigarettes in social situations. The regulation of negative affects factor was characterized by the use of cigarettes as a form of self-medication when confronted by anxiety, sadness, tension, anger, and worries. The hedonism factor was characterized by feelings of pleasure and relaxation while smoking, or derived from the hand gestures associated with smoking. Interactions between gender and other factors emerged. Results for the dependence factor indicate that single males who experience routine boredom and whose friends smoke were more likely to engage in smoking behavior than content, married males whose friends do not smoke. In contrast, women who reported use of stimulants and psychotropic medication were more likely to smoke than women not using these substances. Both male and female smokers who engage in smoking behavior for a greater portion of the day and are either at the "initiation" or "hooked" stage of the smoking cycle were more likely to smoke as a result of dependence. Results for the social integration factor indicate that married men who are high sensation seekers were more apt to smoke as a means of fitting in socially than single, non-sensation seekers. Single women who are highly susceptible to peer pressure were more likely to smoke to attain social integration than their married, autonomous counterparts. Men who smoke as a means of regulating negative affect were more likely to be in the early stages of the smoking cycle and seek high levels of sensation than later stage, nonsensation-seeking smokers.

Women who smoke due to negative affect regulation reported higher levels of anxiety and depression than those women citing other motivations for smoking. Men seeking novel experiences were more likely to smoke for hedonistic reasons than male smokers content with contiguity. In contrast, women who smoke for hedonistic reasons were more likely to report higher levels of extraversion and anxiety than female respondents citing other motivations for smoking.

Depression Issues among Women: Empathy and Depression

Bean, Doutt, Piraino, Schutte, and Chambliss (2007) investigated the relationship between depression and empathy among 167 male and female undergraduate students, who were administered the Beck Depression Inventory (BDI) and the Interpersonal Reactivity Index (IRI: O'Connor, Berry, Weiss, Bush, and Sampson, 1997). A median split was used to create two depression groups (nondepressed and mildly depressed). Directionally adjusted items were totaled to create a summary score on the IRI for all participants, as well as scores on the four empathy subscales of the IRI, Personal Distress (PD), Perspective Taking (PT), Fantasy (F), and Empathic Concern (EC).

A 2 x 2 (sex by depression level) MANOVA revealed significant depression and sex main effects on several of the IRI subscales. Although there was no significant depression main effect on the overall IRI, group differences emerged on three of the four IRI subscales. On the EC subscale, depressed participants' scores were lower than the scores of those participants who were not depressed. (depressed: mean=15.91, s.d.=4.57, n=127 versus nondepressed: mean=16.78, s.d.=3.58, n=105; $F=5.59$, df=1/225, $p<.05$). Also, on the PT subscale, depressed participants' scores were lower than the scores of those participants who were not depressed. (depressed: mean=15.90, s.d.=4.57, n=127 versus nondepressed: mean=16.78, s.d.=3.58, n=105; $F=4.83$, df=1/225, $p<.05$). On the PD subscale, depressed participants' scores were higher than the scores of those participants who were not depressed. (depressed: mean=11.84, s.d.=4.79, n=127 versus nondepressed: mean=9.40, s.d.=4.95, n=105; $F=12.46$, df=1/225, $p<.05$). There was no significant depression main effect on the F subscale of the IRI. In addition, no significant gender by depression interaction effects emerged on any of the measures.

Consistent with results obtained by Andrews, Bean, Doutt, Haas, Schutte, and Chambliss (2007), mildly depressed students gave significantly higher ratings than nondepressed students on Personal Distress subscale items assessing Emergency Anxiety, Emergency Panic, Perceived Helplessness, Emergency Loss of Control and Perceived Fear.

A significant gender main effect was found on the IRI summary measure and three of the subscales. Females' scores were higher on the IRI than males' scores (females: mean=63.39, s.d.=11.72, n=131 versus males: mean=56.57, s.d.=11.36, n=101; $F=16.20$, df=1/163, $p<.000$).

In addition, a significant gender main effect also emerged on the EC subscale. Females' scores were higher on the EC subscale than males' scores (females: mean=17.29, s.d.=3.77, n=131 versus males: mean=15.02, s.d.=4.33, n=101; $F=11.00$, df=1/163, $p<.001$). Similarly, a significant gender main effect was obtained on the PT subscale. Females' scores were higher on the PT subscale than males' scores (females: mean=17.46, s.d.=4.92, n=131 versus males: mean=16.54, s.d.=4.70, n=101; F=4.04, df=1/163, p<.05). Finally, a significant gender main effect emerged on the PD subscale. As on the other subscales, females' scores were higher on the PD subscale than males' scores (females: mean=11.88, s.d.=5.27, n=131 versus males: mean=9.25, s.d.=4.21, n=101; F=10.63, df=1/163, p<.001). No significant sex difference was found on the F subscale.

Bean, et al. (2007) found that undergraduate females showed higher levels of overall empathy than their male peers. In addition, young women displayed greater perspective taking ability and empathic concern about the welfare of others. These women's Personal Distress (PD) scores were also higher, indicating a higher tendency to experience anxiety and panic in emergency situations, greater perceived helplessness and concerns about loss of control, as well as more perceived fear. These factors may play a role in women's greater vulnerability to depression and use of tobacco to regulate negative emotional states. This suggests that college women may be more prone to use cigarettes in order to manage difficult emotional experiences than their male counterparts. Klerman, Weissman, Rounsaville, and Chevron (1984) have reported that interpersonal issues and conflicts figure prominently in the psychopathologies of women. Greater sensitivity to the suffering of others may burden some women and reduce their emotional resilience, leaving them more overwhelmed by destructive extremes of negative affect. Further research exploring the impact of women's higher empathy and personal distress levels on their substance use choices is warranted.

Stress Management Factors

Several psychological and social factors thought to influence college students' smoking were investigated by Bartlett, Brackin, Chubb, Covatta, Ferguson, Hinckley, Hodges, Liberati, Tornetta and Chambliss (1999) by surveying a sample of college students who currently smoke. Personal motivating factors examined were relaxation effects, image effects, competence effects, and stimulant effects. These personal reasons for smoking were indirectly assessed by measuring subjective feeling states that accompany smoking behavior. It was assumed that since many of these states were desirable, they played a role in shaping the smoker's motivation to use tobacco. This means of measuring motivation for smoking was preferable to more direct questions, because it was less susceptible to contamination by social desirability responding or other forms of defensiveness.

In order to assess the importance of different subjective states in maintaining cigarette smoking behavior, the responses of only the smokers in this sample were selectively examined. Their subjective smoking experience was assessed through items rating the subjective impact of smoking cigarettes on the following dimensions: relaxation, contentment, trust, anxiety, jitteriness, perceived attractiveness, sophistication, maturity, alertness, competence, security, intelligence, perceived adequacy, physical fitness, energy, and hunger. These variables were used in order to investigate the importance of four hypothesized motivational factors underlying smoking, relaxation effects, image effects, competence effects, and stimulant effects.

To measure the motivational role of relaxation effects, scores were grouped and averaged for the following feeling items: high levels of relaxation, contentment and trust, and low levels of anxiety and jitteriness. In order to assess the importance of image effects, scores were averaged and grouped for the following feeling items: high levels of attractiveness, sophistication, and maturity. In order to assess the importance of competence effects, scores were grouped and averaged for the following feeling items: high levels of alertness, competence, security, intelligence, and adequacy. In order to assess the importance of stimulant effects, scores were grouped and averaged for the following feeling items: high levels of physical fitness, and energy, and low levels of hunger.

In order to determine if differences existed among the four personal smoking motivation factors, paired sample t-tests were performed on the smokers' factor scores. Significant differences were found between stimulant effects and the other three factors, all $p < .001$. Relaxation effects, image effects, and competence effects were all rated higher than stimulant effects. Smokers reported almost never feeling intelligent, physically fit, or trusting while smoking.

To examine gender differences in personal motivation for smoking, between-group t-tests on the four motivational factor scores were performed, comparing male and female smokers. No significant sex differences emerged.

The results of the Bartlett, Brackin, Chubb, Covatta, Ferguson, Hinckley, Hodges, Liberati, Tornetta, and Chambliss (1999) study suggest that there are three main factors motivating college student to smoke, and that there are negligible differences between men's and women's reasons for smoking. Ratings of the four personal motivation factors underlying both male and female undergraduate smoking placed them in the following descending order of importance: relaxation effects, image effects, competence effects, and stimulant effects. While the strong association between smoking and desired relaxation was not surprising, the highly influential role of social image in college student smoking was unexpected. Although research on younger smokers has clearly documented the importance of peer pressure in fostering smoking, older smokers were presumed to be more immune to these influences. The current findings suggest that concern about appearing sophisticated, mature, and attractive figure prominently in the decision of college students to smoke. College-age students appear to be in a transitory state concerning reasons for smoking; while they enjoy the benefit of relaxation like the older adult population, image is still a crucial factor in smoking motivation, much as it is for the adolescent.

Substance Use Differences between Men and Women

Several studies have noted differences between the ways that men and women make use of psychoactive substances. With the exception of certain sedatives and cocaine, rates of use are significantly higher for men for all types of substances (Sue, Sue, and Sue, 2000). Some research indicates that substances also affect the bodies of men and women differently. For example, the hormonal impact of marijuana has been found to be greater in men; no reproductive effects have been found for nonpregnant women (Jaffe, 1989).

Others have argued that these apparent distinctions are in large part due to differences in willingness to report use, rather than to actual differential substance use. Although studies have shown that women consume less alcohol, when adjustments are made in differences in body size, and ability to absorb alcohol, it turns out the women social drinkers achieve the same blood alcohol levels as men (Vogel-Sprott, 1984).

There is some evidence suggesting that there has been a shift in recent years in gender-linked patterns of abuse. Findings from a cross-cultural study by Helzer, Robins, Przybeck, and Regier (1988) suggest that rates of chemical abuse and dependency will soon be equal in the United States. The current young adult generation seems to endorse more egalitarian attitudes; this cohort was largely born after the feminist movement had challenged many traditional sex role attitudes and reshaped many parents' expectations of their sons and daughters.

Along with more equal opportunities to participate in professional careers and athletics, some young women perceived greater freedom to drink and smoke like men (Fillmore, 1988). Some advertisement campaigns explicitly linked tobacco use and women's rights, asserting that use of a particular tobacco product conveyed a woman's successful liberation. In the 1950s estimates indicated that there were as many as five or six male alcoholics for every female; in the 1960s and 1970s, estimates were about four to one (Gomberg, 1976). By 1994 reports indicate that approximately 12.5% of American men and just over 5% of American women meet the diagnostic criteria for alcohol abuse or dependence (a ratio of 2.4 to 1) (Nelson, Heath, and Kessler, 1998).

Some other recent examinations of group differences in smoking behavior have helped to clarify the impact of gender on decisions to smoke. Dziuban, Moskal, and West (1999) examined the relationship of gender, marital status, and minority status to six smoking behaviors. The behaviors included the following: tried cigarettes, smoking regularly, tried to quit smoking, age when first smoked regularly, number of cigarettes smoked in the last month, and number of days smoked in the past month. Surveys were received from 1,150 Florida University college students. Sixty percent of the respondents were women. Thirty-one percent were 25 years of age or older, 19% were married, and 20% lived on campus.

The results indicated that there were no significant differences between men (79%) and women (78%) in terms of the likelihood of trying smoking. Married students (83%) were more likely than single students (77%) to have tried cigarettes, and Whites (81%) were significantly more likely than minorities (72%) to have smoked.

Despite comparable early experimentation, significantly more women (28%) than men (22%) continued to smoke on a regular basis. Also, married students (37%) were more likely than single students (23%) to smoke on a regular basis, and more White students (81%) smoked than minority students (44%).

In the Dziuban, et al. study, there were no significant differences between the proportions of men and women, or white and minority students, who had tried to quit smoking. However, significantly more single students (48%) had tried to quit, compared to married students (33%). No significant differences emerged when the age at which they first smoked regularly of each demographic group was compared.

Venuti, Conroy, Landis and Chambliss (2000) assessed differential substance use between men and women college students through administration of a detailed survey of recent use of six commonly used psychoactive substances (cigarettes, chewing tobacco, alcohol, marijuana, cocaine, and caffeine). Situational contexts associated with use of particular substances were also investigated, as were motivating factors prompting different types of substance use. The survey also explored the relationships between substance use and participation in college Greek organizations and athletics. Since self-esteem deficits have frequently been assumed to underlie substance use problems, a measure of this variable was included as well.

Respondents were 195 college students (men=69, women=126) from a small liberal arts college from a suburban area in the Northeast United States. The mean age of participants was 19.6 years. A three-page survey, completed by students, consisted of items pertaining to smoking and substance abuse, general attitudes toward these habits, and demographic items assessing membership in Greek life and athletics. Questions as taken from Wechsler et al. (1998) were used to determine cigarette and other drug use in the past 30 days and in the past year. Students were asked to indicate their likelihood of using five specific substances (tobacco, caffeine, alcohol, marijuana, and cocaine) in eight different situational contexts. They were also asked to rate on a four-point Likert scale (1= not at all important, 2= somewhat important, 3= important, and 4= very important) the importance of the motivations for using each of three substances (tobacco, alcohol, and marijuana). Also, questions regarding mental health were asked using a portion of the survey by Fisher and Farina (1979). To measure self-esteem, Rosenberg's (1965) self-esteem survey was also included.

Directionally adjusted items were totaled to create a summary measure of total substance use for each participant. Between-group t-tests were conducted to assess differences associated with gender, involvement in a fraternity or sorority, and participation in collegiate athletics. No significant gender differences were found on total substance use scores. However, males did report greater use of marijuana (males' x= 2.54, s.d.= 1.29, n= 69 versus females' x= 3.95, s.d.= 1.21, n= 126; t= 7.63, df= 1, p <.01), chewing tobacco (males' x= 3.19, s.d.= 1.13, n= 69 versus females' x= 3.95, s.d.= .21, n= 126; t= 54.43, df= 1, p<.001), and other substances (males' x= 3.54, s.d.= .99, n= 69 versus females' x= 3.80, s.d.= .69, n= 126; t= 4.76, df= 1, p <.05).

Significant differences between men and women were found on five of eight items relating to situations associated with substance use. Men reported more use of tobacco to celebrate their achievements (males' x= 1.68, s.d.= 1.24, n= 69 versus females' x= 1.30, s.d.= 1.13, n= 126; t= 4.70, df= 1, p <.05). When compared with females, males reported greater use of alcohol when facing a task requiring creativity (t= 8.37, df= 1, p <.01). Males indicated that they smoke and experiment with other substances as a result of boredom on the weekend more so than women. Males were more likely than females to use marijuana when exhausted or depressed about a bad grade. No significant gender differences emerged in terms of use of substances in situations where students were anxious before a social event, anxious before giving a speech, or angry at their parents. No significant gender differences were found on the items directly assessing conscious motivation underlying use of substances (to fit in with friends; reward for hard work; to feel comfortable with opposite sex; to get away from problems; because everyone else is doing it).

A triunal-split was performed on the summary measure of overall substance use, creating high, moderate, and low use groups. Oneway ANOVA were performed to assess the relationship between amount of substance use and participation in campus Greek organizations (fraternities and sororities) and collegiate athletics and exercise. No significant differences were found. Oneway ANOVA showed no differences among the three substance use groups in terms of their scores on the Rosenberg measure of self-esteem. Correlational analyses corroborated these findings; substance use was not significantly associated with fraternity/sorority membership, athletic participation, or self esteem.

Venuti, Conroy, Landis and Chambliss (2000) found relatively few significant differences emerge between men and women on the substance use measures. Total use did not vary as a function of gender, at least in their sample of undergraduates. Frequency of use of specific substances also did not generally differ by sex, although males reported more use of marijuana. This might reflect greater willingness to report such use, or actual higher preference among males for the effects of this drug.

In considering the reasons why young adults use psychoactive substances, the current findings support the notion that men and women differ in some regards. While no differences emerged on the measures of conscious motivations for substance use, on the majority of items related to situational contexts in which substance use was likely, significant differences were found on all but the items related to anxiety and anger.

When compared to women, men may actually make more instrumental use of psychoactive substances, they may use substances more as a function of situational context, or they may simply be more willing to admit to situational prompts for substance use. For example, males in this sample reported greater use of alcohol as an aid to creativity. It may be more socially acceptable for males to "free" themselves with alcohol. On the other hand, this difference may also be due to males' need for a socially acceptable attribution for being creative, possibly because such behavior is traditionally sex-typed as feminine. Alternatively, it is possible that their socialization makes men less likely to see themselves as creative, which might contribute to their feeling a need for more assistance when faced with a task demanding creativity.

The failure of Venuti, Conroy, Landis and Chambliss (2000) to find any significant differences in substance use as a function of fraternity/sorority membership, athletic participation, or self esteem challenges several common stereotypes. The expectation that fraternity/sorority members use substances more so than nonmembers may be a myth. Similarly, athletes did not differ from nonathletes in their reported substance use. The notion that "losers are users" because of low self esteem was also not supported by the Venuti, Conroy, Landis and Chambliss (2000) data.

It is important to note that although the Dziuban, et al. research showed that women were more likely to continue smoking once they started, and Venuti, et al. found gender differences in situational prompts for smoking, gender differences in cigarette use have not emerged consistently across all studies. For example, Hodges, Srebro, Authier and Chambliss (1999) failed to find significant gender differences on any of the variables they assessed. A similar absence of gender effects was noted by Hu, Zihua, and Keeler (1998).

Conclusion

The findings from several of the empirical investigations summarized in this chapter strongly indicate that the decision to smoke severely handicaps women socially, in addition to placing their health at serious risk. The results of numerous studies, including those completed by Srebro, et al. (1999), Campbell, et al. (2000), Brosh, et al (2003), and Baker, et al. (2004) show that perceptions of smokers are consistently more negative than the perceptions of nonsmokers. Nonsmokers are consistently rated more positively than smokers, whether male or female, on various dimensions, including intelligence, ambition, artistic creativity, conscientiousness, consideration, hostility, independence, and judgment.

Because of all of the highly publicized health risks associated with this habit, it is perhaps not surprising that smokers are viewed as less intelligent, and as showing poor judgment. Research detailing the risks of second hand smoke may help to account for why smokers are seen as less considerate, less conscientious, and more hostile. The findings related to ambition and artistic creativity are a bit more puzzling. It is possible that since smoking has become increasingly rare among highly educated, economically successful adults, those who smoke are more apt to be seen as lacking the positive attributes usually associated with social success.

Several studies have established that negative attitudes about smokers are not limited to adults. Adolescent and young adult samples express views paralleling those of older adults, suggesting that individuals absorb critical ideas about those who smoke early on. Among both high school and college samples, participants' smoking status was found to influence the ratings of individuals. Nonsmokers were rated most positively out of all of the targets. These findings challenge the common assumption that high school students begin smoking because they and their peers universally view smokers positively. In fact, the majority of students and teachers in high schools today seem to hold very critical attitudes toward cigarette smoking.

Interestingly, both smokers and nonsmokers were found to rate those who smoke more negatively than others who do not smoke, although this was somewhat less pronounced among the high school students who regularly smoke. Future research should seek to clarify why high school students' negative news of smokers fail to offer more of a deterrent to their smoking.

The research also indicates that women who quit smoking at least partially restore their image; while smoking cessation failed to erase stigma entirely, it did appear to alleviate it. On the majority of personal qualities assessed, former smokers were rated more positively than current smokers. Because quitting the smoking habit suggests that the individual acknowledged the health risks involved, and successfully acted upon that knowledge, it makes sense that subjects would adjust their perception of a smoker in a more positive direction when the smoker quits. However, since the former smokers' reputation is not fully restored (nonsmokers are still viewed more favorably), the implication is clear that it is best for a young woman to never start smoking. In addition, these findings suggest that in some social situations, it may be wise to conceal one's former use of cigarettes in order to avoid negative stereotyping.

In trying to design more effective prevention programs, it may be useful to build upon existing anti-smoking norms among the student population. In this regard, it is especially interesting to note that the high school females comprised the subgroup showing the most pronounced tendency to evaluate nonsmokers positively. This could be due to many factors. The masculine ideal precludes fear, dependence, and compliance with authority, and instead embraces courage, thrill-seeking, and autonomy. Because of the health risks associated with smoking behavior, the decision to smoke permits boys an opportunity to prove their fearlessness. Since underage smoking is illegal, it also provides a means of rebelling. In these ways, adolescent smoking embodies the "masculine" traits of bravery and deviance. As a consequence, many high school females may perceive smoking as a somewhat masculine behavior, and subsequently may be more likely to reject the activity because of the social implications attached to violating sex-role norms. Furthermore, it is more socially acceptable for females to acknowledge fears and avoid encounters with feared stimuli. Therefore, females are may find it more socially accepted to refrain from smoking as a means of avoiding illness and to share this motivation with others. For boys, however, being afraid runs counter to the masculine ideal. Females are also generally less challenging of adult authority, which may allow them to internalize and act upon anti-smoking health messages more completely. These ideas gain support from the finding that a higher percentage of males than females smoked in many of the research high school and college samples. Interestingly, among those girls strongly valuing androgyny, the same factors linking cigarette use with masculinity may regrettably actually promote smoking behavior. Broadening expectations of girls may make them more vulnerable to this habit.

It is important to note that if the high school females' male peers realized the extent to which many of their female peers perceived smokers negatively, more boys might be dissuaded from starting to engage in this habit. Without being aware of it, boys who begin smoking in high school may face some dire social consequences (e.g., rejection by many females). Future prevention programs might make more methodical and strategic use of such targeted peer pressure.

Messages about the health risks associated with cigarette smoking seem to account for why the majority of young women today refrain from smoking. Perhaps those who ignore the extant communications about these risks need to be reached in more creative ways. Although the empirical findings have been somewhat equivocal, it appears that many young women smoke cigarettes due to concerns about becoming overweight. If instead of viewing cigarette smoking young women as chic and slim, college students were encouraged to imagine such women as having bleak futures, marred by premature aging and often compromised by agonizing early terminal illnesses such as lung cancer and emphysema, the decision to smoke in college might be viewed as a social and sexual impediment. During this developmental period, many women and men start to consider making long term relationship commitments. Poised for the first time to contemplate growing old with prospective partners, they may be especially sensitive to information about the cruel long term impact of this habit. If their sexual attractiveness was obviously at stake, possibly far fewer college women would light up at campus parties.

In addition to disseminating information about how smoking impairs one's desirability as a future spouse, campus programs should share findings about the career and academic hazards associated with cigarette use. Myriad studies have firmly established the growing prejudice and discrimination directed against young smokers in American workplace and academic milieus. Ambitious, career-focused college women may be deterred from smoking if they were to realize how this behavior might handicap them and neutralize all their hard work and accomplishments in the eyes of prospective employers. Although currently campuses rightly emphasize the values of diversity and tolerance, they are arguably failing to prepare undergraduate females for the realities these women will face if the growing, widespread social biases against those who smoke cigarettes are not fully disclosed and discussed.

Lastly, it may be informative for students participating in prevention programs to explore the paradox that smokers indulge "to relax" by inhaling a substance that is actually physiologically arousing. While nicotine is pharmacologically a stimulant, most smokers don't realize this, rationalizing their choice to smoke by emphasizing tobacco's power to relax them. It might deter potential smokers if they realize that tobacco does not actually relax a non-addicted person, because it actually increases blood pressure, accelerates heart rate, and often produces jitteriness. Smokers who have become dependent on nicotine experience agitation upon withdrawal, which can be reversed by smoking. Understanding that it is this alleviation of withdrawal-related "stress" that smokers typically experience as "relaxing" might reduce the appeal of smoking to the novice.

Understanding this paradoxical use of a psychoactive stimulant in order to relax requires a recognition of how easily attributional errors can arise. Smoking generally occurs within a situational context that promotes misattribution of relaxation effects to tobacco and nicotine. Although nicotine itself is pharmacologically stimulating, typically smokers administer this drug by breathing more slowly, and deeply inhaling warm smoke, often while taking a break from stressful activities. The relaxation associated with this is probably more due to the deep breathing, slowed pace, and absence of stressful distractions than to the substances in cigarettes themselves. Similarly, many people report finding drinking hot coffee relaxing, although caffeine itself produces stimulant effects somewhat similar to those of nicotine. Cigarette marketers promote such misattributions by describing their product as responsible for pleasurable, relaxed feelings.

Realizing that the "relaxation" that female smokers experience in conjunction with smoking seems primarily to involve cessation of unpleasant withdrawal symptoms may reduce smoking among those seeking to self medicate. Rather than providing female smokers with a valuable means of coping with unwanted anxiety, this substance actually aggravates their baseline level of distress, while tricking them into thinking it has a salutary impact. Informing potential users about the actual pharmacologic stimulant effects of nicotine may reduce smoking if it succeeds in challenging the assumption that this drug is a useful tool for reducing unpleasant arousal.

Prevention programs can also gently help young women to view cigarette marketers as villains, exploitatively trying to create lifelong addiction to their expensive product. Like others who profit from addictive drug sales, cigarette manufacturers benefit each time another young woman chooses to make her brain dependent on nicotine. Most who experiment for any length of time will become a long term customer, worth tens of thousands of dollars in lifetime revenue.

Young women who might otherwise smoke in order to rebel and assert their autonomy should respond especially strongly to this notion that cigarette companies are hoping to manipulate and control young women. The anti-authority stance of these women may make them particularly loathe to succumb to such corporate pressures.

Developing multiple messages addressing the variable motivations for smoking should enhance the effectiveness of prevention programs. In addition, young women need to be more fully informed about the whole range of social, financial, and physical hazards associated with tobacco use. Finally, young women must be equipped with reliable alternative strategies to enhance their image, assert their autonomy, maintain a healthy weight, counter anxiety and depression, and manage stress, in order to guard against their making foolish, counterproductive choices that may haunt them and their families for years.

References

Altman, D.G., Levine, D.W., Coeytaux, R., Slade, J., and Jaffe, R. (1996). Tobacco promotion and susceptibility to tobacco use among adolescents aged 12 through 17 years in a nationally representative sample. *American Journal of Public Health, 86* (11), 1590-1593.

Altman, D.G., Slater, M.D., Albright, C.L., and Maccoby, N. (1987). How an unhealthy product is sold: Cigarette advertising in magazines. 1960-1985. *Journal of Communication, 37* (4), 95-106.

American Lung Association. (1998). Quit smoking action plan. (National Publications). New York: New York.

Anda, R.F., Williamson, D.F., Escobedo, L.G., Mast, E.E., Giovino, G.A., and Remington, P.L. (1990). Depression and the dynamics of smoking: A national perspective. *Journal of the American Medical Association, 264*, 1541-1545.

Andrews, J., Bean, K., Doutt,A., Haas,S., Schutte, J. and Chambliss, C (2007, March) *The Relationship Between Depression and Empathy in Mildly Depressed and Nondepressed Male and Female College Students.* Poster session presented at the 78th Annual Meeting of the Eastern Psychological Association, Philadelphia, Pennsylvania. Ashley, M.J. (1996). Support among smokers and nonsmokers for restrictions on smoking. *Journal of the American Medical Association, 11*, 283-287.

Austin, M., Brosh, J. and Chambliss, C. (2002). An Exploration of Paradox: High School and College Students' Self-Reported Motivations for Smoking. Resources in Education, ERIC/CASS,CG031872.

Austin, M., Brosh,J., Dous, J.A., Iannella, G., Outten, R., Rowles, P. and Chambliss, C.A. (2003). The relationship between personality and self reported substance use: Exploring the implications for high school and college educational programs, Resources in Education, ERIC/CASS, CG032168.

Authier, C., Hodges, J.,Srebro, K., and Chambliss, C. (1999). Faculty and Student Views of College Student Smokers. *Resources in Education*, ERIC/CASS, CG029394.

Baer, J.S. (2002). Student Factors: Understanding individual variation in college drinking. Special Issue: College drinking, what it is, and what to do about it: Review of the state of the science. *Journal of Studies on Alcohol, 14*, 40-53.

Baker, K., Katona, C., Brosh, J., Shull, M., and Chambliss, C. (2004). The vilification of smokers: High school and college students' perceptions of current smokers, former smokers, and nonsmokers. *Resources in Education*, ERIC/CASS, CG032693.

Bandura, A. and Walters, R.H. (1963). *Social Learning and Personality Development*. New York, Holt, Rinehart, and Winston.

Barnett, R. C. (2004). Women and multiple roles: Myths and reality. *Harvard Review of Psychiatry, 12,* 158-164.

Bartlett, A., Brackin, T., Chubb, J., Covata, S., Ferguson, L., Hinckley, A., Hodges, J., Liberati, C., Tornetta, J., and Chambliss, C. (1999). Factors influencing and motivating smoking among college students. *Resources in Education,* ERIC/CASS, ED440323

Bartlett, A., Brackin, T., Chubb, J., Covata, S., Ferguson, L., Hinckley, A., Hodges, J.,

Liberati, C., Tornetta, J., and Chambliss, C. (2000). Correcting Media Mis-education: The Portrayal of Smokers and Smoking in Top Grossing Films. *Resources in Education,* ERIC/CASS, CG029857.

Barton, J., Chassin, L., and Presson, C. C. (1982). Social image factors as motivators of smoking initiation in early and middle adolescence. *Child Development, 53,* 1499-1511.

Bean, K., Doutt, A., Piraino, D., Schutte, J. and Chambliss, C. (2007). Empathy in mildly depressed and nondepressed male and female college students. Twenty-Second Annual LVAIC Undergraduate Psychology Conference, Muhlenberg College, April 28, 2007.

Bergman, M.M., and Scott, J. (2001). Young adolescents' wellbeing and health-risk behaviours: gender and socio-economic differences. *Journal of Adolescence,24,* 183-197.

Bleda, P. R. and Bleda, S.E. (1978). The effects of sex and smoking on reactions to spatial invasion at a shopping mall. *Journal of Social Psychology, 104,* 311-312.

Bleda, P. R.and Sandman, P.H. (1977). In smoke's way: Socioemotional reactions to another's smoking. *Journal of Applied Psychology, 52,* 452-458.

Brehm, S. S. and Brehm, J. W. (1981). *Psychological reactance: a theory of freedom and control.* NY: Academic Press.

Brannon, L.and Feist, J. (1992). Smoking Tobacco. *Health Psychology, 2nd ed.* (pp.317-349). CA:Wadsworth

Brennan, A.F., Walfish, S., and AuBuchon, P. (1986). Alcohol use and abuse in college students: I. A review of individual and personality correlates. *Int. Journal of Addiction, 21,* 475-493.

Brenner, H., Born, J., Novack, P., and Wanek, V. (1997). Smoking behavior and attitude toward smoking regulations and passive smoking in the workplace. *Preventative Medicine, 26,* 138-143.

Brickman, J.C. and D'Amato, B. (1975). Exposure effects in a free-choice situation. *Journal of Personality and Social Psychology, 32,* 415-20.

Brigham, J., Gross, J., Stitzer, M.L., and Felch L.J. (1994). Effects of a restricted work-site smoking policy on employees who smoke. *American Journal of Public Health, 84,* 773-778.

Brook, J.S., Whiteman, M., Czeisler, L.J., Shapiro, J., and Cohen, P. (1997). Cigarette smoking in young adults: childhood and adolescent personality familial, and peer antecedents. *Journal of Genetic Psychology, 158,* 172-189.

Brooks, A. (1998).Teenage Girls Start Smoking to Lose Weight. *British Medical Journal (International)*, 317: 366, August 8, 1998.

Brosh, J., Austin, M. and Chambliss, C. (2003). High school and college students' perceptions of current smokers, former smokers, and nonsmokers, *Perceptual and Motor Skills*, 97, 1200-1202, 2003.

Brynin, M. (1999). Smoking behaviour: predisposition or adaptation? *Journal of Adolescence, 22*, 635-646.

Burton, D., Sussman, S., Hansen, W.B., Johnson, C. A., and Flay, B.R. (1989). Image attributions and smoking among seventh-grade students. *Journal of Applied Psychology, 19,* 656-664.

Campbell, M., Bartlett, A., Liberati, C., Tornetta, J., and Chambliss, C. (2000). Educational Discrimination Against Smokers: Evidence of Student and Faculty Prejudice. *Resources in Education,* ERIC/CASS, CG030121.

Campbell, R. L., Svenson, L. W., Jarvis, G. K. (1993). Age, gender, and location as factors in permission to smoke among university students. *Psychological Reports, 72,* 1231-1234.

Campion, E. W. (1997). Can house calls survive? *The New England Journal of Medicine, 337* (25), 1840-1841.

Cawley, J., Markowitz, S., and Tauras, J. (2005). *Body Weight, Cigarette Prices, Youth Access Laws and Adolescent Smoking Initiation.* presented at the 2005 ASSA Meetings.

Chambliss, C.A. (2004) High school, college, and professional school faculty members' perceptions of current smokers, former smokers, and nonsmokers. *Perceptual and Motor Skills, 99,* 629-632.

Chambliss, C., Austin, M., Brosh, J., Iannella, G., Outten, R., Rowles, M..(2005). The relationship between substance use and scores on the mini markers five factors personality scale in college and high school students. *Journal of Alcohol and Drug Education, 49,* 1, 21- 31.

Chambliss, C., Shull, M., Baker, K., Burton, C., Nesbit, M., Weir, C., Wilson, F., Katona, C. and Brosh, J. (2006). The social hazards of smoking in academic contexts: Students and teachers' attitudes about student smokers. *Journal of Alcohol and Drug Education, 50, 3,* 21-31.

Chambliss, C. and Murray, E. (1979). Cognitive Procedures for Smoking Reduction: Symptom Attribution Versus Efficacy Attribution. *Cognitive Therapy and Research,* 3 (1): 91-95.

Chassin, L., Presson, C.C., and Sherman, S.J. (1990). Social psychological contributions to the understanding and prevention of adolescent cigarette smoking. *Personality and Social Psychology Bulletin, 16,* 133-151.

Chassin, L., Presson, C.C., Rose, J.S., and Sherman, S.J. (1996). The natural history of cigarette smoking from adolescence to adulthood: Demographic predictors of continuity and change. *Health Psychology, 15* (6), 478-484.

Chaudhary, V. (1997, August 7). Front door smokers stubbed out. *The Guardian.* p.1, 9.

Cherlin, A., and Walters, P. B. (1981).Trends in United States men's and women's sex-role attitudes: 1972-1978. *American Sociological Review, 46,* 453- 460.

Cinciripini, P. M., Lapitsky, L.G., Wallfisch, A., Mace, R., Nezami, E., and Van Vunakis, H. (1994). An evaluation of a multicomponent treatment program involving scheduled smoking and relapse prevention procedures: Initial findings. *Addictive Behaviors, 19,* 13-22.

Clark, R. R. (1978). Reactions to other people's cigarette smoking. *The International Journal of Addictions, 13 (8),* 1237-1244.

Clausen, J.A. (1987). Health and the life course: Some personal observations. *Journal of Health and Social Behavior, 28,* 337-344.

Cochran, S., Filipkowski, J.N., Cooper, E., Egresitz,A., King, A., Mack, A., Piraino, D., Sills, E., Bisinger, N., and Chambliss, C. (2007) The relationship between maternal employment history and young adults' attitudes about maternal work status and career aspirations. 78th Eastern Psychological Association meeting, Philadelphia, PA March 2007.

Comeau, N., Stewart, S. H., and Loba, P. (2001). The relations of trait anxiety, anxiety sensitivity, and sensation seeking to adolescents' motivations for alcohol, cigarette, and marijuana use. *Addictive Behaviors, 26,* 803-825.

Compas, B. E., Haaga, D. A., Keefe, F. J., Leitenberg, H., and Williams, D. A. (1998). Sampling of empirically supported psychological treatments from health psychology: Smoking, chronic pain, cancer, and bulimia nervosa. *Journal of Consulting and Clinical Psychology, 66 (1),* 89-112.

Costa, P. T., Jr., and McCrae, R. R. (1997). Longitudinal stability of adult personality. *Handbook of personality psychology,* 269-291.

Dalton, M.A., Sargent, J.D., Beach, M.L., Titus-Ernstoff, L.,Gibson, J.J., Aherns, M.B.,Tickle, J.J., and Heatherton, T.F. (2003).Effect of viewing smoking in movies on adolescent smoking initiation: A cohort study. *Lancet , 362,* 9380.

Davis, R. M., Boyd, G. M., and Schoenborn, C. A. (1990). "Common courtesy" and the elimination of passive smoking. *Journal of the American Medical Association,* 2208-2210.

Department of Health and Human Services. (1994). Preventing tobacco use among young people: A report of the surgeon general. Washington, DC: U.S. Government Printing Office.

Dermer, M. L. and Jacobsen, E. (1986). Some potential negative consequences of cigarette smoking: marketing research in reverse. *Journal of Applied Social Psychology, 16,* 702-725.

Douglas, L., Allen, P., Arian, G., Crawford, M. A., Headen, S., Spigner, C., Tassler, P., and Ureda, J. (2001). Teens' images of smoking and smokers. *Public Health Reports, 116,* 194-207.

Duryea, E. J. and Martin, G. L. (1981). The distortion effect in student perceptions of smoking prevalence. *Journal of School Health, 51,* 115-118.

Dziuban. C. D., Moskal, P. D., West, G. B. (1999) Examining the Use of Tobacco on College Campuses. *Journal of American College Health, 47,* p 260.

Emmons, K. M., Wechsler, H., Dowdall, G., and Abraham, M. (1998). Predictors of smoking among US college students. *American Journal of Public Health, 88* (1), 104-107.

Eysenck, H. (1967). The Biological Basis of Personality. Springfield:Charles C. Thomas.

Flay, B.R., Hu, F.B., Siddiqui, O., Day, L.E., Hedeker, D., Petraitis, J., Richardson, J., and Sussman, S. (1994). Differential influence of parental smoking and friends' smoking on adolescent initiation and escalation of smoking. *Journal of Health and Social Behavior, 35,* 248-265.

Garfinkel, L. (1997). Trends in cigarette smoking in the United States. *Preventive Medicine, 26,* 447-450.

Geist, C. R. and Herrmann, S. M. (1990). A comparison of the psychological characteristics of smokers, exsmokers, and nonsmokers. *Journal of Clinical Psychology, 46,* 102-105.

Gibson, B. (1997). Smoker-nonsmoker conflict: Using a Social psychological framework to understand a current social controversy. *Journal of Social Issues, 53,* 1, 97-112.

Gibson, B. and Werner, C. M. (1992). The decision to attempt interpersonal control: the case of nonsmoker-smoker interaction. *Basic and Applied Social Psychology, 13,* 269-284.

Gibson, B. and Werner, C. M. (1994). The airport as a behavior setting: the role of legibility in communicating the setting program. *Journal of Personality and Social Psychology, 66,* 1049-1060.

Gilbert, D.G. (1979). Paradoxical tranquilizing and emotion-reducing effects of nicotine. *Psychological Bulletin, 86,* 643-661.

Gilbert, D.G. (1988). EEG and personality differences between smokers and nonsmokers. *Personality and Individual Differences, 9,* 659-665.

Gillard, J. and Bruchon-Schweitzer, M. (2001). Development and validation of a multidimensional smoking behaviour questionnaire. *Psychological Reports, 89,*499-509.

Glassman, A.H., Helzer, J.E., Covey, L.S., Cottler, L.B., Stetner, F., Tipp, J.E., and Johnson, J. (1990). Smoking, smoking cessation, and major depression. *Journal of the American Medical Association, 264,* 1546-1549.

Glassman, A.H., Stetner, F., Walsh, T.B., Raizman, P.S., Fleiss, J.L., Cooper, T.B., and Covey, L.S. (1988). Heavy smokers, smoking cessation, and clonidine: Results of a double-blind, randomized trial. *Journal of the American Medical Association, 259,* 2863-2866.

Goldstein, J. (1991). The stigmatization of smokers: an empirical investigation. *Journal of Drug Education, 21,* 167-182.

Gomberg, E. (1976) "The Female Alcoholic," in Ralph E. Tarter and A. Arthur Sugerman, Alcoholism: Interdisciplinary Approaches to an Enduring Problem (Reading, MA: Addison-Wesley, 1976), pp. 605-607

Gonzalez, G.M. (1889). Early onset of drinking as a predictor of alcohol comsumption and alcohol-related problems in college. *Journal of Drug Education, 19,* 225-230.

Green, G., MacIntyre, S., West, P., and Erob, R. (1990). Do children of lone parents smoke more because their mothers do? *British Journal of Addiction, 85,* 1497-1500.

Greenberger, E., and Goldberg, W. A. (1989). Work, parenting, and the socialization of children. *Developmental Psychology, 25,* 22-35

Grube, J. W., McGree, S., and Morgan, M. (1986). Beliefs related to cigarette smoking among Irish college students. *The International Journal of Addictions, 21 (6),* 701-706.

Hanson, G., and Venturelli, P. (1998). *Drugs and society. (5th ed.)* Boston, MA: Jones and Campbell.

Hazan, A.R., Lipton, H.L., and Glantz, S.A. (1994). Popular films do not reflect current tobacco use. *American Journal of Public Health, 84* (6), 998-1000.

Helzer, J.E., Robins L.N., Przybeck T.R., and Regier D.A. (1988). "Alcoholic Disorders in the Community: A Report from the Epidemiologic Catchment Area," in Robert M. Rose and James E. Barrett (eds.) Alcoholism: Origins and Outcome (New York: Raven Press, 1988), pp.15

Hemenway, D., Solnick, S.J., and Colditz, G.A. (1993). Smoking and suicide among nurses. *American Journal of Public Health, 83,* 249-251.

Hill, J. L., Waldfogel, J., Brooks-Gunn, J., and Han, W. (2005). Maternal employment and child development: A fresh look using newer methods. *Developmental Psychology, 41,* 833-850.

Hines, D., Fretz, A., and Nollen, N. L. (1998). Regular and occasional smoking by college students: Personality attributions of smokers and nonsmokers. *Psychological Reports, 83,* 1299-1206.

Hock, E., Gnezda, M. T., and McBride, S. L. (1984). Mothers of infants: Attitudes toward employment and motherhood following birth of first child. *Journal of Marriage and the Family, 46,* 425-431.

Hobson, K. (2006). Conquering craving. *U.S.News and World Report*, October 23, p.64.

Hodges, J., Srebro, K., Authier, C., and Chambliss, C. (1999). Why Do Undergraduates Smoke? Subjective Effects of Cigarette Smoking. *Resources in Education,* ERIC/CASS, CG029396.

Hoffman, L. W. (1998). The effects of the mother's employment on the family and the child. *Parenthood in America.*

Hu, T., Zihua, L. and Keeler, T. (1998), Teenage smoking: Attempts to quit and school performance, *American Journal of Public Health,* 88, 6 : 940–943.

Hughes, J.R., Higgins, S.T., and Hatsukami, D. (1990). Effects of abstinence from tobacco: A critical review. In L.T. Kowzlowski and H.M. Annis (Eds.). *Recent advances in alcohol and drug problems* (Vol.10, pp. 317-398). New York: Plenum.

Jacobson, P. D., Wasserman, J., and Raube, K. (1992). *The political evolution of antismoking legislation.* Santa Monica, CA: Rand.

Jaffe, J.H. (1989). Drug dependence: Opiods, nonnarcotics, nicotine (tobacco), and caffeine. In H.I. Kaplan and B.J. Sadock (Eds.), Comprehensive textbook of psychiatry, 5th ed. Baltimore: Williams and Wilkins.

Janiszewski, C. (1993). Preattentive mere exposure effects. *Journal of Consumer Research, 20* (3), 376-417.

Jason, L. A. and Lonak, C. A. (1990). A survey of corporate smoking policies. *Evaluation and the Health Professions, 13,* 405-411.

Jeffrey, R., Kelder, S., Forster, J., French, S., Lando, H., Baxter, J. (1994). Restrictive smoking policies in the workplace: effects on smoking prevalence and cigarette consumption. *Preventive Medicine*, 23: 78-82.

Jones, J. W. and Bogat, G. A. (1978). Adverse emotional reactions of nonsmokers to secondary cigarette smoke. *Environmental Psychology and Nonverbal Behavior, 3,* 125

Kane, J., Hodges, J., Srebro, K., Authier, C. and Chambliss, C. Individualized Attempts to Reduce Cigarette Smoking Among College Students. ERIC/CASS, CG029312, 1999.

Kane, J., Hodges, J., Srebro, K., Fruhwirth, M. and Chambliss, C. (1999) Attempts to reduce cigarette smoking among college students: A pilot study. Resources in Education, ERIC/CASS, ED430190.

Kaufman, M. Teens Who See Smoking in Movies More Likely to Light Up. *Washington Post*, June 10, 2003; p. A07.

Kawabata, T., Cross, D., Nishioka, N., and Shimai, S. (1999). Relationship between self-esteem and smoking behavior among Japanese early adolescents: initial results from a three-year study. *Journal of School Health, 69,* 280-290.

Klerman, G., Weissman, M., Rounsaville, B., and Chevron, E. (1984). Interpersonal Psychotherapy of Depression. New York: Basic Books.

Kliff, S. Failing the health test. *Newsweek*, July 2, 2007; p. 16.

Kingsbury, A. Admittedly unequal. *U.S. News and World Report*, June 25, 2007; p. 50-51.

Lee, C. (1989). Stereotypes of smokers among health science students. *Addictive Behaviors, 14,* 327-333.

Leventhal , H. and Cleary, P. (1980). The smoking problems: A review of the research and theory in behavioral risk modification. *Psychological Bulletin, 88,* 370-405.

Longo, D., Brownson, R., Johnson, J., Hewett, J., Kruse, R., Novotny, T., and Logan, R. (1996). Hospital smoking bans and employee smoking behavior: results of a national survey. *The Journal of the American Medical Association., 275,* 1252-1257.

Lloyd, B. and Lucas, K. (1997). *Smoking in adolescence: Images and identities.* London: Routledge.

Lucas, K. and Lloyd, B. (1999). Starting smoking: girls' explanations of the influence of peers. *Journal of Adolescence, 22,* 647-655.

Malouff, J., Schutte, N. S., and Kenyon, A. (1991). Negative social effects of being a smoker. *Journal of Drug Education, 21,* 293-302.

Mason, K. O., and Lu, Y. (1988). Attitudes toward U.S. women's familial roles, 1977-1985. *Gender and Society, 2,* 39-57.

McCrae, R. R, and Costa, P. T. (1989). The structure of personality traits: Wiggins' circumplex and the five-factor model. *Journal of Personality and Social Psychology, 56,* 586-595.

McKillip, J., and Vierke, M. S. (1980). College smokers: Worried, sick but still puffing. *Journal of the American College Health Association, 28,* 280-282.

Moore, E. (1998, March 10). Kicking the habit despite the dangers, twelve million people in the UK smoke. *The Guardian*, 8.

National Center for Education Statistics (2005). Digest of education statistics tables and figures 2005*: Degrees conferred by degree-granting institutions, by level of degree and sex of student.* Retrieved on June 13, 2007 from http://nces.ed.gov /programs /digest/d05 /tables/dt05_246.asp

Nelson, Heath, and Kessler, 1998; Temporal progression of alcohol dependence symptoms in the U.S. household population: Results from the National Comorbidity Survey. *Journal of Consulting and Clinical Psychology, 66,* 474-483.O'Connor, L.E., Berry, J.W., Weiss, J., Bush, M, and Sampson, H. (1997). Interpersonal guilt:development of a new measure. *Journal of Clinical Psychology, 53,* 73-89.

O'Connor, Lynn E., Berry, Jack W., Weiss, Joseph, and Gilbert, Paul. (2002). Guilt, fear, submission, and empathy in depression. *Journal of Affective Disorders, 71,* 19-27.

Office of the U.S. Surgeon General. (1988*). Nicotine addiction.* Washington, DC: US Government Printing Office.

Ouellette, J. A., and Wood, W. (1998). Habit and intention in everyday life: The multiple processes by which past behavior predicts future behavior. *Psychological Bulletin, 124* (1), 54-74.

Outten,R., Rowles, P and Chambliss, C.A. Faculty members' attitudes toward students who smoke: The last permitted type of discrimination, Resources in Education, ERIC/CASS, CG032546, 2004.

Page, R. M. (1998). College students' distorted perception of the prevalence of smoking. *Psychological Reports, 82,* 474.

Parrott, A.C. (1999). Does cigarette smoking cause stress? *American Psychologist, 54* (10), 817-820.

Parrott, A.C. and Garnham, N.J. (1998). Comparative mood states and cognitive skills of cigarette smokers, deprived smokers, and nonsmokers. *Human Psychopharmacology, 13,* 367-376.

Pechmann, C., and Shih, C. (1999). Smoking scenes in movies and antismoking advertisements before movies: effects on youth. *Journal of Marketing, 63* (3), 1. Retrieved September 22, 1999 from Expanded Academic ASAP (InfoTrac) on the World Wide Web; http://www.infotrac.galegroup.com/itweb

Pechmann, C., Ratneshwar, S. (1994). The effects of anti-smoking and cigarette advertising on young adolescents' perceptions of peers who smoke. *Journal of Consumer Research,* 21, 236-252.

Polivy, J., Hackett, R., and Bycio, P. (1979). The effect of perceived smoking status on attractiveness. *Personality and Social Psychology Bulletin, 5,* 401-404.

Potkin, S.G. (2004). The association between anger and susceptibility to nicotine. In L. Neergaard, Some predisposed to smoking. *Miami Herald* (p. 3A). February 17, 2004.

Potts, H., Gillies, P., and Herbert, M. (1986). Adolescent smoking and opinion of cigarette advertisements. *Health Education Research: Theory and Practice, 1* (3), 195-201.

Price, J. H., Beach, P., Everett, S., Telljohann, S. K., and Lewis, L. (1998). Evaluation of a three-year urban elementary school tobacco prevention program. *Journal of School Health, 68,1,26-31.*

Reid, D. (1985). Prevention of smoking among school children: Recommendations for policy development. *Health Education Journal, 44* (1), 3-12.

Rigotti, N.A., Lee, J.E., and Wechsler, H. (2000). US college students' use of tobacco products: the results of a national survey. *The Journal of the American Medical Association, 284,* 699.

Rosal, M. C., Ockene, J. K., Hurley, T. G., and Hebert, J. R. (1998). Effectiveness of nicotine-containing gum in the physician delivered smoking intervention study. *Preventive Medicine, 27,* 262-267.

Rosenberg, M. (1965). Society and the adolescent self-image. Princeton, Princeton University.

Rubin, L. B. (1994). *Families on the Fault Line.* New York: Harper Collins Publishers.

Rutledge, P.C. and Sher, K.J. (2001). Heavy drinking from the freshman year into early young adulthood: The role of stress, tension-reduction drinking motives, gender, and personality. *Journal of Studies on Alcohol, 62(4),* 457.

Sarason, I.G., Mankowski, E.S., Peterson, A.V., Jr., and Dinh, K.T. (1992). Adolescents' reasons for smoking. *Journal of School Health, 62,* 185-191.

Saucier, G. (1992). Mini-Markers: A brief version of Goldberg's unipolar Big-Five markers. *Journal of Personality, 63,* 506-512.

Schooler, C., Feighery, E., and Flora, J.A. (1996). Seventh graders' self-reported exposure to cigarette marketing and its relationship to their smoking behavior. *American Journal of Public Health, 86* (2), 225-230.

Scott, J. W., and Tilly, L. A. (1975). Women's work and the family in nineteenth-century Europe. *Comparative Studies in Society and History, 17,* 36-64.

Seltzer, C. C. and Oeschsli, F. W. (1985). Psychological characteristics of adolescent smokers before they started smoking: evidence of self-selection. *Journal of Chronic Disorders, 38,* 17-26.

Shogren, E. (1997). Hollywood is urged to act on smoking. *Los Angeles Times,* p.A25.

Special Report: State Tobacco Settlement. (2002, January 15). Report Shows most states falling short in using tobacco settlement funds for prevention. Prepared by the Campaign for Tobacco Free Kids, American Heart Association, American Cancer Society, and American Lung Association. Retrieved July 15,2002 from Campaign for Tobacco Free Kids on the World Wide Web; http://www.tobaccofreekids.org/reports/settlement

Srebro, K., Hodges, J., Authier, and Chambliss, C. (1999). Views of College Student

Smoking: A Comparison of Smokers and Nonsmokers. Resources in Education, ERIC/CASS, CG029395.

Stein, J. A., Newcomb, M. D., and Bentler, P. M. (1996). Initiation and maintenance of tobacco smoking: Changing personality correlates in adolescence and young adulthood. *Journal of Applied Social Psychology, 26* (2), 160-187.

Stronks, K., van de Mheen, D., Looman, C.W.N., and Mackenbach, J.P. (1997). Cultural, material, and psychosocial correlates of the socioeconomic gradient in smoking behavior among adults. *Preventive Medicine, 26,* 754-766.

Sue, D., Sue, L., and Sue, S. (2000). *Abnormal Psychology.* New York: Houghton Mifflin.

Thomson, P., and Graham, J. (2005). *A Woman's place is in the boardroom.* London: Palgrave Macmillan.

Tomeo, C.A., Field, A., Berkey, C.S., Colditz, G.A., and Frazier, A.L. (1999). Weight Concerns, Weight Control Behaviors, and Smoking Initiation. *Pediatrics.* 104: 918-24.

Torrey, G. Fuller. (1999). *Treating Schizophrenia.* Hyperion: New York.

Trends in cigarette smoking among high school students—United States, 1991-2001. (2002). *The Journal of the American Medical Association,* 288, 308-310.

U. S. Department of Health and Human Services. (1985) Cancer and chronic lung disease in the workplace: A report of the Surgeon General. Rockville, MD: U. S. Department of Health and Human Services, Office on Smoking and Health.

U.S. Department of Health and Human Services. (1986). The health consequences of involuntary smoking, a report of the Surgeon General (DHHS Publication No. 87-8309). Washington, DC: U. S. Government Printing Office.

U.S. Department of Health and Human Services. (1989). Reducing the Health Consequences of Smoking: 25 Years of Progress: A Report of the Surgeon General 1989. (DHHS Publication No.89-8411) Atlanta, GA: Office on Smoking and Health, Centers for Disease Control and Prevention.

United States Department of Labor. (2007). *News: Bureau of Labor Statistics. Employment characteristics of families in 2006.* Retrieved June 25, 2007, from http:// www. bls. Gov /cps/.

van Roosmalen, E. H. and McDaniel, S. A. (1989) Peer group influence as a factor in smoking behavior of adolescents. *Adolescence*, 24, 801–816.

van Roosmalen, E. H. and McDaniel, S. A. (1992) Adolescent smoking intentions: gender differences in peer context. *Adolescence*, 27, 87–105.

Venuti, J. P., and Chambliss, C. (2000). Effects of Substance Use Education Programs. *Resources in Education,* ERIC/CASS, CG030259.

Venuti, J. P., Conroy, M., Landis, P. and Chambliss, C.A. (2000). Subjective Determinants of Substance Use: Gender Differences in Student Substance Use, *Resources in Education*, ERIC/CASS, CG030260.

Venuti, J., Conroy, M., Bucy, P., Landis, P., and Chambliss, C., (2002). The Relative Stigma Associated with Smoking, Obesity, and Criminality, *Resources in Education*, ERIC/CASS, CG031614.

Venuti, J.P., and Chambliss, C. (2000). Effects of substance use education programs: Cultural Differences in College Substance Use, Resources in Education, ERIC/CASS, CG030259.

Venuti, J.P., Conroy, M., Bucy, P., Landis, P.L., Chambliss, C. (2000). Prejudice against cigarette smokers in higher education, *Resources in Education*, ERIC/CASS, CG030261.

Vogel-Sprott, M. (1984) Response measures of social drinking: Research implications and applications. Journal of Studies on Alcohol, 44, 817-836.

Wagner, M.K. (2001). Behavioral characteristics related to substance abuse and risk-taking, sensation-seeking, anxiety sensitivity, and self-reinforcement. *Addictive Behaviors, 26*, 115-120.

Wechsler, H., Rigotii, N.A., Gledhill-Hoyt, J., and Lee, H. (1998). Increased levels of cigarette use among college students: A cause for national concern. *Journal of the American Medical Association, 280* (19), 1673-1678.

Wills, T.A., Sandy, J.M., and Yaeger, A.M. (2002). Stress and smoking in adolescence: a test of directional hypotheses. *Health Psychology, 21,* 122-130.

Zinser, O., Kloosterman, R., and Williams, A. (1991). Perceptions of cigarette advertisements by college student smokers, former smokers, and nonsmokers. *Journal of Social Behavior and Personality, 6* (2), 355-366.

Zinser, O., Kloosterman, R., and Williams, A. (1994). Advertisements, volition, and peers among other causes of smoking: Perceptions of college student smokers. *Journal of Alcohol and Drug Education, 39* (3), 13-26.

Zuckerman, M. (1994). *Behavioral Expressions and Biosocial Bases of Sensation Seeking,* New York: Cambridge University Press.

In: Smoking and Women's Health
Editors: M.K. Wesley and I.A. Sternbach, pp.69-108

ISBN 978-1-60456-148-7
© 2008 Nova Science Publishers, Inc.

Chapter 2

Tobacco Use and Dependence: Health Impact on Women

***Taru Kinnunen [1], Tellervo Korhonen[2], Petra Miesmaa[1]
and Donna M. Terwal[1]***
1.Harvard University, Faculty of Medicine, School of Dental Medicine
Tobacco Dependence Treatment and Research, Department of Oral Health Policy and
Epidemiology, Boston, Massachusetts, USA
2.University of Helsinki, Department of Public Health, Helsinki, Finland

Abstract

Every year nearly one million women die from tobacco-induced diseases worldwide. The majority of tobacco-related deaths are due to cardiovascular diseases followed by lung cancer. Although smoking related cancer deaths are decreasing among men, they are increasing among women – 90 % of female lung cancer deaths are attributable to smoking. Moreover, smoking contributes to osteoporosis, breast cancer, and pregnancy complications. Because prevalence of smoking has not decreased as successfully among women as men, we can expect that smoking-related illnesses will continue to increase among women. Health burden is further enhanced by the fact that the current female smokers are more likely to have other co-morbidities (high nicotine dependence, depression, physical inactivity, low education) contributing to more severe and chronic conditions. Smoking cessation is the most rapid way to decrease tobacco related morbidity and mortality. Although majority of tobacco users would like to quit, less than 10% succeed in a given year. Weight concerns, stress, depression, lack of social support, and low education level are some of the factors contributing to poorer outcome in cessation treatments for women than men. Women report also greater physical and emotional dependence on tobacco than men do. Successful treatment for tobacco dependence among women should include both pharmacological and non-pharmacological components. Pharmacological tobacco dependence treatments have been actively developed during the past decade. They include wide selection of nicotine replacement therapies, bupropion, and varenicline. Non-pharmacological treatment includes behavioral interventions such as relapse prevention or cognitive-behavioral counseling and should always be added to pharmacotherapy. Hindrances to success come from findings that nicotine replacement therapy alone may not be as effective for women as for men, and that none of the pharmacological treatments are recommended for pregnant or breastfeeding women. Cognitive-behavioral therapies addressing negative affectivity and weight concerns have been found promising. Similarly, exercise has been tested as a novel and particularly suitable treatment for female smokers. In order to reduce the health burden of tobacco among women worldwide a lot more work needs to be done both in prevention and cessation. First, we need to find ways to reduce the initiation and development of dependence of tobacco use among young women. Second, we need continue to develop treatments that offer social support as well as address weight concerns and negative affect. Third, we need to identify and remove barriers preventing women from utilizing treatments.

1. Introduction

There are more than 200 million female smokers in the world. Tobacco companies are targeting women and girls worldwide with aggressive campaigns to recruit more new customers. Until today, cultural constraints have kept the level of female tobacco use relatively low in developing countries. Unfortunately, smoking prevalence is beginning to rise in the developing world as well due to rapid economic and cultural changes. Currently, every fifth woman in the United States is a smoker. Young women too often start smoking because they desire to be thin. Tobacco companies design misleading messages in which smoking facilitates weight control. Nicotine, the addictive substance in tobacco, has an addictive potential comparable to heroin and methadone. Tobacco and nicotine dependence has been officially recognized as a chronic disease. It fulfills dependence criteria such as compulsion to smoke, difficulty controlling smoking, smoking despite harmful health effects and withdrawal symptoms during abstinence. Once addicted to tobacco, women tend to have more difficulties quitting than men. It has been suggested that the slower decline in smoking prevalence among women may partially be explained by lower smoking cessation rates in women than in men. In this chapter we will review the epidemiology of female smoking and also provide evidence on its essential adverse health consequences. The constantly increasing body of evidence regarding the disproportional health risks of environmental tobacco smoke for women will be reviewed. Conversely, we will highlight the major health gains obtained by stopping tobacco use. Further, we will also discuss those barriers to smoking cessation typically faced by women. Finally, we will discuss evidence and share our own clinical experience on multi component smoking cessation trials tailored for women, focusing on exercise as a behavioral adjunct to standard smoking cessation treatment.

2. Epidemiology of Smoking among Women

2.1. Historical Trends of Female Smoking Habits

In the nineteenth century and beginning of the twentieth century smoking was the exclusive privilege of men. Usually men smoked in designated male areas such as cafes, places of entertainment and offices. Women who smoked were considered immoral both by men and women (Haustein, 2003). The First World War was a turning point in women's smoking habits in the Western World. Women started claiming the right to wear pants and smoke during The American Women's Movement and their influence spread fast to Europe. Smoking became a symbol of independence, power and liberation for women (Vierola, 1998). During the Second World War smoking consumption quadrupled worldwide. While men were in the battle fields, women had to do their jobs on the home front. This was an opportunity for women to take up manly habits, including smoking. It became acceptable for women to smoke in public just as men had done for decades (Haustein, 2003; Vierola, 1998).

The prevalence of cigarette smoking in the USA peaked in the 1940s and 1950s for men, when 67% of the male population smoked. Women reached their peak in the 1960s, with a maximum prevalence of 44% (Tolley, Crane, and Shipley, 1991). Since then the smoking prevalence has decreased, thanks to the massive anti-smoking campaigns of the 1970s (Haustein, 2003). However, the decline has been greater among men than among women. Moreover, in the 1990s the decline in smoking rates among adult women stalled while smoking rates rose steeply among teenaged girls (U.S. Department of Health and Human Services [USDHHS], 2001).

Currently, about 21% of women in the US smoke. Smoking prevalence is slightly higher for Caucasian women (23%) and much higher for the American Indian/Alaskan Native racial group (37%) (National Women's Law Center and Oregon Health and Science University [NWLCandOHandSU], 2003). Other high risk groups include women with low education and low income, and young women (USDHHS, 2007).

Popular culture has had a profound impact on women's smoking habits. Movies, magazines and other media have portrayed smoking as a symbol of attractiveness, sophistication, independence and liberation of convention (Haustein, 2003; USDHHS, 2007). Moreover, the aggressive campaigning targeting women by the cigarette companies has influenced the habits of countless women.

Since the 1920s, the cigarette companies have exploited the values of the Women's Movement in its advertising directed to women. Women in the smoking ads are displayed as empowered and independent. Another popular but false message targeting women has been that smoking helps control weight (Haustein, 2003; NWLCandOHandSU, 2003; Vierola, 1998). After it became acceptable for women to smoke in public the cigarette companies realized a lot of money could be made by increasing women's smoking prevalence. They studied the female preferences and created special brands and attractive packaging for women. Many familiar cigarette features, such as filtered, mentholated, light and king-size cigarettes, were initiated because the cigarette companies thought that they would attract more female smokers (Carpenter, Ferris, and Connolly, 2005; Haustein, 2003;

NWLCandOHandSU, 2003; Vierola, 1998). Unfortunately, brand development and marketing efforts paid off as can be seen in women's increasing smoking prevalence.

While the US and the European Union now have restrictions on cigarette advertising (the EU has a total ban on cigarette advertising), the same marketing techniques that were used in developed countries until the 1970s to promote smoking among women and girls are now being used in the new democracies of Central and Eastern Europe and many developing countries around the world (Vierola, 1998). In addition to the marketing campaigns, rapid cultural and economic changes have increased women's smoking rates globally (USDHHS, 2007).

2.2. Stages of Smoking Behavior

Stages of smoking behavior – initiation, daily smoking, tobacco dependence, and quitting – are influenced by genetic and environmental factors as well as interactions between those factors. The shared and unique environmental factors have the strongest influence in smoking initiation, but genetic factors are more important in determining which individuals become persistent daily smokers, develop tobacco dependence and who will quit smoking or not. Somewhat lower heritability for smoking initiation (Pomerleau et al., 2007) and smoking cessation has been observed in women than in men (Broms, Silventoinen, Madden, Heath, and Kaprio, 2006), suggesting that the influence of environmental factors in smoking behavior may be more important for women than for men. However, the heritable tendency to become a daily smoker after initiation does not seem to be modified by gender (Hamilton et al., 2006).

Smoking Initiation
Smoking initiation is the first phase of a longitudinal process where one gradually proceeds from experimentation to regular smoking (Haustein, 2003). Many start smoking and become addicted to nicotine as teenagers and some 25% report having their first cigarette already before the age of 10 (Mackay, Eriksen, and Shafey, 2006). Step-by-step, the self-image of a smoker develops leading to regular smoking. Recently, the rapid onset of nicotine dependence has been confirmed among adolescent smokers (DiFranza et al., 2007). However, some may not become daily smokers but smoke only on weekends (Mayhew, Flay, and Mott, 2000).

For some adolescents smoking initiation may be related to the socializing process, such as imitating adult behavior or complying with peer pressure. Further, some may initiate smoking in order to alleviate negative moods (Dani and Harris, 2005). Concerning the decision to smoke or not to smoke, less than 20% of the gender differences can be explained by different background characteristics of men compared to women (Bauer, Gohlmann, and Sinning, 2007). Advertisement of tobacco products has been used as a powerful tool in motivating women especially to start smoking. The tobacco companies also launched several cigarette brands specifically targeted for women. For example, brand names such as 'Lucky Strike', 'Virginia Slim' and 'Silva Thin' have been promoted by suggesting that keeping a slender figure would be better achieved through smoking than eating sweets (Haustein, 2003). The first wave of smoking initiation among young women of higher socioeconomic status emerged in the mid-1920s, coincident with the 'Lucky Strike' women's marketing campaigns. In the second wave during the late 1960s, smoking uptake among young females increased rapidly again coincident with large-scale marketing of women's brands, such as 'Virginia Slim' (Pierce and Gilpin, 1995).

Daily Smoking

Regular or daily smoking among adults is usually defined as having smoked at least 100 cigarettes during their lifetime and smoking currently daily or almost daily. Progression to daily smoking after initiation may be more rapid among female than male adolescents. The average time interval between age at first cigarette and age at daily smoking was significantly shorter for girls (0.9 years) than for boys (1.5 years) (Thorner, Jaszyna-Gasior, Epstein, and Moolchan, 2007). The relative influence of factors for maintaining smoking after initiation may differ between men and women (Perkins, Jacobs, Sanders, and Caggiula, 2002). Maintenance of tobacco use and proceeding to regular daily smoking is affected mainly by positive and negative reinforcements elicited by nicotine in cigarette smoke or snuff. An example of positive reinforcement is mild euphoria, whereas relief from withdrawal illustrates negative reinforcement (Royal College of Physicians of London [RCPL], 2000). However, it is shown that the dose effect of nicotine on smoking reinforcement is smaller in women than in men (Perkins et al., 2002). Conditioned learning, social aspects of smoking, psychosocial factors, psychiatric conditions, and other addictions further contribute to maintenance of regular smoking (RCPL, 2000). Some of those subjectively perceived aspects, smoking-associated environmental cues, and reinforcing effects of 'non-nicotine' stimuli may be more important for women than men (Perkins, 2001). Once a regular daily smoker, more than 90% of the gender differences in the number of cigarettes smoked per day may be due to different behavior patterns. The remaining 10% may be explained by differences in the observed background characteristics, such as education, type of job, income, and marital status (Bauer, Gohlmann, and Sinning, 2007).

Occasional Smoking

In addition to regular or daily smokers, the concept of a 'smoker' can include a variety of other smoking patterns, such as occasional smoking as well as light and intermittent smoking (LITS) (National Cancer Institute [NCI], 2007). Several terms are used for this kind of smoking pattern, such as light smoking (consistently low levels of cigarette consumption, i.e. maximum of 10 cigarettes per day) (Okuyemi et al., 2002), intermittent smoking (smoked 100 cigarettes or more, but never smoked daily) (Husten, McCarty, Giovino, Chrismon, and Zhu, 1998), occasional smoking (smoking only on some days of the week) (Hennrikus, Jeffery, and Lando, 1996), and 'chipping' (smoking five or fewer cigarettes per day on at least five days a week) (Shiffman and Paty, 2006). It is important to recognize LITS as an alternative pattern of smoking behavior. Although the overall prevalence of tobacco smoking in the United States is decreasing, the proportion of light smokers is increasing, particularly among vulnerable groups such as adolescents, ethnic minorities, and women, especially those who continue smoking during pregnancy at a reduced level (Okuyemi et al., 2002). Moreover, there is growing evidence that light smokers experience significantly higher health risks compared to non-smokers (NCI, 2007).

Tobacco Dependence

Nicotine is the addictive substance in tobacco. Its addictive potential is comparable to heroin and methadone (West, 2006). Cigarette smoking is the most efficient device for becoming dependent on tobacco and nicotine (Benowitz, 1999). Tobacco dependence (ICD-10) and nicotine dependence (DSM-IV-TR) (American Psychiatric Association [APA], 2000), both fulfilling certain dependence criteria, have been officially recognized as chronic diseases. (N.B. Although ICD refers to 'tobacco dependence', whereas DSM refers to 'nicotine dependence', for brevity we use the former phrase). Most of the established dependence criteria apply for smoking: difficulty controlling the habit, keeping up the habit despite harmful health effects, and withdrawal symptoms during abstinence. However, other dependence criteria, such as spending large amounts of time to obtain the substance and recovering from use are not common for smokers (Hughes, Helzer, and Lindberg, 2006). Tobacco dependence is not only a physical phenomena, i.e. neurobiological adaptation to nicotine, it is also a psychological condition that includes impaired behavioral control related to personality and coping skills as well as social components. For example, psychological dependence may develop so that one smokes to cope with emotionally difficult situations or as a reward from stressful events (Kassel, Stroud, and Paronis, 2003). Tobacco dependence is among the most common mental disorders. The lifetime prevalence is around 30% in people who have ever smoked and 50% in current smokers. These rates are as high for women than for men (Hughes, Helzer, and Lindberg, 2006) although smoking exposure measured by nicotine levels adjusted for body volume, is less in women (Perkins, 2001). This suggests that women become more dependent on tobacco than men from the same or lesser exposure.

Smoking Cessation

Many smokers would like to quit, but it is often difficult, mostly because of dependence and withdrawal symptoms (Fiore et al., 2000). The likelihood of successful quitting without treatment is less than 10% (Hughes, Keely, and Naud, 2004), whereas with pharmacological and non-pharmacological treatments the likelihood is up to 30% (Fiore et al., 2000). Many smokers cycle through multiple quit attempts, lapse, relapse and remission (Fiore et al., 2000). Relapse after a quit attempt is a quite rapid process; some 75% of relapse occurs within the first week. When progressing from a lapse to relapse, smoking behavior is marked by bouts of abstinence followed by slowly escalating smoking (Shiffman, 2006). The difficulty in quitting smoking even when there are compelling reasons to do so is a key feature of dependence (Benowitz, 1999). Furthermore, tolerance to nicotine may remain even after long term smoking cessation. If one starts smoking again after several weeks of abstinence one can get back to the previous level of consumption in a few days (Perkins et al., 2001a).

It has been suggested that less favorable development in smoking prevalence among women than men may partially be explained by lower smoking cessation rates in women (Bolego, Poli, and Paoletti, 2002). Although women are as motivated as men to quit and are more likely to seek assistance with quitting than men, surprisingly, women are consistently less likely to be asked about their smoking behavior and advised to quit by their physician than men (Perkins, 2001). Although the evidence that women were less successful in quitting than men is not consistent, several studies show that women face more difficulties in quitting than men do (Abrams et al., 2003). Among reasons for inconsistent findings are that male relapse rates may be artificially lowered due to their switch to smokeless tobacco or that there has been lack of statistical power to detect significant differences in abstinence rates across gender (Perkins, 2001). It has been suggested that some specific factors, such as post-cessation weight gain among women concerned about their weight (Abrams et al., 2003), higher depressiveness or stress levels and lower self-confidence are determinants of early relapse more commonly among women (Perkins, 2001). Further, women may not be as responsive to nicotine replacement treatments as men are and pregnant smokers who try to quit cannot even utilize all pharmacological smoking cessation aids. Moreover, as a function of menstrual cycle phase, mood related symptoms may have a stronger impact on smoking cessation among women (Perkins, 2001). There is limited evidence on other factors, such as socio-cultural influences, which might explain potential gender differences in the risk for relapse or in response to tobacco dependence treatments (Abrams et al., 2003). However, some non-nicotine medications and adjunct behavioral treatments, such as counseling tailored to women, might reverse their poorer outcome compared to men (Perkins, 2001). More research is needed to evaluate the effectiveness of more specific adjunct behavioral interventions, such as physical activity in smoking cessation (Ussher, 2005), especially whether this behavioral treatment would be particularly helpful for female smokers trying to quit.

2.3. Co-Morbidities of Tobacco Dependence in Women

Persistent smokers tend to have more co-morbidities than people who never smoked. For example, smokers tend to report more depressive symptoms (Morrell and Cohen, 2006), have lower educational status (Bolego, Poli, and Paoletti, 2002), or be engaged in less physical activity (Schumann, Hapke, Rumpf, Meyer, and John, 2001).

Depressive Symptoms
Smokers are more likely to have a history of lifetime depression or current depressive symptoms than non-smokers, and *vice versa*, smoking habit remains particularly common among persons with depressive disorders (Morrell and Cohen, 2006). For example, smoking prevalence in the United States reaches nearly 40% among persons with lifetime major depression compared to some 20% among those without depression history (Lasser et al., 2000). Moreover, co-morbidity of smoking and depression has become more common with time. From the 1950s to 1970s that association was not significant, but in the1990s the odds for a smoker to be depressed were three times the odds of a nonsmoker to be depressed (Murphy et al., 2003). While the prevalence of smoking in general is lower among women than men (World Health Organization [WHO], 1997) the prevalence of depression is higher among women than men (WHO, 2001a). Further, the association between smoking and depressive symptoms may be modified by gender (Korhonen et al., 2007).

Although many risk factors for smoking initiation during adolescence seem to be similar for girls and boys, girls appear to be especially affected by the perception that smoking provides relief from negative mood states, such as depression, anxiety and tensions

(Christen and Christen, 2003; USDHHS, 2004). Both smoking initiation and tobacco dependence among women have been associated with history of mood disorders even after controlled for genetic influences (Kendler et al., 1999). More specifically, current female smokers in a population-based study had higher mean depression scores than former female smokers and those women who had never smoked, and depression scores among current smokers correlated to the amount of smoking (Haukkala, Uutela, Vartiainen, McAlister, and Knekt, 2000). One possible explanation is that negative affect associated to continuing smoking is more common among women than among men (Perkins, 2001). Negative affect is a potential barrier for women trying to quit smoking (Schmitz, 2003). Although female smokers with elevated depressive symptoms seem to be more motivated to quit smoking (Haukkala et al., 2000), their depressive symptoms inhibit their quit attempts and increase the likelihood of relapse (Doherty, Kinnunen, Militello, and Garvey, 1995; Kinnunen, 2001).

Low Educational Status

Populations at the greatest risk for tobacco dependence and tobacco-related diseases include women with low levels of education (USDHHS, 2004). Also, when looking at socioeconomic status (SES) that includes education, income, and occupation, tobacco use in the USA and most of the industrialized world is the highest among those with the lowest SES. In addition to these traditional measures of SES, gender often appears as an important characteristic of low SES (McLellan and Kaufman, 2006). Depending on which stage of the smoking epidemic the country is in, the differences in smoking prevalence vary according to educational level in women *versus* men (Bolego, Poli, and Paoletti, 2002).

Women's smoking patterns usually lag 10–20 years behind those of men. In the first stage, smoking is rare and mainly a behavior of men in higher socio-economic groups. In the second stage, male smoking becomes more common and the differences between educational groups diminish, whereas women from higher socioeconomic groups start adopting the habit. In the third stage, smoking prevalence decreases in men, with women following the trend 10-20 years later. Finally, in stage 4, prevalence keeps declining in both genders and smoking becomes more and more a habit of lower educated men and women (Bolego, Poli, and Paoletti, 2002). This general pattern was confirmed by an international comparison of 12 European countries in various stages of the smoking epidemic in 1990 (Cavelaars et al., 2000). The notion that the association between smoking and socioeconomic status may not be immutable is supported by an analysis conducted in the US with surprising results. Namely, from 1992 to 2002 smoking prevalence among low educated women declined at a greater rate than among more highly educated women, in contrast with trends of earlier periods. It was also suggested that some tobacco control policies, such as media campaigns targeting low education women, may make inroads in reducing the smoking prevalence of this vulnerable population (Levy, Mumford, and Compton, 2006).

Smoking initiation and tobacco dependence among women are associated with low levels of education (Kendler et al., 1999). Women's smoking behavior in early adulthood seems to be influenced not only by current social disadvantage, such as low educational status, but also by longer term background, such as childhood social disadvantage (Graham, Inskip, Francis, and Harman, 2006). Additionally, lower educated women may be at higher risk for passive smoking exposure both at home and work, because they often live in households with smokers or work at jobs where smoking is permitted (Shavers et al., 2006). Moreover, children of women of low SES tend to be at higher risk to start smoking (McLellan and Kaufman, 2006). According to the 2001 Surgeon General's Report on Women and Smoking, high education is a good predictor of success in smoking cessation among women (USDHHS, 2001). This conclusion has been more recently supported in a European twin study, where indicators of socioeconomic status such as low education and social class were strong and independent predictors of smoking cessation. More specifically, highly educated women were more likely to be successful in their smoking cessation attempt than women with low education and the difference in the success rate between the two educational groups was almost twice as high as men's (Broms, Silventoinen, Lahelma, Koskenvuo, and Kaprio, 2004). In other words, women who continue to smoke and those who fail at attempts to stop smoking tend to have lower education and employment levels than women who quit smoking successfully (USDHHS, 2004).

Physical Inactivity

Participation in leisure-time physical activity seems to be associated with tobacco-free life style (Johnson, Boyle, and Heller, 1995). Likewise, smoking seems to play a central role in the associations between health behaviors, such as the co-morbidity between smoking and physical inactivity (Laaksonen, Luoto, Helakorpi, and Uutela, 2002). Persistent physical inactivity in adolescence predicts subsequent smoking initiation, even after familial factors are taken into account (Kujala, Kaprio, and Rose, 2007). Those adult smokers who are highly dependent on tobacco tend to do less physical activity than smokers with low dependence (Schumann et al., 2001). Particularly, consonant female smokers, i.e. those who would not like to quit, tend to be more sedentary than dissonant female smokers, i.e. those who would like to quit (Haukkala, Laaksonen, and Uutela, 2001). The presence of multiple health risk behaviors such as smoking and sedentary lifestyle seems to be related to more serious problems with smoking, such as dependence and lower self-efficacy from refraining from smoking. However, this co-morbidity does not seem to affect prognosis for smoking cessation (Sherwood, Hennrikus, Jeffery, Lando, and Murray, 2000).

There is evidence indicating that physical activity may delay the occurrence of disease and premature death initiated by smoking. Thus, increasing physical activity among sedentary smokers may be an important intervention in the future (Ferrucci et al., 1999). Moreover, because regular exercise has many positive effects related to the smoking cessation process (Haus, Hoerr, Mavis, and Robison, 1994), physical activity may become a promising treatment, particularly for women who want to quit smoking (Marcus et al., 1999). However, there are concerns regarding the feasibility of physical activity as a 'harm reduction' strategy (deRuiter and Faulkner, 2006).

2.4. False Beliefs of Smoking Among Women

Since the 1920s the tobacco industry has targeted women and girls with exclusive female brands, aggressive marketing, advertising and promotional campaigns. Several studies have established that industry efforts have resulted in elevated smoking rates, increased smoking-related morbidity and mortality, and false beliefs about cigarettes among women (Amos and Haglund, 2000; Ernster, 1986; Ernster, Kaufman, Nichter, Samet, and Yoon, 2000; O'Keefe and Pollay, 1996; Richmond 1997).

In their review of previously secret tobacco industry documents Carpenter, Ferris, and Connolly (2005) discovered that the tobacco industry has conducted extensive research on female smoking patterns and product preferences, and has intentionally modified product design to attract female smokers. Cigarette manufacturers started focusing on social and health matters because women tend to be more concerned about these issues than men (NWLCandOHandSU, 2003). The resulting products exploit mistaken health notions about the relative safety of light cigarettes, create false perceptions of social and health effects through reduced side stream smoke and improved aroma and aftertaste; match female taste preferences through flavoured, smooth and mild-tasting cigarettes; and target physiological and inhalation differences with greater ease of draw, increased sensory pleasure and altered tar and nicotine levels (Carpenter, Ferris, and Connolly, 2005).

The marketing strategies of the tobacco industry targeting women have contributed to the association of smoking with appealing attributes such as liberation, glamour, success and thinness (Carpenter, Ferris, and Connolly, 2005; Haustein, 2003; Vierola, 1998). Aggressive marketing campaigns have lead to two stubborn misconceptions of smoking among women: light cigarettes are less harmful than regular cigarettes and smoking cigarettes helps staying slim.

Light Cigarettes are Less Harmful?

Light and ultra light cigarettes have lower concentrations of toxic substances (nicotine, tar, carbon monoxide etc.) but as the tobacco industry realised early on, these brands are smoked differently from regular cigarettes (Creighton, 1978). Dependent smokers immediately detect the modified release pattern of nicotine from the light cigarettes. Cigarettes with a reduced nicotine yield are inhaled more deeply and in many cases more cigarettes are used to obtain the same nicotine dose (Greig, 1970). As a result of a different smoking pattern, light cigarettes are not less harmful than regular cigarettes. In addition, increased sucking to obtain a desired amount of nicotine may cause more wrinkles around the mouth which is an unwanted side effect of smoking for many women.

Smoking Cigarettes Keeps You Slim?

The issue of smoking and weight is complicated. Studies have found that smokers weigh less than former smokers or those who have never smoked. The weight differences increase with age –a finding that suggests that smoking may inhibit weight gain over relatively long periods of time. Recent studies indicate that smoking initiation may not be related to short-term changes in body weight (USDHHS, 2001). However, smoking seems to promote negative body image. White and Hispanic women who smoke are more likely than women who have never smoked to perceive themselves as overweight (NWLCandOHandSU, 2003). A recent study of the White female population found that daily smokers were more likely than occasional, former and non-smokers to have tried to lose weight regardless of their weight status (Saarni, Silventoinen, Rissanen, Sarlio-Lahteenkorva, and Kaprio, 2004). Despite all this, concern about body weight is related to smoking initiation, especially among women and girls (Austin and Gortmaker, 2001; Camp, Klesges, and Relyea, 1993; French, Perry, Leon and Fulkerson, 1994; Fulkerson and French, 2003).

It has been established that smoking cessation may result in weight gain. Furthermore, continued smoking may promote a harmful pattern of body fat distribution. Abdominal obesity refers to a pattern of body fat distribution characterized by excess subcutaneous or visceral fat in the abdominal region. This type of obesity is a risk factor for several medical conditions, including type 2 diabetes mellitus, stroke, coronary artery disease, and is associated with increased total mortality among men and women. Many studies have reported a positive association of smoking with high waist-to-hip ratio among women. The relationship between smoking and waist-to-hip ratio may be stronger among women than among men (USDHHS, 2001).

2.5. Young Women and Smoking

According to the Global Youth Tobacco Survey (GYTS) one quarter of young people smoke their first cigarette before the age of 10 (Mackay, Eriksen, and Shafey, 2006). Although men's overall smoking rate is higher than women's, the difference in smoking rates between girls and boys is almost non-existent. In half of the countries surveyed in the GYTS, there were no differences in boys' and girls' smoking rates. Worldwide, tobacco use among girls is increasing and in parts of Europe and South America girls' smoking rates are higher than boys'. As with boys, the overwhelming majority of female smokers use tobacco before they reach adulthood (Mackay, Eriksen, and Shafey, 2006). In the United States, one in four female high school students have smoked during the past 30 days (NWLCandOHandSU, 2003) and the rate is higher in most European countries and Australia (Mackay, Eriksen, and Shafey, 2006).

The factors that have influenced adolescent's tobacco prevalence include promotion by tobacco companies; easy access to tobacco products; low prices; peer pressure; tobacco use by parents, siblings and peers; wide approval of tobacco use in the society; and the misperception that smoking enhances social popularity (Mackay, Eriksen, and Shafey, 2006). Also, young women are motivated by the misconception that smoking helps one to stay thin. However, cigarette smoking is not associated with lower body mass index (BMI) in younger women (Mackay, Eriksen, and Shafey, 2006) In addition, girls appear to be more affected by the perception that smoking provides relief from negative mood states, such as depression, anxiety and tensions than are boys (Christen and Christen, 2003; USDHHS, 2004).

While the most serious health effects of tobacco consumption normally occur after decades of smoking, tobacco also causes immediate effects for young smokers. Perhaps more importantly, children and teenagers who experiment with smoking at an early age have an especially high risk of becoming regular smokers later in life. If nicotine dependence sets in at early age, smoking cessation is extremely hard to achieve (Haustein, 2003; Mackay, Eriksen, and Shafey, 2006). As a result, smokers who become addicted to tobacco in their youth face the greatest risk of eventually contracting diseases caused by smoking, such as cancer, emphysema and heart disease (Mackay, Eriksen, and Shafey, 2006).

As smoking initiation occurs earlier and earlier, tobacco-use prevention programs for school children have a critical role in the worldwide anti-tobacco campaign. Tobacco-use prevention education should be provided in kindergarten through 12th grade, with particularly intensive instruction in the early school grades. Prevention programs should provide training for teachers and involve students' parents and families. An effective prevention program includes instruction about short- and long-term negative consequences of tobacco use; social influences of tobacco use; peer norms regarding tobacco use; and refusal skills. In addition, support should be provided for students and school staffs who wish to make a smoking cessation attempt (CDCP, 1994).

3. Health Consequences of Smoking Among Women

3.1. Smoking-Related Disease Epidemic

Every year, tobacco-related illnesses prematurely claim the lives of nearly one million women worldwide. The majority of these deaths are due to coronary heart disease, stroke and increasingly, lung cancer. Moreover, smoking may increase women's vulnerability to gender-specific health consequences such as osteoporosis and pregnancy complications (e.g., miscarriages, low birth weight, Sudden Infant Death Syndrome, pulmonary diseases, and otitis media). Despite these risks, smoking-related illnesses are becoming more, rather than less, prevalent and will continue to increase among women (USDHHS, 2001). When analyzing heart disease risk and the prevalence of associated conditions in women, smoking seems to be the key preventable factor. Physical inactivity and obesity are also very significant factors (Schnohr, Jensen, Scharling, and Nordestgaard, 2002).

3.2. Cancers

Tobacco use has been linked unequivocally to myriad cancers. The most recent report (USDHHS, 2007) listed the following organs where tobacco is a causative or contributory agent: lung, trachea, bronchus, esophagus, oral cavity, lip, nasopharynx, nasal cavity, larynx, paranasal sinuses, stomach, bladder, kidney, pancreas, uterine cervix, and acute myeloid leukaemia as a condition. Nowadays, about 70 of approximately 4,000 chemicals in tobacco smoke are known carcinogens (USDHHS, 2007). Tobacco use is not only a primary cause of cancers but exacerbates the problem if continued after cancer diagnosis. Compared to those who quit smoking after diagnosis, cancer treatment may not be as effective for continued smokers, survival time is shorter and disease reoccurrence and second primary tumors are more frequent. Nevertheless, 23% to 35% of head neck cancer patients and 13% to 20% of lung cancer patients continue to smoke after diagnosis and during treatment (Schnoll et al., 2002).

Lung Cancer

Cigarette smoking is the leading cause of lung cancer among women. The current lung cancer rates among women vary dramatically between countries, reflecting historical differences in cigarette smoking across populations. Lung cancer rates are intermediate or low in female populations where smoking is still relatively uncommon or was adopted later than in Western countries (WHO, 2001b). However, the rates of tobacco-related cancers among US women have soared. Since 1950, women's lung cancer mortality rates have increased 600 percent (USDHHS, 2007). Among US female smokers about 90% of all lung cancer deaths are attributable to smoking. In 1950, lung cancer accounted for only 3% of all cancer deaths among women. However, by 2000, lung cancer accounted for an estimated 25% of female cancer deaths. Smoking-related cancer deaths are decreasing among men, while in women they are increasing (USDHHS, 2001). In female smokers the risk of developing lung cancer is about 13 times higher compared with lifelong non-smokers (USDHHS, 2007).

Breast Cancer

Until recently it was thought that tobacco use contributed very little to the risk of developing breast cancer. Although not recognized as a condition where tobacco is a causative or contributory agent (USDHHS, 2007), the breast cancer and tobacco link may deserve more attention. Literature addressing this question has been mixed, and the question has seldom been examined in large prospective study designs. However, based on longitudinal data, Reynolds and co-authors (2004) have suggested that active smoking may increase breast cancer risk, particularly among women without familial risk. The risk is further increased for women who use tobacco prior to or during adolescence. These data raise public health concerns related to cigarette smoking as the current trend for women is to initiate smoking at increasingly younger ages. Further research into the connection is warranted, especially with respect to genetic susceptibilities (Reynolds et al., 2004).

3.3. Cardiovascular-Related Diseases

Two-thirds of heart disease deaths in US women under 50 are tobacco related (USDHHS, 2001).

Women who smoke have an increased risk of cardiovascular disease (CVD), including coronary heart disease, ischemic stroke and subarachnoid hemorrhage (WHO, 2001b). For example, smoking in women is associated with a two to six-fold increased risk for myocardial infarction (heart attack), threefold increased risk of incident angina (chest pain), six to 30-fold increased risk of peripheral vascular disease, and two to threefold increased risk of stroke. Even when age, education, and other CVD risk factors were taken into account, smoking related CVD risk was higher among women than men (Prescott, Hippe, Schnohr, Hein, and Vestbo, 1998).

Gender Specific Cardiovascular Mechanisms

Endogenous estrogen is thought to provide women with some protection from CVD. However, tobacco use reduces that benefit. Thus, it is important to keep in mind that the protective effects of estrogen before menopause are conditional on being a non-smoker. Further, smoking is not simply a single independent risk factor. Rather, smoking interacts with many other CVD risk factors, imperiling especially those women with coronary risk factors (Prescott et al., 1998) such as high cholesterol and low physical activity level.

Coronary Heart Disease

Smoking is one of the major causes of coronary heart disease in women. Relative risks associated with smoking seem to be greater for younger than for older women. For example, in the 1980s, evidence suggested that smoking may account for the majority of coronary heart disease cases among US women under the age of 50 (Rosenberg et al., 1985). Risk of coronary heart disease increases with number of cigarettes smoked daily and with duration of smoking. Current smokers who had begun to smoke before the age of 15 years had an estimated relative risk of about 9 in comparison with those who have never smoked (WHO, 2001b). Although the risk for smoking-related complications generally increases linearly with the number of cigarettes smoked, even smoking only 1-4 cigarettes per day actually doubles or triples coronary risk in women (Bjartveit and Tverdal, 2005).

Women who use oral contraceptives have a particularly elevated risk of coronary heart disease if they smoke. Use of oral contraceptives alone is associated with a moderate increase in coronary heart disease risk. However, that risk is 20- to 40-fold greater among women who both use oral contraceptives and smoke heavily compared to women with neither of those exposures. Lower dose formulations show overall risk of coronary heart disease associated with oral contraceptive use to be less than was observed with the first-generation formulations. However, the relative risk among heavy smokers who use oral contraceptives is still markedly elevated compared with that among non-smokers who do not use oral contraceptives. Thus, it is particularly important that women who are planning to use oral contraceptives are informed of these risks and are strongly encouraged not to smoke (WHO, 2001b).

Other Cardiovascular Diseases

Beyond coronary heart disease, women who smoke also have elevated risks of other CVDs, such as ischemic stroke and subarachnoid hemorrhage (WHO, 2001b). Risk of stroke among female smokers has been reported to be 1.7- fold greater than never smokers (Shinton and Beevers, 1989). Among women younger than 65 years about half of cerebrovascular deaths have been shown to be attributed to smoking (CDC, 1989). Women who smoke also have significantly increased risks of carotid atherosclerosis, peripheral vascular atherosclerosis, and death from ruptured abdominal aortic aneurysm (WHO, 2001b).

3.4. Chronic Obstructive Pulmonary Disease

In the coming years, the burden of chronic obstructive pulmonary disease (COPD) will increase as the population ages. Smoking is the most important preventable risk factor of

COPD, ahead of air pollution (Mannino and Buist, 2007). Nearly 90% of COPD among women is caused by tobacco use (Peto et al., 2000). Historically, COPD has been far more frequent in men than in women, primarily due to patterns of smoking (Mannino, Homa, Akinbami, Ford, and Redd, 2002). However, in high-income countries where smoking habits are more similar between the sexes, COPD seems to become more equally prevalent in women and men. Further, some evidence lends support to a hypothesis that women are more susceptible to development of COPD than men, although this is still an issue for further investigation (Buist et al., 2007). This is noteworthy since women in countries of low income have historically had a low smoking prevalence, but are increasingly targeted by advertising campaigns to increase their cigarette consumption (Mannino and Buist, 2007). Fortunately, many of the adverse effects of smoking, such as the decline of lung function, can be slowed by stopping smoking (Peto et al., 2000).Thus, smoking cessation is becoming an increasingly urgent objective, particularly for an ageing female population.

3.5. Reproductive Health

According to the National Women's Law Center and Oregon Health and Science University (2003), 12% of the women in the United States continue to smoke through pregnancy. The smoking during pregnancy rate is even higher in Caucasian (16%) and American Indian/Alaskan Native (20%) racial groups, among teenagers (18%) and women with no more than high school level education (23%). However, 92% of American women are aware that smoking while pregnant can lead to complications in pregnancy (Roth, Taylor, and Hugh, 2001).

Tobacco use contributes to an increased risk for conception delay as well as primary and secondary infertility. Women who continue to smoke close to the time of conception take significantly longer to become pregnant than women who never smoked or stopped smoking before the year during which they attempted to conceive. Shuttleworth (2004) reported that women who smoke have up to 40% lower chance of getting pregnant per cycle than their non-smoking counter-parts. Several studies have reported trends in increasing time to conception with increasing number of cigarettes smoked (Bolumar, Olsen, and Bolsen, 1996; Curtis, Savitz, and Arbuckle, 1997; Howe, Westoff, Vessey, and Yeates, 1985; Hull, North, Taylor, Farrow, and Ford, 2000).

An association between spontaneous abortion (miscarriage) and maternal smoking has been suspected since the early 1960s (DiFranza and Lew, 1995) but early epidemiological studies had inconsistent findings (USDHHS, 1980). Current data provide evidence that there is in fact a higher risk for spontaneous abortion among smokers than non-smokers (Eskenazi et al., 1995; Wilcox, Weinberg, and Baird, 1990). However, the risk of former smokers seems to be similar to that of non-smokers (Stein, Kline, Levin, Susser, and Warburton, 1981).

Similarly, many adverse pregnancy outcomes are observed more frequently in tobacco users. The report of the Surgeon General (USDHHS, 2001) concluded that smoking during pregnancy increases the risk for premature birth. The U.S. Department of Health, Education, and Welfare (USDHEW, 1979), estimated that 11 to 14% of all premature births are attributable to smoking during pregnancy. Some studies also show that the risk of premature birth increases with the quantity of cigarettes smoked and mother's age but the findings have been inconsistent (Cnattingius, Forman, Berendes, Graubard, and Isotalo, 1993; Olsen et al., 1995; Wisborg, Henriksen, Hedegaard, and Secher, 1996; USDHEW, 1979). Smoking cessation during pregnancy reduces the risk for premature birth. The risk for premature delivery among women who discontinue smoking during the first trimester is similar to that among women who have never smoked (Mainous and Hueston, 1994).

An association between stillbirth and maternal smoking has been suspected and studied since the late 1950s. The early investigators did not always find a positive relationship between stillbirth and smoking because their studies were often statistically underpowered and did not control for known risk factors (DiFranza and Lew, 1995). More recent studies have found an increased risk for stillbirth among women who smoke during pregnancy (USDHHS, 2001). Wu, Buck, and Mendola (1998) suggest that the use of multivitamins and mineral supplements during pregnancy significantly reduces the rate of stillbirths among women who smoke.

For more than 40 years, it has been known that babies born to smoking mothers weigh less than babies born to nonsmoking mothers (USDHHS, 1980). Low birth weight is of concern because it has been associated with neonatal and perinatal mortality and infant morbidity (USDHHS, 2001). Cigarette smoking during pregnancy is the number one preventable risk factor associated with low birth weight in the United States. Twenty percent or more of the incidents where newborn babies' weight fall below a defined criterion for gestational age are attributable to cigarette smoking (CDC, 1990; Roquer, Figueras, Botet, and Jimenez, 1995).

To date, most studies have not found an association between cigarette smoking during pregnancy and the overall risk for birth defects (USDHHS, 2001). Some investigators have suggested that the lack of effect on birth defects can be explained by the increased risk for spontaneous abortion and stillbirth among smokers (Kallen, 1998; Li et al., 1996; Shiono, Klebanoff, and Brendes, 1986; Van den Eeden, Karagas, Daling, and Vaughan, 1990). These outcomes would prevent a deformed fetus from being born alive and recognized as having a birth defect. Nonetheless, in utero exposure to tobacco smoke has been associated with reduced lung function, developmental delay, and biochemical changes in the infant's brain (USDHHS, 2001). In addition, smoking may be modestly related to an increased risk for oral clefts, limb reductions, and urogenital or gastrointestinal defects (USDHHS, 2001).

Finally, smoking is associated with more severe menstrual and menopausal symptoms. Several studied have shown that prevalence of pain and discomfort during menstruation is higher among smokers than former smokers and women who never smoked (Paparazzini et al., 1994; Sundell, Milsom, and Andersch, 1990; Teperi and Rimpela, 1989). Menstrual irregularity, intermenstrual bleeding, and short or varied length of menstrual cycle have also been associated with smoking (Brown, Vessey, and Stratton, 1988; Hornsby, Wilcox, and Weinberg, 1998; Windham, Elkin, Swan, Waller, and Fenster, 1999). Smoking is associated with age at natural menopause. The mechanisms by which cigarette smoking might lead to an early menopause are not clear but studies have consistently shown that menopause occurs one or two years earlier among smokers than among nonsmokers (Andersen, Transbol, and Christiansen, 1982; Jick, Porter, and Morrison, 1977; Lindquist and Bengtsson, 1979). Although data on the association between smoking and menopausal symptoms is limited, there are some studies that have linked smoking and more severe menopausal symptoms, such as hot flashes (Dennerstein et al., 1993; Hellström-Lindahl and Nordberg, 2002; USDHHS, 2001).

3.6. Benefits of Quitting Smoking

Quitting smoking significantly reduces the risk of many diseases, including the above reviewed conditions. For example, those who quit smoking cut their risk for lung cancer by one-half to two-thirds after 10 years of abstinence, compared to continued smokers (USDHHS, 2001). Anthonisen and co-authors (2005) compared long term (15 years) risks of death from lung cancer, CVD and respiratory disease between three groups of ever smokers. They demonstrated a linearly decreasing trend of mortality risk when moving from continuing smokers to intermittent quitters and further to sustained quitters.

Quitting smoking seems to significantly reduce the risk of lung cancer. However, it is beneficial to quit smoking even after cancer diagnosis. Nevertheless, many patients continue to smoke after diagnosis and during treatment. Continuing smoking after a cancer diagnosis seems to shorten survival time, reduce treatment efficacy, and increase treatment complications. A study with cancer patients suggested that smoking and lower readiness to quit was associated with having smoking relatives, greater nicotine dependence, lower self-efficacy, fatalistic beliefs, and emotional distress (Schnoll et al., 2002).

Quitting smoking decreases the CVD risk by half in a year. That risk drops to levels close to those of non-smokers by 2 to 5 years following smoking cessation (USDHHS, 2001). More specifically, the risk of coronary heart disease is reduced by 25-50 percent within 1-2 years of smoking cessation, followed by a continued, yet more gradual, reduction to that of non-smokers by approximately 10-15 years following cessation (WHO, 2001b). Furthermore, even among elderly women with coronary artery disease, smoking cessation improves survival and decreases the chance of re-infarction and improves quality of life. Thus, smoking cessation appears to be one of the most effective ways to reduce further cardiac events (USDHHS, 2001). Stroke risk among smokers also reverses with quitting, with the estimated amount of time needed for risks to approximate those of never smokers ranging from less than 5 years to some 15 years of abstinence (WHO, 2001b). Clearly, developing treatments specifically tailored for women seems to be an important component of reducing the smoking-related CVD health burden in the United States and globally.

Finally, the benefits of smoking cessation are observable also in relation to reproductive health. Namely, among former smokers, age at menopause is between that of women who had never smoked and that of current smokers (Adena and Gallagher, 1982).

3.7. Health Consequences of Environmental Tobacco Smoke

Non-smokers may be exposed to environmental tobacco smoke (ETS) in a number of places: in their homes, workplaces, restaurants, public buildings and social gatherings. Overall, it has been estimated that more than 126 million people in the U.S. are exposed to

ETS (USDHHS, 2007). ETS, also referred to as second-hand smoke, passive smoking, and involuntary smoking, contains smoke from two sources: side stream and exhaled mainstream smoke. Side stream smoke that comes from the burning tip of a cigarette or a cigar is known to be more toxic than exhaled mainstream smoke because many harmful chemicals are emitted at higher levels in the side smoke than in the main smoke (Haustein, 2003). Exposure to ETS can be objectively detected by biochemical markers, such as plasma cotinine levels, as reported by the NHANES III Study (Pirkle et al., 1996). While levels of non-smokers and passive smokers were clearly lower than those of smokers, cotinine was detected in small amounts both in passive smokers and non-smokers. For example, among non-smoking ETS-exposed women an increase in cotinine levels of 5 ng / mg was predicted by exposure to 7.2 cigarettes/8 hours/40 m^3 from the husband and 17.9 cigarettes/8 hours/40 m^3 in the workplace (Riboli et al., 1990). Unfortunately, smoking in restaurants and bars is still allowed in many countries. Thus, restaurant and bar workers, a relatively high proportion of them young women, constitute a high risk group of passive smokers (Haustein, 2003).

ETS causes a variety of adverse health effects in non-smokers (Mackay, Eriksen, and Shafey, 2006). ETS is a significant contributor to lung cancer as well as cardiac, respiratory, and other diseases in individuals exposed to it. In total, ETS exposure claims the lives of approximately 38,000 non-smokers annually (USDHHS, 2007). Several changes at the molecular and cellular levels have been described as mechanisms explaining harmful effects of ETS on health. Such changes include elevations of plasma fibrinogen and platelet reactivity, damages in endothelial cells, and inflammatory responses leading to oxidative membrane damage (Haustein, 2003). Scientific evidence indicates that there is no risk-free level of exposure to ETS (USDHHS, 2006).

Lung Cancer

ETS has been established as a cause of approximately 3,000 lung cancer deaths each year among non-smokers in the United States (USDHHS, 2007). Since the 1980s, the association between passive smoking and lung cancer has been examined epidemiologically (Taylor, Najafi, and Dobson, 2007). At least one of the metabolites of tobacco smoke showing direct aetiological association with lung cancer is found both in side and main stream smoke (Denissenko, Pao, Tang, and Pfeifer, 1996). In terms of occupational exposure to carcinogens, in Europe, ETS is considered the second most common exposure after solar radiation (Haustein, 2003) and the situation is likely to be similar in the United States. Taylor et al. published a review of earlier meta-analyses and their own meta-analysis of 55 studies conducted on passive smoking and lung cancer during 1981-2006. More precisely, they estimated relative risk of lung cancer associated with exposure to passive smoking in women who had never smoked but had smoking spouses. There was evidence of a causal dose-response relationship between passive smoking and lung cancer, the pooled risk of lung cancer being elevated by about 30% among those exposed to spousal ETS compared to those not exposed. This seemed to be a consistent finding across continents (North America, Asia, Europe) and study type (cohort study, case-control study) (Taylor, Najafi, and Dobson, 2007).

Breast Cancer

So far the evidence of association between ETS and breast cancer is less consistent than that of ETS and lung cancer among women. The link between ETS and breast cancer has been characterized as suggestive but not sufficient to infer a causal relationship and additional research is needed to clarify this issue (USDHHS, 2007). Although a causal association has not been proved, there are several findings that indicate that an association exists (Haustein, 2003). ETS exposure may need to occur at a relatively early age, shortly before the development of breast tissue, in order to induce mitogenic changes consistent with carcinogenesis (Wartenberg et al., 2000). For example, women exposed to ETS before the age of 12 were 4.5 times more likely than women not exposed to ETS to get breast cancer, whereas that relative risk among active smokers was 7.5 (Lash and Aschengrau, 1999).

Other Adverse Health Effects

On adults, exposure to ETS has immediate adverse effects on the cardiovascular system and long-term exposure causes coronary heart disease (USDHHS, 2006). Non-smokers exposed to ETS have a 25% increased risk of heart disease (Mackay, Eriksen, and Shafey, 2006). Recently, it has been suggested that exposure to ETS would, at least partly, explain why COPD is found among people who have never smoked (Menezes and Hallal, 2007). This has been demonstrated in a large population study, including over 15,000 non-smokers, 90% of them being women. Those non-smokers who were exposed to ETS more than 40 hours per week for more than 5 years were 48% more likely to present with COPD than were unexposed non-smokers (Yin et al., 2007). Finally, in addition to harming the expecting mother, ETS during pregnancy is linked to health problems in the foetus and infant (Mackay, Eriksen, and Shafey, 2006). Children who are exposed to ETS are also at increased risk for sudden infant death syndrome, low birth weight, acute respiratory infections, ear problems, and severe asthma (USDHHS, 2006).

Prevention Of Environmental Tobacco Smoke

Although substantial progress in tobacco control has introduced smoke free restaurants and bars in several European countries, California and many US cities (New York City, Boston etc.), approximately 30 percent of indoor workers in the United States are not covered by smoke-free workplace policies (USDHHS, 2006). Clearly, more government control and regulations are needed to tackle this serious health issue. Only elimination of smoking in indoor spaces fully protects nonsmokers from exposure to secondhand smoke. Separating smokers from nonsmokers, cleaning the air, and ventilating buildings cannot eliminate exposures of nonsmokers to secondhand smoke. Conventional air cleaning systems can remove large particles, but not the smaller particles or the gases found in secondhand smoke. Routine operation of a heating, ventilating, and air conditioning system can make things worse and distribute secondhand smoke throughout a building (USDHHS, 2006). In addition, restaurants and bars are not the only places where people get exposed to ETS. Private homes and cars are another place where especially children breathe in most of their secondhand smoke. Therefore, it is to be hoped that the national legislators follow the example set by Louisiana, Arkansas, Puerto Rico and Bangor, Maine that have recently enacted laws banning smoking in cars when children are present.

4. Women and Smoking Cessation

4.1. Why Might Quitting Smoking be Harder for Women?

Despite widely employed tobacco control efforts, every fifth woman in the United States continues to smoke. Annual tobacco-related mortality has reached almost 200,000 in the US (NWLCandOHandSU, 2003). Effective cessation would significantly reduce this public health problem. However, most standard smoking cessation methods, such as counseling and nicotine replacement therapy (NRT) have not been as effective for women as for men (Cepeda-Benito, Reynoso, and Erath, 2004; Gritz et al., 1998; Leventhal et al., 2007; Perkins, Levine, Marcus, and Shiffman, 1997; USDHHS, 2001). Further, women may experience higher desire to relieve withdrawal distress and have more severe withdrawal, particularly negative affectivity symptoms (Leventhal et al., 2007). Negative affectivity and depression in general are major hindrances for quitting success and women are twice as likely to experience these in lifetime as men. Similarly, hormonal changes during the menstrual cycle can exacerbate withdrawal symptom (Perkins, 2001). An additional component that often hinders successful cessation among women is the concern about weight gain (Perkins et al., 1997; Perkins et al., 2001b; Wee, Rigotti, Davis, and Phillips, 2001; Wetter et al., 1999). It has been suggested that treatment tailored for women should include factors that would reduce withdrawal distress and negative affect, address weight concerns, and provide social support (Cepeda-Benito, Reynoso, and Erath, 2004; Leventhal et al., 2007; Wetter et al., 1999). Finally, women have shown to be more ambivalent about giving up tobacco use than men. Because high motivation and confidence are strong predictors of success, increasing women's commitment and decision for smoke free life remains a challenge (Perkins, Conklin, and Levine, 2007).

4.2. Standard Treatment for Tobacco Dependence: Pharmacotherapy and Counseling

The Clinical Guideline (Fiore et al., 2000) suggests that each treatment for tobacco dependence should include both pharmacotherapy and behavioral counseling. Currently there are several first-line pharmacological treatments for smoking cessation: nicotine patch, nicotine gum, nicotine inhaler, nicotine lozenge, nicotine sublingual tablet, and nicotine nasal spray. As non-nicotinic medicines, dopamine-noradrenalin reuptake inhibitor bupropion (HCL, SR, and XL) and nicotinic receptor partial agonist, varenicline, are available by prescription. Only the nicotine patch and gum are available over the counter (OTC) in the US and the nicotine sublingual tablet is not available at all.

In general, the nicotine patch has attained highest compliance rates (Hajek et al., 1999) and subsequent nicotine replacement levels mainly because of its ease of use. Although it is not clear how much nicotine patch treatment helps with the prevention of weight gain, some research reports have indicated at least a short-term prevention in weight gain (Dale et al., 1995; Jorenby et al., 1996; Moffatt, Biggerstaff, and Stamford, 2000) and a decrease in hunger as a withdrawal symptom (Moffatt, Biggerstaff, and Stamford, 2000). In regards to negative affect, some studies have found the nicotine patch alleviates dysphoric mood (Westman, 2001), although the results have been inconsistent (Fiore, Smith, Jorenby, and Baker, 1994a). Adjunct behavioral interventions, such as relapse prevention counseling (Fiore et al., 1994b; 2000; Cepeda-Benito, Reynoso, and Erath, 2004) or cognitive-behavioral counseling (Hall, Tunstall, Ginsberg, Benowitz, and Jones, 1987; Hall et al., 1998), have been found to increase cessation rates when added to pharmacotherapy. Moreover, it seems that the effectiveness of NRT among women is dependent on the level of adjunct treatment. Thus, to obtain the maximum benefits from the NRT, women may need more intensive adjuncts than men (Cepeda-Benito, Reynoso, and Erath, 2004).

Bupropion as a pharmaco-agent was first used for depression. Since it also has been shown to minimize the post-cessation weight gain, it seemed to be an ideal treatment for female smokers. It has been shown to be at least as, but not more effective for women than men (Scharf and Shiffman, 2004). Finally, the most recent addition to FDA approved pharmacological choices, varenicline, is not expected to be more beneficial for men than women, but there is insufficient data to draw any conclusions. Two additional therapies may be available in the future. Naltrexone, a mu-opioid receptor antagonist approved for opioid and alcohol dependencies, is one pharmacotherapy that has shown in a few studies to be more effective for women than men (King et al., 2006). Rimonabant is a selective endocannoboid receptor antagonist that also affects fat cells. It has been approved in Europe for weight loss purposes, while some data for smoking cessation indications exist as well. If medically safe, it may eventually provide yet another option for those women who delay cessation because of feared or actual weight gain.

In regards to the counseling component, women seem to need more intensive counseling than men (Perkins, Conklin, and Levine, 2007; Senore et al., 1998), and the social support plays an important role (Cepeda-Benito, Reynoso, and Erath, 2004). Two interventions that target issues pertaining to women – weight concerns and negative affectivity – have been developed and studied among female smokers. Cognitive-behavioral therapy treating the negative thoughts and attitudes about smoking related weight concerns among women have shown to be very promising (Perkins, Conklin, and Levine, 2007). Second, an exercise intervention as an adjunct to standard smoking cessation counseling and pharmacotherapy is yet another avenue for women to conquer negative affect and weight concerns associated with smoking cessation. Certainly, additional gender-specific therapies exist and are being developed, but we are examining the two approaches that have the most scientific data available and are safe and easily adapted into practice.

4.3. Cognitive-Behavioral Therapy for Women: Successful Approach for Weight Concerns

One of the main impediments to successful cessation for women is the fear of weight gain. On average, women gain approximately 8 pounds (lbs) during the first year after quitting. However, some 13% of female quitters gain more than 28 lbs (Fiore et al., 2000). The gain is faster during the first weeks of cessation and gradually levels off. There is large individual variability both in how much weight each woman gains and how much weight women are comfortable gaining. Some women also report using smoking as a way to control their hunger and appetite. Various approaches have been examined to alleviate either the fear and/or actual weight gain. The general conclusion is that dieting while quitting smoking leads to failure in both the smoking cessation and the weight control. It seems to be more important to deal with the attitudes associated with weight and smoking rather than the behavior itself during the quitting process. The basic rationale underlying the cognitive behavioral therapy (CBT) approach for weight-concerned women is that if one wants to promote her health and longevity by quitting smoking, continuing to smoke for weight control is irrational (Perkins et al., 2007). While it is important to educate a smoker about the plausible weight gain, a reminder that in order to negate the health benefits of quitting smoking one would have to gain over 80 lbs has to be delivered repeatedly. A successful CBT includes a through assessment of each individual's fears and concerns as well as past experiences. It stresses that changing two behaviors at once is rarely successful, i.e., dieting while quitting is not recommended. The core of the therapy focuses on the attitudes about body shape and weight and the dysfunctional thoughts surrounding them. These may include unrealistic expectations set by the media and attitudes held by a smoker trying to quit. Finally, it must be kept in mind that while restricted eating is forbidden, information and support around making healthy nutritional choices, moderate portions and regular physical activity are encouraged during smoking cessation. Cognitive behavior therapy can be used independently or as an adjunct to the standard smoking cessation treatment and may be one of the few choices available to those for whom medication is contraindicated or prefer not to use them, e.g., pregnant women.

What types of results can be expected with CBT therapy? Perkins et al., (2001b) conducted a study involving 219 women with weight concerns who wanted to quit smoking. In addition to regular state-of-the-art smoking cessation, they were randomly assigned either to a CBT therapy, a behavioral weight control, or a control condition adjunct. No pharmacotherapy was provided for the participants. At the end of the one month treatment, those who received CBT as an adjunct had quit rates of 56%, those receiving behavioral weight control therapy had 44% and those in the control group had 31%. More importantly, the one-year abstinences rates were 21%, 13%, and 9%, respectively. CBT resulted in the sustained quitting. In regards to actual weight gain, those in the CBT group gained the least amount of weight; i.e. 5.5 lbs at the end of the year. Initially the women in behavioral weight control were able to slow down the weight gain but during the remainder of the year they had gained as much as those in the control group (11.9 lbs and 16.9 lbs, respectively.) Interestingly, when weight concerns were assessed before and after treatment there was very little change among those women who had been completely abstinent from cigarettes. On the other hand, weight concerns decreased slightly among those who had resumed smoking. It has not been studied whether those who relapsed but whose weight concerns were reduced during the cessation program might have successfully quit later in life.

4.4. Effectiveness of Exercise in Smoking Cessation among Women

Hindrances to successful smoking cessation among women include weight concerns, severe withdrawal symptoms, stress, depression, and lack of social support. Since exercise promotes emotional well-being, healthy weight and cardiovascular function, it has the potential to be a far-reaching adjunct to standard care for tobacco dependence (USDHHS, 1996). There are factors that make exercise or increased physical activity level an appealing component to a comprehensive tobacco dependence treatment program. Evidence suggests that exercise may help with weight control (Haus et al., 1994; Katoh, Hara, and Narutaki, 1994; National Institutes of Health, 1998) and weight concerns, particularly for women (Bock, Marcus, King, Borrelli, and Roberts, 1999), both of which are often cited as a reason for smoking among younger women (Wee et al., 2001). It has not yet been determined whether an aerobic exercise program can eliminate the weight gain usually associated with smoking cessation, but it appears to at least delay it (Marcus et al., 1999) and may decrease the general concerns about smoking. Smoking cessation programs implementing a weight control component have often interfered with the cessation process and resulted in lower abstinence rates, while exercise has not been shown to have a detrimental effect. Aerobic exercise decreases negative affect, boosts self-confidence, and reduces tension, all of which may assist with smoking cessation (Perkins, 1993).

Although exercise presents itself as a promising and appropriate treatment for smoking cessation, there is scarcity of valid research about its effectiveness. Most studies have had either small sample sizes or insufficient exercise interventions in length or adherence to produce improvement in functional fitness levels. A critical review of the trials conducted before 2004 (Ussher, 2005) revealed that among 11 trials which fulfilled all criteria for a controlled design, only one gave reliable evidence that exercise has a positive impact on smoking cessation abstinence at one year follow-up (Marcus et al.,1999). A more recent study reported by Marcus and co-authors (2005) compared smoking cessation rates between a group receiving cognitive-behavioral counseling together with moderate exercise and a group receiving counseling only. At three month follow-up, the results indicated that those in the exercise group had higher rates of cessation. However, this difference was lost at one year follow-up. Interestingly, within the exercise group, compliance was associated with abstinence. Although there is still insufficient evidence to support the long-term effectiveness of moderate exercise programs, this study highlighted the importance of compliance to treatment success (Marcus et al., 2005). The most recent published study by Prapavessis and colleagues (2007) investigated whether exercise and cognitive behavioral therapy produced similar effects on cessation and whether NRT increased the effects of exercise. Although the effect did not reach statistical significance, their findings suggested that exercise facilitated smoking cessation (Prapavessis et al., 2007). Hence, there is a need for more research with larger samples and well-defined exercise interventions, which include a sufficient duration and intensity of exercise to produce changes in fitness levels. This is very important in smoking cessation research, because a dose response relationship between treatment success and dose of the intervention appears to exist. Further, trials should assess adherence to the exercise regimen in order to determine if exercise represents an adjunct treatment option to which women will adhere (Kinnunen Mustonen, 2005a).

Recent clinical trials funded by the National Institute of Health and conducted at Harvard University have tested exercise intervention as a behavioral adjunct to the standard treatment for tobacco dependence, which consists of pharmacotherapy (e.g. NRT) and brief counseling (Fiore et al. 2000). The main objectives of these novel trials have been to find the optimal combinations of exercise and behavioral counseling in order to improve exercise adherence and smoking cessation. The aim of the first randomized controlled trial was to examine exercise as an adjunct to nicotine gum therapy and brief smoking cessation counseling while also controlling for equal contact (i.e. social support). The participants were randomized into one of three conditions, with each lasting a total of 19 weeks. The first was the "exercise group", consisting of supervised sessions taking place under the direction of an exercise physiologist. Participants were also encouraged to take part in home-based exercise sessions. The second "wellness group" was an equal contact control group consisting of health and wellness lectures. These sessions were of equal duration and frequency as the supervised exercise sessions, but included no tangible cessation help, focusing instead on activities ranging from aromatherapy and self-defense to first aid and facial massage. Thus, the wellness group was used to control for positive effects related to social support known to be present in group counseling therapies. The final group was a standard care control involving the same nicotine gum and brief behavioral counseling that participants in the other two groups also received. Overall, the relapse rates were high; at the end of the treatment 24% of the exercise group, 23% of the wellness group, and 15% of the standard care group remained abstinent. At the end of the follow up the abstinence rates were 10%, 12% and 6%, respectively. Both the exercise and wellness groups almost doubled the cessation rates over the standard group (Kinnunen Mustonen, 2005a). Additionally, depressive symptoms decreased and positive affect increased among those who abstained for at least four months and exercised regularly, whereas among those in the control group negative affect increased (Kinnunen and Korhonen, 2004). Exercise adherence was particularly low among women, whose cardiovascular risk was already elevated (high body mass index, nicotine dependence, depression, stress) before the quit attempt (Kinnunen Mustonen, 2005a). It appeared that exercise may aid smoking cessation among women, but it seemed critical to create ways to increase adherence to exercise. Similarly, it seemed important to understand what would be the level and type of structure needed to produce exercise effects, smoking cessation effects, and short- and long-term adherence to exercise.

4.5. Exercise as A Harm Reduction Strategy

In tobacco control, harm reduction can be defined as any process or program that reduces harm in continuing tobacco users. The term can be applied to methods for reducing toxins in tobacco smoke, to programs promoting conversion to smokeless tobacco, to the long-term complete substitution of nicotine as replacement therapy for tobacco (Gray and Henningfield, 2006). A further harm reduction strategy is to reduce the use of tobacco – with or without conjoint use of pharmacotherapy (Fiore et al., 2000). With the possible exception of medicinal nicotine products, so far no scientific evidence exists that these harm reduction strategies reduce tobacco-related exposure, morbidity, or mortality (Godtfredsen, Prescott,

Vestbo, and Osler, 2006; McNeill, 2004; Tonnesen, 2002). It has been suggested that a broader range of potentially effective harm reduction strategies should be considered. A recent review has suggested that regular exercise could be potentially considered an additional harm reduction strategy (DeRuiter and Faulkner, 2006). There are at least two types of smokers which may comprise harm reduction target groups for exercise interventions (DeRuiter and Faulkner, 2006). The first group involves those who are not interested in quitting abruptly. The second are those who would like to quit and have tried several times, but are unable to do so (Fagerstrom, 2005). In reference to the health promoting effects of exercise it is logical to believe that the detrimental effects associated with tobacco use could be partly compensated for through regular exercise. According to the review by DeRuiter and Faulkner (2006), exercise seems to at least partially fulfill the criteria of a potential novel harm reduction approach. For example, an innovative exposure reduction approach should reduce the occurrence of disease and death; not present additional health or safety risks; not reduce the likelihood of eventual cessation; not increase the level of tobacco dependence; and allow smokers to become free of tobacco and nicotine. DeRuiter and Faulkner (2006) considered that exercise criterion could be fulfilled at least via positive effects on other variables that protect against smoking relapse, such as stress, anxiety and weight concerns as well as additional health benefits obtained from exercise. In the proposed study we are able to measure subjective, self-reported changes in tobacco exposure-- and objective via biomarkers--and examine how exercise affects these changes.

4.6. Challenges of Multiple Behavior Changes

When using increased level of physical activity to support and enhance the smoking cessation process, women face the challenges inherent in multiple behavior changes. One is asked to change two health behaviors concurrently: to start exercising on a regular basis and to stop smoking for good. However, because both smoking and sedentary lifestyle are the main CVD risk factors (Schmitz, 2003; Schnohr et al., 2002) it is of crucial importance to include these behavior changes in interventions aiming to decrease morbidity and mortality of CVD among women. Unfortunately, as described in section 1.3., many of these women suffer from comorbid depressive symptoms, which in turn are also a risk factor for development of CVD (Musselman, Evans, and Nemeroff, 1998). Hence, these facts raise a further question whether multiple risk behavior interventions should be combined to reduce the total burden of those comorbid CVD risk factors. It has been suggested that change in one risk behavior may relate to change in another. For example, the cognitive mechanisms associated with changes in smoking behavior are related to the cognitive variables which have been shown to predict changes in other behaviors (King, Marcus, Pinto, Emmons, and Abrams, 1996). The readiness to change multiple risk behaviors was studied among nicotine and alcohol dependent outpatients (Stotts, Schmitz, and Grabowski, 2003). Patients reported higher confidence to abstain from alcohol than from cigarettes. Those with high motivation for changing alcohol use and low motivation to quit smoking remained in the program longer, whereas those with high motivation for changing both behaviors dropped out early. It seems that, in spite of readiness to change dual-dependency behaviors, actual quitting both simultaneously may prove difficult. Smoking cessation in dual-dependence programs may be less successful than in interventions targeting smoking only. However, in terms of total cardiovascular risk profile, some combined interventions may produce higher public health impact. For example, smoking cessation together with exercise may have significant combined effects, although the absolute quit rates would not be highest.

5. Conclusion

The former Surgeon General David Satcher accurately expressed the alarming state of female smoking:

"When calling attention to public health problems, we must not misuse the word 'epidemic.' But there is no better word to describe the 600 % increase since 1950 in women's death rates for lung cancer, a disease primarily caused by cigarette smoking. Clearly, smoking-related disease among women is a full-blown epidemic."

Unfortunately, smoking-related illnesses such as lung cancer and cardiovascular disease are becoming more prevalent among women. The only known ways of reducing tobacco-caused morbidity and mortality among women are through prevention and cessation of tobacco use as well as by eliminating environmental tobacco smoke exposure. Because regular cigarette smoking is usually initiated early in the teenage years, effective smoking prevention and cessation programs for adolescent girls and young women are urgently needed. Women have been suggested to have different determinants for successful smoking cessation than for men. Weight concerns, stress, depression, lack of social support, and low education level are among the factors contributing to poorer outcome in cessation treatment for women. Treatment of tobacco dependence is among the most cost-effective health interventions. Thus, smoking cessation programs should be accessible to all female smokers and health insurance plans should cover such services. Smoking cessation treatments need to become more available to women so they can enjoy the relatively immediate benefits of quitting. Efforts to maximize smoking cessation among women before, during, and after pregnancy deserve high priority. Further, we need to identify and remove barriers that prevent women from utilizing effective tobacco dependence treatments. Programs that have been particularly successful for women have offered social support and pharmacotherapy while addressing weight concerns and negative affect. Exercise is one example of a behavioral adjunct to pharmacotherapy that would also positively impact other CVD risk factors and health-compromising behaviors. However, how to address tobacco dependence among women more effectively remains a global challenge.

6. Acknowledgments

The authors would like to thank Mr. Eliot Baker, M.S., for proofreading the submitted manuscript. The first and second author would like to acknowledge the funding agencies

(NIH-DA12503 for Dr. Kinnunen; and Academy of Finland #200075, #103650 for Dr. Korhonen).

7. References

Abrams, D. B., Niaura, R., Brown, R. A., Emmons, K. M., Goldstein, M. G., and Monti, P. M. (2003). *The tobacco dependence treatment handbook: A guide to best practices* (1st ed.). New York NY: The Guilford Press.

Adena M. A., and Gallagher H. G. (1982). Cigarette smoking and the age at menopause. *Annals of Human Biology,* 9(2):121-130.

American Psychiatric Association [APA]. (2000). *Diagnostic and statistical manual of mental disorders* (4th ed.). Washington, DC: Author.

Amos A., and Haglund M. (2000). From social taboo to 'torch of freedom': the marketing of cigarettes to women. *Tobacco Control,* 9, 3-8.

Andersen, F. S., Transbol, I., and Christiansen, C. (1982). Is cigarette smoking a promoter of the menopause? *Acta Medica Scandinavica,* 212(3), 137-139.

Anthonisen, N.R., Skeans, M.A., Wise, R.A., Manfreda, J., Kanner, R.E., and Connet, J.E. (2005). The effects of a smoking cessation intervention on 14.5-year mortality: A randomized clinical trial. *Annals of Internal Medicine,* 142, 233-239.

Austin, S. B., Gortmaker, S. L. (2001). Dieting and smoking initiation in early adolescent girls and boys: a prospective study. *American Journal of Public Health.* 91, 446-50.

Bauer, T., Gohlmann, S., and Sinning, M. (2007). Gender differences in smoking behavior. *Health Economics,* 16(9), 895-909.

Benowitz, N. L. (1999). Nicotine addiction. *Primary Care,* 26(3), 611-631.

Bjartveit, K., and Tverdal, A. (2005). Health consequences of smoking 1–4 cigarettes per day. *Tobacco Control,* 14, 315–320.

Bock, B. C., Marcus, B. H., King, T. K., Borrelli, B., and Roberts, M. R. (1999). Exercise effects on withdrawal and mood among women attempting smoking cessation. *Addictive Behaviors,* 24(3), 399-410.

Bolego, C., Poli, A., and Paoletti, R. (2002). Smoking and gender. *Cardiovascular Research,* 53(3), 568-576.

Bolumar F., Olsen J., and Boldsen, J. (1996). Smoking Reduces Fecundity: A European multicenter study on infertility and subfecundity. The European Study Group on Infertility and Subfecundity. *American Journal of Epidemiology,* 143(6), 578-587.

Broms, U., Silventoinen, K., Lahelma, E., Koskenvuo, M., and Kaprio, J. (2004). Smoking cessation by socioeconomic status and marital status: The contribution of smoking behavior and family background. *Nicotine and Tobacco Research,* 6(3), 447-455.

Broms, U., Silventoinen, K., Madden, P. A., Heath, A. C., and Kaprio, J. (2006). Genetic architecture of smoking behavior: A study of Finnish adult twins. *Twin Research and Human Genetics,* 9(1), 64-72.

Brown S., Vessey S., and Stratton, I. (1988). The influence of method of contraception and cigarette smoking on menstrual patterns. *British Journal of Obstetrics and Gynecology,* 95(9), 905-910.

Buist, A.S., McBurnie, M.A. Vollmer, W.M., Gillespie, S., Burney, P., Mannino, D.M., Menezes, A.M., Sullivan, S.D., Lee, T.A., Weiss, K.B., Jensen, R.L., Marks, G.B., Gulsvik, A., Nizankowska-Mogilnicka, E., and BOLD Collaborative Research Group. (2007). International variation in the prevalence of COPD (the BOLD Study): a population-based prevalence study. *Lancet,* 370 (9589), 741-750.

Camp, D.E., Klesges, R.C., and Relyea, G. (1993). The relationship between body weight concerns and adolescent smoking. *Health Psychology.* 12, 24-32.

Carpenter, C. M., Ferris, W.G., and Connolly, G.N., (2005). Designing cigarettes for women: New findings from the tobacco industry documents. *Addiction* ,100, 851-873.

Cavelaars, A. E., Kunst, A. E., Geurts, J. J., Crialesi, R., Grotvedt, L., Helmert, U., (2000). Educational differences in smoking: International comparison. *British Medical Journal (Clinical research ed.), 320*(7242), 1102-1107.

Centers for Disease Control [CDC]. (1989). Reducing the health consequences of smoking: 25 years of progress: A report of the surgeon general. Rockville, MD: Author.

Centers for Disease Control [CDC]. (1990). Effects of maternal cigarette smoking on birth weight and preterm birth- Ohio, 1989. *Morbidity and Mortality Weekly Report*, 39(38), 662-665.

Centers for Disease Control and Prevention [CDCP]. (1994). Guidelines for school health programs to prevent tobacco use and addiction. *Morbidity and Mortality Weekly Report*, 43(RR-2), 1-9.

Cepeda-Benito, A., Reynoso, J. T., and Erath, S. (2004). Meta-analysis of the efficacy of nicotine replacement therapy for smoking cessation: Differences between men and women. *Journal of Consulting and Clinical Psychology, 72*(4), 712-722.

Christen, A. G., and Christen, J. A. (2003). The female smoker: From addiction to recovery. *The American Journal of the Medical Sciences, 326*(4), 231-234.

Cnattingius, S., Forman, M. R., Berendes, H. W., Graubard, B. I., and Isotalo, L. (1993). Effect of age, parity, and smoking on pregnancy outcome: a population based study. *American Journal of Obstetrics and Gynecology, 168*(1 Pt 1),16-21.

Creighton, D. E. (1978). Compensation for changed delivery. Trail exhibit 11089. 27-6-1978. BAT.

Curtis, K. M., Savitz, D. A., and Arbuckle, T. E. (1997). Effects of cigarette smoking, caffeine consumption and alcohol intake on fecund ability. *American Journal of Epidemiology*, 146(1), 32-41.

Dale, L. C., Hurt, R. D., Offord, K. P, Lawson, G. M., Croghan, I. T., and Schroeder, D. R. (1995). High-dose nicotine patch therapy: Percentage of replacement and smoking cessation. *Journal of the American Medical Association*, 274, 1353-1358.

Dani, J. A., and Harris, R. A. (2005). Nicotine addiction and comorbidity with alcohol abuse and mental illness. *Nature Neuroscience, 8*(11), 1465-1470.

Denissenko, M. F., Pao, A., Tang, M., and Pfeifer, G. P. (1996). Preferential formation of benzo[a]pyrene adducts at lung cancer mutational hotspots in P53. *Science (New York, N.Y.), 274*(5286), 430-432.

Dennerstein, L., Smith, A. M., Morse, C., Burger, H., Green, A., Hopper, J., and Ryan, M. (1993). Menopausal symptoms in Australian women. *Medical Journal of Australia,* 159(4), 232-236.

DeRuiter, W., and Faulkner, G. (2006). Tobacco harm reduction strategies: The case for physical activity. *Nicotine and Tobacco Research, 8*(2), 157-168.

DiFranza, J. R., and Lew, R. A. (1995). Effect on maternal cigarette smoking on pregnancy complications and sudden infant death syndrome. *Journal of Family Practice*, 40(4), 385- 394.

DiFranza, J. R., Savageau, J. A., Fletcher, K., O'Loughlin, J., Pbert, L., Ockene, J. K., McNeill, A.D., Hazelton, J., Friedman, K., Dussault, G., Wood, C., and Wellman,R.J. (2007). Symptoms of tobacco dependence after brief intermittent use: The development and assessment of nicotine dependence in youth-2 study. *Archives of Pediatrics and Adolescent Medicine,* 161(7), 704-710.

Doherty, K., Kinnunen, T., Militello, F. S., and Garvey, A. J. (1995). Urges to smoke during the first month of abstinence: Relationship to relapse and predictors. *Psychopharmacology,* 119(2), 171-178.

Ernster, V. L. (1986). Women, smoking, cigarette advertising and cancer. *Women Health* 11, 217-35.

Ernster, V, Kaufman, N, Nichter, M, Samet, J, and Yoon, S. Y. (2000). Women and tobacco: Moving from policy to action. *Bulletin of the World Health Organization.* 78, 891-901.

Eskenazi, B., Gold, E. B., Lasley, B. L., Samuels, S. J., Hammond, S. K., Wight, S., Rasor, M., Hines, C.J., Schenker, M.B. (1995). Prospective monitoring of early fetal loss and clinical spontaneous abortion among female semiconductor workers. *American Journal of Industrial Medicine* 28(6), 833-846.

Fagerstrom, K. O. (2005). Can reduced smoking be a way for smokers not interested in quitting to actually quit? *Respiration*, 72(2), 216-220.

Ferrucci, L., Izmirlian, G., Leveille, S., Phillips, C. L., Corti, M. C., Brock, D. B., et al. (1999). Smoking, physical activity, and active life expectancy. *American Journal of Epidemiology, 149*(7), 645-653.

Fiore, M. C., Bailey, W. C., Cohen, S. J., Dorfman, S. F., Goldstein, M. G., Gritz, E. R., Heyman, R.B., Holbrook, J., Jaen, C.R., Kottke, T.E., Lando, H., Mecklenburg, A., Mullen, P.D., Nett, L.M., Robinson, L., Stitzer, M., Tommasello, A.C., Villejo, L., and Wewers, M.E. (2000). *Treating tobacco use and dependence. Clinical practice guideline.* Rockville, MD: U.S. Department of Health and Human Services.

Fiore, M. C., Kenford, S. L., Jorenby, D. E, Wetter, D. W., Smith, S. S., and Baker, T. B. (1994b). Two studies of the clinical effectiveness of the nicotine patch with different counseling treatments. *Chest,* 105(2), 524-33.

Fiore, M. C., Smith, S. S., Jorenby, D. E, and Baker, T. B. (1994a). The effectiveness of the nicotine patch for smoking cessation: A meta-analysis. *Journal of the American Medical Association*, 271(24), 1940-1947.

French, S. A., Perry, C. L., Leon, G. R., and Fulkerson, J. A. (1994). Weight concerns, dieting behavior, and smoking initiation among adolescents: a prospective study. *American Journal of Public Health.* 84, 1818-1820.

Fulkerson, J. A., and French, S. A. (2003). Cigarette smoking for weight loss or control among adolescents: gender and racial/ethnic differences. *American Adolescent Health*, 32, 306-313.

Godtfredsen, N. S., Prescott, E., Vestbo, J., and Osler, M. (2006). Smoking reduction and biomarkers in two longitudinal studies. *Addiction*, 101, 1516-1522.

Graham, H., Inskip, H. M., Francis, B., and Harman, J. (2006). Pathways of disadvantage and smoking careers: Evidence and policy implications. *Journal of Epidemiology and Community Health, 60 (Suppl 2)*, 7-12.

Gray, N., and Henningfield, J. (2006). Dissent over harm reduction for tobacco. *Lancet*, 368, 899- 901.

Greig, C. C. (1970). Structured creativity group, thoughts by CC Greig – RandD Southampton marketing scenario, 1: low CO product; 2: high expanded tobacco cigarette. Trail exhibit 10683. 1970. BAT.

Gritz, E. R., Thompson, B., Emmons, K., Ockene, J. K., McLerran, D. F., and Nielsen, I. R. (1998). Gender differences among smokers and quitters in the Working Well Trial. *Preventive Medicine, 27*(4), 553-561.

Hajek, P., West, R., Foulds, J., Nilsson, F., Burrows, S., and Meadow, A. (1999). Randomized comparative trial of nicotine polacrilex, a transdermal patch, nasal spray, and an inhaler. *Archives of Internal Medicine, 159*(17), 2033-2038.

Hall, S. M., Reus, V. I., Munoz, R. F., Sees, K. L, Humfleet, G., Hartz, D. T., Frederick, S., and Triffleman, E. (1998). Nortriptyline and cognitive-behavioral therapy in the treatment of cigarette smoking. *Archives of General Psychiatry, 55*(8), 683-690.

Hall, S. M., Tunstall, C. D, Ginsberg, D., Benowitz, N. L, and Jones, R. T. (1987). Nicotine gum and behavioral treatment: a placebo controlled trial. *Journal of Consulting and Clinical Psychology*, 55(4),603-605.

Hamilton, A. S., Lessov-Schlaggar, C. N., Cockburn, M. G., Unger, J. B., Cozen, W., and Mack, T. M. (2006). Gender differences in determinants of smoking initiation and persistence in California twins. *Cancer Epidemiology, Biomarkers and Prevention, 15*(6), 1189-1197.

Haukkala, A., Laaksonen, M., and Uutela, A. (2001). Smokers who do not want to quit--is consonant smoking related to lifestyle and socioeconomic factors? *Scandinavian Journal of Public Health, 29*(3), 226-232.

Haukkala, A., Uutela, A., Vartiainen, E., McAlister, A., and Knekt, P. (2000). Depression and smoking cessation: The role of motivation and self-efficacy. *Addictive Behaviors, 25*(2), 311-316.

Haus, G., Hoerr, S. L., Mavis, B., and Robison, J. (1994). Key modifiable factors in weight maintenance: Fat intake, exercise, and weight cycling. *Journal of the American Dietetic Association, 94*(4), 409-413.

Haustein, K. O. (2003). *Tobacco or health? Physiological and social damages caused by tobacco smoking* (1st ed.). Berlin, Germany: Springer.

Hellström-Lindahl, E. and Nordberg, A. (2002). Smoking during pregnancy: A way to transfer the addiction to the next generation. *Respiration*, 69, 289-293.

Hennrikus, D. J., Jeffery, R. W., and Lando, H. A. (1996). Occasional smoking in a Minnesota working population. *American Journal of Public Health, 86*(9), 1260-1266.

Horsnby, P. P, Wilcox, A. J., and Weinberg, C. R. (1998). Cigarette smoking and disturbance of menstrual function. *Epidemiology,* 9(2), 193-198.

Howe, G., Westoff, C., Vessey, M., and Yeates, D. (1985). Effects of age, cigarette smoking and other factors on fertility: Findings in a large prospective study. *British Medical Journal, 290*(6483), 1697-1700.

Hughes, J. R., Helzer, J. E., and Lindberg, S. A. (2006). Prevalence of DSM/ICD-defined nicotine dependence. *Drug and Alcohol Dependence, 85*(2), 91-102.

Hughes, J. R., Keely, J., and Naud, S. (2004). Shape of the relapse curve and long-term abstinence among untreated smokers. *Addiction, 99*(1), 29-38.

Hull, M. G. R., North, K., Taylor, H., Farrow, A., and Ford, W. C. L. (2000). The Avon Longitudinal Study on Pregnancy and Childhood Study Team. Delayed conception and active passive smoking. *Fertility and Sterility*, 74(4), 725-733.

Husten, C. G., McCarty, M. C., Giovino, G. A., Chrismon, J. H., and Zhu, B. (1998). Intermittent smokers: A descriptive analysis of persons who have never smoked daily. *American Journal of Public Health, 88*(1), 86-89.

Jick, H., Porter, J., and Morrison, A. S. (1977). Relation between smoking and age of natural menopause. *Lancet*, 1(8026), 1354-1355.

Johnson, N. A., Boyle, C. A., and Heller, R. F. (1995). Leisure-time physical activity and other health behaviours: Are they related? *Australian Journal of Public Health, 19*(1), 69-75.

Jorenby, D. E., Hatsukami, D. K., Smith, S. S., Fiore, M. C., Allen S., Jensen J, and Baker, T.B. (1996). Characterization of tobacco withdrawal symptoms: Transdermal nicotine reduces hunger and weight gain. *Psychopharmacology, 128*(2), 130-138.

Kallen, K. (1998). Maternal smoking, body mass index, and neural tube defects. *American Journal of Epidemiology*, 147(12), 1103-1111.

Kassel, J. D., Stroud, L. R., and Paronis, C. A. (2003). Smoking, stress, and negative affect: Correlation, causation, and context across stages of smoking. *Psychological Bulletin, 129*(2), 270-304.

Katoh, J., Hara, Y., and Narutaki, K. (1994). Cardiorespiratory effects of weight reduction by exercise in middle-aged women with obesity. *Journal of International Medical Research,* 22, 160-164.

Kendler, K. S., Neale, M. C., Sullivan, P., Corey, L. A., Gardner, C. O., and Prescott, C. A. (1999). A population-based twin study in women of smoking initiation and nicotine dependence. *Psychological Medicine, 29*(2), 299-308.

King, A., de Wit, H., Riley, R.C., Cao, D., Niaura, R., and Hatsukami, D. (2006). Efficacy of naltrexone in smoking cessation: A preliminary study and an examination of sex differences. *Nicotine and Tobacco Research*, 8, 671-682.

King, T. K, Marcus, B. H., Pinto, B. M., Emmons, K. M., and Abrams, D. B.(1996). Cognitive- behavioral mediators of changing multiple behaviors: Smoking and a sedentary lifestyle. *Preventive Medicine*, 25, 684-691.

Kinnunen, T. (2001). Integrating hypnosis into a comprehensive smoking cessation intervention: Comments on past and present studies. *The International Journal of Clinical and Experimental Hypnosis, 49*(3), 267-271.

Kinnunen, Mustonen, T. (b) (2005). [Abstract] Exercise in treating tobacco dependence among women. *Annals of Behavioral Medicine, 29*, S043.

Kinnunen, T., and Korhonen, T. (2004). Weight concerns and negative affectivity in tobacco dependence among women: Is exercise a solution? *Proceedings of The 5th Annual Women's Health Research Conference*, Boston, Unites States.

Korhonen, T., Broms, U., Varjonen, J., Romanov, K., Koskenvuo, M., Kinnunen, T., and Kaprio, J. (2007). Smoking behaviour as a predictor of depression among Finnish men and women: A prospective cohort study of adult twins. *Psychological medicine, 37*(5), 705-715.

Kujala, U. M., Kaprio, J., and Rose, R. J. (2007). Physical activity in adolescence and smoking in young adulthood: A prospective twin cohort study. *Addiction, 102*(7), 1151-1157.

Laaksonen, M., Luoto, R., Helakorpi, S., and Uutela, A. (2002). Associations between health-related behaviors: A 7-year follow-up of adults. *Preventive Medicine, 34*(2), 162-170.

Lash, T. L., and Aschengrau, A. (1999). Active and passive cigarette smoking and the occurrence of breast cancer. *American Journal of Epidemiology, 149*(1), 5-12.

Lasser, K., Boyd, J. W., Woolhandler, S., Himmelstein, D. U., McCormick, D., and Bor, D. H. (2000). Smoking and mental illness: A population-based prevalence study. *Journal of the American Medical Association, 284*(20), 2606-2610.

Leventhal, A. M., Waters, A. J., Boyd, S., Moolchan, E. T., Lerman, C., and Pickworth, W. B. (2007). Gender differences in acute tobacco withdrawal: Effects on subjective, cognitive, and physiological measures. *Experimental and Clinical Psychopharmacology,* 15(1), 21-36.

Levy, D. T., Mumford, E. A., and Compton, C. (2006). Tobacco control policies and smoking in a population of low education women, 1992-2002. *Journal of Epidemiology and Community Health, 60 (Suppl 2)*, 20-26.

Li, D. K., Mueller, B. A., Hickok, D. E., Daling, J. R., Fantel, A. G., Checkoway, H. G, and Weiss, N. S. (1996). Maternal smoking during pregnancy and the risk of congenital urinary tract anomalies. *American Journal of Public Health*, 86(2), 249-253.

Lindquist, O., and Bengtsson, C. (1979). Menopausal age in relation to smoking. *Acta Medica Scandinavica, 205*(1-2), 73-77.

Mackay, J., Eriksen, M., and Shafey, O. (2006). *The tobacco atlas* (2nd ed.). Atlanta: The American Cancer Society.

Mainous, A. G., and Hueston, W. J. (1994). Passive smoke and low birth weight: Evidence of a threshold effect. *Archives of Family Medicine*, 3(10), 875-878.

Mannino, D.M., and Buist, A.S. (2007). Global burden of COPD: Risk factors, prevalence, and future trends. *Lancet*, 370 (9589), 765-773.

Mannino, D.M., Homa, D.M., Akinbami, L.J., Ford, E.S., Redd, S.C. (2002). Chronic obstructive pulmonary disease surveillance--United States, 1971-2000. *Respiratory Care,* 47 (10), 1184-1199.

Marcus, B. H., Albrecht, A. E., King, T. K., Parisi, A. F., Pinto, B. M., Roberts, M., Niaura, R.S., Abrams, D.B. (1999). The efficacy of exercise as an aid for smoking cessation in women: A randomized controlled trial. *Archives of Internal Medicine,* 159(11), 1229-1234.

Marcus, B. H., Albrecht, A. E., Niaura, R. S., Taylor, E. R., Simkin, L. R., Feder, S. I., Abrams, D.B., and Thompson, P.D. (1995). Exercise enhances the maintenance of smoking cessation in women. *Addictive Behaviors*, 20, 87-92.

Marcus, B. H., Lewis, B. A., Hogan, J., King, T.K., Albrecht, A.E., Bock, B., Parisi, A.F., Niaura, R., and Abrams, D.B. (2005). The efficacy of moderate-intensity exercise as an aid for smoking cessation in women: A randomized controlled trial, *Nicotine and Tobacco Research*, 7, 871-80.

Mayhew, K. P., Flay, B. R., and Mott, J. A. (2000). Stages in the development of adolescent smoking. *Drug and Alcohol Dependence*, 59 (Suppl 1), S61-81.

McLellan, D. L., and Kaufman, N. J. (2006). Examining the effects of tobacco control policy on low socioeconomic status women and girls: An initiative of the tobacco research network on disparities (TReND). *Journal of Epidemiology and Community Health*, 60 (Suppl 2), 5-6.

McNeill, A. (2004). ABC of smoking cessation: Harm reduction. *British Medical Journal*, 328, 885-887.

Menezes, A. M., and Hallal, P. C. (2007). Role of passive smoking on COPD risk in non-smokers. *Lancet, 370*(9589), 716-717.

Moffatt, R. J., Biggerstaff, K. D., and Stamford, B. A. (2000). Effects of the transdermal nicotine patch on normalization of HDL-C and its subfractions. *Preventive Medicine*, (2 Pt 1):148- 152.

Morrell, H. E. R., and Cohen, L. M. (2006). Cigarette smoking, anxiety and depression. *Journal of Psychopathology and Behavioral Assessment, 28*(4), 283-297.

Murphy, J. M., Horton, N. J., Monson, R. R., Laird, N. M., Sobol, A. M., and Leighton, A. H. (2003). Cigarette smoking in relation to depression: Historical trends from the Stirling County study. *The American Journal of Psychiatry*, 160(9), 1663-1669.

Musselman, D. L., Evans, D. L., and Nemeroff, C. B. (1998). The relationship of depression to cardiovascular disease: Epidemiology, biology, and treatment. *Archives of General Psychiatry*, 55, 580-592.

National Cancer Institute [NCI]. (2007). *What's in a name? Examination of light and intermittent smokers.* Author.

National Institutes of Health (1998). *Clinical guidelines on the identification, evaluation, and treatment of overweight and obesity in adults.* (NIH Publication No. 98-4083) Washington, DC: U.S. Author.

National Women's Law Center and Oregon Health and Sciences University [NWLCandOHandSU]. (2003). *Making the grade on women's health: Women and smoking, a national and state-by-state report card.* Author.

Perkins, K. A. (1993). Weight gain following smoking cessation. *Journal of Consulting and Clinical Psychology*, 61(5), 768-77.

O'Keefe, A. M., and Pollay, R. W. (1996). Deadly targeting of women in promoting cigarettes. *Journal of the American Medical Women's Association.* 51, 67-69.

Okuyemi, K. S., Harris, K. J., Scheibmeir, M., Choi, W. S., Powell, J., and Ahluwalia, J. S. (2002). Light smokers: Issues and recommendations. *Nicotine and Tobacco Research, 4* (Suppl 2), S103-12.

Olsen, P., Laara, E., Rantakallio, P., Jarvelin, M. R., Sarpola, A., and Hartikainen, A. R. (1995). Epidemiology of preterm delivery in two birth cohorts with an interval of 20 years. *American Journal of Epidemiology*, 142(11), 1184-1193.

Paparazzini, F., Tozzi, L., Mezzopane, R., Luchini, L., Marchini, M., and Fedele, L. (1994). Cigarette smoking, alcohol consumption, and risk of primary dysmenorrheal. *Epidemiology* 5(4), 469-472.

Perkins, K. A. (2001). Smoking cessation in women: Special considerations. *CNS Drugs*, 15(5), 391-411.

Perkins, K.A., Concklin, C.A., and Levine, M.D. (2007). *Cognitive-behavioral therapy for smoking cessation: A practical guidebook to the most effective treatments*. New York, NY: Taylor and Francis Group, LLC.

Perkins, K. A., Gerlach, D., Broge, M., Sanders, M., Grobe, J., Fonte, C., Cherry, C., Wilson, A., and Jacob, R. (2001a). Quitting cigarette smoking produces minimal loss of chronic tolerance to nicotine. *Psychopharmacology, 158*(1), 7-17.

Perkins, K. A., Jacobs, L., Sanders, M., and Caggiula, A. R. (2002). Sex differences in the subjective and reinforcing effects of cigarette nicotine dose. *Psychopharmacology, 163*(2), 194-201.

Perkins, K. A., Levine, M. D., Marcus, M. D, and Shiffman, S. (1997). Addressing women's concerns about weight gain due to smoking cessation. *Journal of Substance Abuse Treatment*, 14, 173-182.

Perkins, K. A, Marcus, M. D, Levine, M. D., D'Amico, D., Miller, A., Broge, M., Ashcom, J., and Shiffman, S. (2001b). Cognitive–behavioral therapy to reduce weight concerns improves smoking cessation outcome in weight-concerned women. *Journal of Consulting and Clinical Psychology*, 69 (4), 604–613.

Peto, R., Darby, S., Deo, H., Silocks, P., Whitley, E., Doll, R. (2000). Smoking, smoking cessation, and lung cancer in the UK since 1950: combination of national statistics with two case-control studies. *British Medical Journal*, 321, 323-329.

Pierce, J. P., and Gilpin, E. A. (1995). A historical analysis of tobacco marketing and the uptake of smoking by youth in the United States: 1890-1977. *Health Psychology, 14*(6), 500-508.

Pirkle, J. L., Flegal, K. M., Bernert, J. T., Brody, D. J., Etzel, R. A., and Maurer, K. R. (1996). Exposure of the US population to environmental tobacco smoke: The third national health and nutrition examination survey, 1988 to 1991. *Journal of the American Medical Association, 275*(16), 1233-1240.

Pomerleau, O. F., Burmeister, M., Madden, P., Long, J. C., Swan, G. E., and Kardia, S. L. (2007). Genetic research on complex behaviors: An examination of attempts to identify genes for smoking. *Nicotine and Tobacco Research, 9*(8), 883-901.

Prapavessis, H., Cameron, L., Baldi, J. C., Robinson, S., Borrie, K., Harper, T., and Grove, J. R. (2007). The effects of exercise and nicotine replacement therapy on smoking rates in women. *Addictive Behaviors*, *32*, 1416-1432.

Prescott, E., Hippe, M., Schnohr, P., Hein, H. O., and Vestbo, J. (1998). Smoking and risk of myocardial infarction in women and men: Longitudinal population study. *British Medical Journal*, 316(7137), 1043-1047.

Reynolds, P., Hurley, S., Goldberg, D.E., Anton-Culver, H., Bernstein, L., Deapen, D., Horn-Ross, P.L., Peel, D., Pinder, R., Ross, R.K., West, D., Wright,W.E., and Ziogas,A. (2004). Active smoking, household passive smoking, and breast cancer: Evidence from the California Teachers Study. *Journal of the National Cancer Institute*, 96, 29-37.

Riboli, E., Preston-Martin, S., Saracci, R., Haley, N. J., Trichopoulos, D., Becher, H., Burch, J.D., Fontham, E.T., Gao,Y.T., and Jindal,S.K. (1990). Exposure of non-smoking women to environmental tobacco smoke: A 10-country collaborative study. *Cancer Causes and Control, 1*(3), 243-252.

Richmond, R. L. (1997). How women and youth are targeted by the tobacco industry. *Monaldi Archives of Chest Diseases.* 52, 384-389.

Roth, L. K., Taylor, and Hugh, S. (2001). Risks of smoking to reproductive health: Assessment of women's knowledge. *American Journal of Obstetrics and Gynecology*, 184(5), 934-939.

Roquer, J. M., Figueras, J., Botet, F., and Jimenez, M. (1995). Influence on fetal growth of exposure to tobacco smoke during pregnancy. *Acta Pediatrica*, 84(2), 118-121.

Rosenberg, L., Kaufman, D.W., Helmrich, S.P., Miller, D.R., Stolley, P.D., and Shapiro, S (1985). Myocardial infarction and cigarette smoking in women younger than 50 years of age. *Journal of the American Medical Association,* 253, 2965-2969.

Royal College of Physicians of London [RCPL]. (2000). *Nicotine addiction in Britain.* London, UK: Author.

Saarni, S. E., Silventoinen, K., Rissanen, A, Sarlio-Lahteenkorva, S., and Kaprio, J. (2004). Intentional weight loss and smoking in young adults. *International Journal of Obesity.* 28, 796-802.

Scharf, D. and Shiffman, S. (2004). Are there gender differences in smoking cessation, with and without bupropion? Pooled-and meta-analyses of clinical trials of bupropion SR. *Society for the Study of Addiction* 99, 1462-1469.

Schmitz, J. M. (2003). Smoking cessation in women with cardiac risk. *The American Journal of the Medical Sciences, 326*(4), 192-196.

Schnohr, P., Jensen, J. S., Scharling, H., and Nordestgaard, B. G. (2002). Coronary heart disease risk factors ranked by importance for the individual and community: A 21 year follow-up of 12 000 men and women from The Copenhagen City Heart Study. *European Heart Journal,* 23, 620-626.

Schnoll,R.A.; Malstrom,M.; James,C.; Rothman,R.L.; Miller,S.M.; Ridge,J.A.; Movsas,B.; Unger,M.; Langer,C.; Goldberg,M. (2002). Correlates of tobacco use among smokers and recent quitters diagnosed with cancer. *Patient Education and Counseling,* 46(2), 137-145.

Schumann, A., Hapke, U., Rumpf, H. J., Meyer, C., and John, U. (2001). The association between degree of nicotine dependence and other health behaviours: Findings from a German general population study. *European Journal of Public Health, 11*(4), 450-452.

Senore, C., Battista, R. N., Shapiro, S. H., Segnan, N., Ponti, A., Rosso, S., and Aimar, D. (1998). Predictors of smoking cessation following physicians' counseling. *Preventive Medicine,* 27, 412-421.

Shavers, V. L., Fagan, P., Alexander, L. A., Clayton, R., Doucet, J., and Baezconde-Garbanati, L. (2006). Workplace and home smoking restrictions and racial/ethnic variation in the prevalence and intensity of current cigarette smoking among women by poverty status, TUS-CPS 1998-1999 and 2001-2002. *Journal of Epidemiology and Community Health,* (60 Suppl 2), 34-43.

Sherwood, N. E., Hennrikus, D. J., Jeffery, R. W., Lando, H. A., and Murray, D. M. (2000). Smokers with multiple behavioral risk factors: How are they different? *Preventive Medicine, 31*(4), 299-307.

Shiffman, S. (2006). Reflections on smoking relapse research. *Drug and Alcohol Review, 25*(1), 15-20.

Shiffman, S., and Paty, J. (2006). Smoking patterns and dependence: Contrasting chippers and heavy smokers. *Journal of Abnormal Psychology, 115*(3), 509-523.

Shinton, R., and Beevers, G. (1989). Meta-analysis of relation between cigarette smoking and stroke. *British Medical Journal,* 298,789-794.

Shiono, P. H., Klebanoff, M. A., and Brendes, H. W. (1986). Congenital malformations and maternal smoking during pregnancy. *Teratology,* 34(1), 65-71.

Shuttleworth, J. (2004). *Tobacco FactFile: Smoking and Reproductive Life.* Brittish Medical Association Tobacco Control Resource Center.

Stein, C., Kline, J., Levin, B., Susser, M., and Warburton, D. (1981). Epidemiologic studies of environmental exposure in human reproduction. In: Berge CG, Maillie HD, editors. *Measurement of Risks.* New York: Plenum Press, 163-183.

Stotts, A. L, Schmitz, J. M., and Grabowski, J. (2003). Concurrent treatment for alcohol and tobacco dependence: Are patients ready to quit both? *Drug Alcohol Depend,* 69, 1-7.

Sundell, G., Milsom, I., and Andersch, B. (1990). Factors influencing the prevalence and severity of dysmenorrhea in young women. *British Journal of Obstetrics and Gynecology,* 97(7), 588-594.

Taylor, R., Najafi, F., and Dobson, A. (2007). Meta-analysis of studies of passive smoking and lung cancer: Effects of study type and continent. *International Journal of Epidemiology,* doi:10.1093/lje/dym158.

Teperi, J., and Rimpela, M. (1989). Menstrual pain, health and behavior in girls. *Social Science and Medicine,* 29(2), 163-169.

Thorner, E. D., Jaszyna-Gasior, M., Epstein, D. H., and Moolchan, E. T. (2007). Progression to daily smoking: Is there a gender difference among cessation treatment seekers? *Substance Use and Misuse, 42*(5), 829-835.

Tolley, H. D., Crane, L., and Shipley, N. (1991). Smoking Prevalence and Lung Cancer Death Rates, pp.75-144. In: *Strategies to control tobacco use in the United States: A blueprint for public health action in the 1990s.* Bethesda, MD: US Department of Health and Human Services, Public Health Service, National Institutes of Health, National Cancer Institute. NIH publication no. 92-3316.

Tonnesen, P. (2002). Smoking reduction for smokers not able or motivated to quit? *Respiration,* 69(6), 475-478.

U.S. Department of Health and Human Services [USDHHS]. (1980). *The health consequences of smoking for women: A report of the surgeon general.* Washington: Author. Public Health Service, Office of the Assistant Secretary for Health, Office on Smoking and Health.

U.S. Department of Health and Human Services [USDHHS]. (1996). *Physical activity and health: A report of the surgeon general.* Atlanta, GA: Author, Centers for Disease Control and Prevention, National Center for Chronic Disease Prevention and Health Promotion.

U.S. Department of Health and Human Services [USDHHS]. (2001). *Women and smoking: A report of the surgeon general,* Atlanta, GA: Author, Centers for Disease Control and Prevention, National Center for Chronic Disease Prevention and Health Promotion, Office on Smoking and Health.

U.S. Department of Health and Human Services [USDHHS]. (2004). *Women, tobacco, and cancer: An agenda for the 21st century.* National Institutes of Health, National Cancer Institute.

U.S. Department of Health and Human Services [USDHHS] (2006). *The health consequences of involuntary exposure to tobacco smoke: A report of the surgeon general.* Rockville, MD; Washington, DC: Author. Public Health Service, Office of Surgeon General, Office on Smoking and Health.

U.S. Department of Health and Human Services [USDHHS]. (2007). *Promoting healthy lifestyles: Policy, program and personal recommendations for reducing cancer risk.* 2006-2007 Annual Report of President's Cancer Panel. Washington, DC: Author. National Institutes of Health, National Cancer Institute.

U.S. Department of Health, Education and Welfare [USDHEW]. (1979). *Smoking and health: A report of the surgeon general.* Washington: Author. Public Health Service, Office of the Assistant Secretary for Health, Office on Smoking And Health, DHEW Publication No PHS 79-50066.

Ussher, M. (2005). Exercise interventions for smoking cessation. *Cochrane database of systematic reviews (Online : Update Software), (1)*(1), CD002295.

Van den Eeden, S. K., Karagas, M. R, Daling, J. R., and Vaughan, T. L. (1990). A case-control study of maternal smoking and congenital malformations. *Paediatric and Perinatal Epidemiology,* 4(2), 147-155.

Vierola, H. (1998). *Tobacco and women's health.* Helsinki, Finland: Art House Oy.

Wartenberg, D., Calle, E. E., Thun, M. J., Heath, C. W.,Jr, Lally, C., and Woodruff, T. (2000). Passive smoking exposure and female breast cancer mortality. *Journal of the National Cancer Institute, 92*(20), 1666-1673.

Wee, C. C. Rigotti, N. A., Davis, R. B. and Phillips, R. S. (2001). Relationship between smoking and weight control efforts among adults in the United States. *Archives of Internal Medicine,* 161(4), 546-550.

West, R. (2006). *Theory of addiction.* Oxford, UK: Blackwell Publishing.

Westman, E. C. (2001). Review: Nicotine replacement treatments achieve smoking abstinence at 6-12 months. *Evidence Based Mental Health,* 4(1):21.

Wetter, D. W., Kenford, S. L., Smith, S. S., Fiore, M. C., Jorenby, D. E, Baker, T. B. (1999). Gender differences in smoking cessation. *Journal of Consulting Clinical Psychology,* 67(4), 555-62.

Wilcox, A. J., Weinberg, C. R., and Baird, D. D. (1990). Risk factors for early pregnancy loss. *Epidemiology* 1(5), 382-385.

Windham, G. C, Elkin, E. P, Swan, S. H, Waller, K. O, and Fenster, L. (1999). Cigarette smoking and effects on menstrual function. *Obstetrics and Gynecology*, 93(1), 59-65.

Wisborg, K., Henriksen,T. B., Hedegaard, M., and Secher, N. J. (1996). Smoking during pregnancy and preterm birth. *British Journal of Obstetrics and Gynecology*, 103(8), 800-805.

World Health Organization [WHO]. (1997). *Tobacco or health: A global status report.* Geneva, Switzerland: Author.

World Health Organization [WHO] (2001a). *The world health report 2001 - mental health.* Geneva, Switzerland: Author.

World Health Organization [WHO]. (2001b). *Women and the tobacco epidemic: Challenges for the 21st century.* Canada: Author.

Wu, T., Buck, G., and Mendola, P.(1998). Maternal cigarette smoking, regular use of multivitamin/mineral supplements, and risk of fetal death: The 1988 National Maternity and Infant Health Survey. *American Journal of Epidemiology*, 148(2), 215-21.

Yin, P., Jiang, C. Q., Cheng, K. K., Lam, T. H., Lam, K. H., Miller, M. R., Zhang, W.S., Thomas, G.N., and Adab, P. (2007). Passive smoking exposure and risk of COPD among adults in China: The Guangzhou Biobank cohort study. *Lancet, 370*(9589), 751-757.

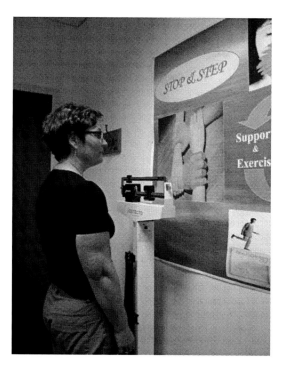

Photo 1. (Woman and the scale) Many women are concerned about gaining weight after quitting smoking and most people do gain weight during the first year of cessation. The weight gained does not, however, negate the health benefits of quitting.

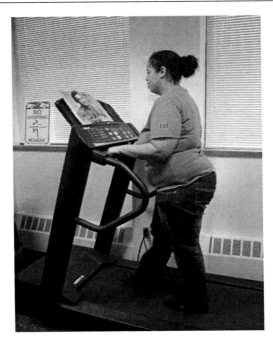

Photo 2. (Woman on the treadmill) Aerobic exercise as an adjunct to regular smoking cessation program promotes quitting and may be an appropriate choice for women with depression or fearful of gaining weight.

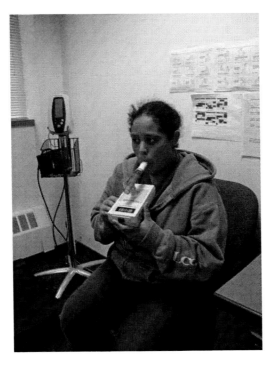

Photo 3. (Woman and the CO-machine) Carbon monoxide can be easily assessed with various devices. It is a convenient tool to verify biochemically abstinence from cigarettes during clinical trials as well as to provide biofeedback for smokers regarding their tobacco exposure level.

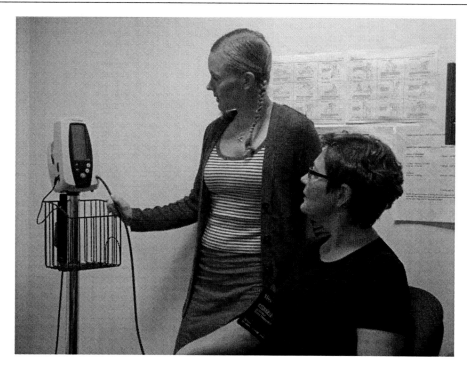

Photo 4. (Woman and a counsellor) Women can reduce their cardiovascular risk by quitting smoking. Successful cessation requires pharmacotherapy and counselling. Women need more intensive counselling and social support than men.

In: Smoking and Women's Health   ISBN 978-1-60456-148-7
Editors: M.K. Wesley and I.A. Sternbach, pp.109-120   © 2008 Nova Science Publishers, Inc.

Chapter 3

Smoking and Women's Health Research

Monica Ortendahl[2]
Royal Institute of Technology, Stockholm, Sweden

Smoking is a critical hazard for women in their reproductive years, particularly when they are pregnant (1). It is a well-established fact that smoking is very detrimental to health, and for pregnant woman smoking is detrimental also to the health of the fetus, the newborn and the infant (2). Smoking in early gestation and through pregnancy is associated with adverse outcomes, and some of these effects can be avoided by reducing smoking or quitting entirely (3). Research on the health consequences of smoking has obtained results indicating that smoking is associated, among other things, with early pregnancy loss and complications of labor and delivery, preterm delivery, stillbirth, high rates of sudden infant death syndrome (SIDS), and low birth weight, (4) in addition to intrauterine growth retardation (5).

Research over the years has clearly established both short- and long-term benefits for women who do not smoke during pregnancy. Therefore, it is an important task of health professionals to influence people's smoking behavior and to disburse information about the negative effects of smoking on health. However, achieving changes in smoking behavior in pregnant women is not an easy task (6). Of women who quit smoking spontaneously, i.e., persons who stopped smoking before entering prenatal care, many went into relapse and resumed smoking sometime before obstetrical delivery (7, 8). Similar patterns of resumption are noted with both sudden cessation and gradual reduction in smoking (9). Persons with a more positive attitude toward smoking cessation more often intend to quit smoking (10). Therefore, smokers' intent to quit smoking should receive additional support (11).

An increasing number of health care professionals recognize the problem of smoking during pregnancy (12) and workers in health education have developed several smoking cessation programs for pregnant women with the expectation that these educational projects would produce positive results in terms of behavior change (13). Subsequent evaluations of the programs, however, suggest that behavioral change often is temporary (14). When it

2 Mail address: monicaortendahl@hotmailcom, August 2007-08-26.

comes to health and preventive programs, the difficulty of improving future health status is a well-established fact. The likelihood of persuading mothers to quit is not always promising, especially with regard to heavy smokers (15). Apparent expectations to quit are not always followed by behavioral change (16).

Time Preference and Smoking

The problem related to behavior change and its maintenance is an important challenge to domains dealing with health-related behaviors, like professional health care services. This applies to such addictive habits as smoking because most cessation programs are generally effective only temporarily in helping people in their struggle against the addictive quality of (nicotine) smoking.

One possible explanation for these discouraging results is that many health programs and medical preventive situations involve an exchange of costs in the present for benefits in the future (17). The preventive programs are intended to alter behavior in the present and to save for the future rather than consume in the present. This implies a relative evaluation of immediate and delayed outcome. Despite the relevance of time in decision making, the psychology of human decision making has not paid much attention to this factor. Instead, this field of research has focused on the importance of values and beliefs in decisions.

Health and addictive behavior like smoking could be regarded as a temporal preference, where the immediate pleasure of the addictive behavior is preferred to the distant and hard to imagine benefit of non-addictive behavior (18). Current smokers have been found to be more impulsive than ex-smokers (19). Impulsiveness, with difficulty working toward long-term goals, may predict perceptions of positive and negative reinforcement from smoking. In another study (20) it was found that greater impulsivity predicted more rapid relapse to smoking. The conclusion was that targeted treatments were needed that address the special needs of smokers high in impulsivity.

The value a person places on the future vs. the present is called time preference or time discounting; this represents the weight he/she places on the future relative to the present when he/she makes decisions that have future consequences (21). In addictive behavior there is a discounting effect, as the value of the non-addictive behavior diminishes as a function of the time distance (22). A positive discount rate for health outcomes would imply that a healthy state many years ahead has such a small value that it will be very hard to get people engaged in a preventive behavior like quitting smoking. The low value of a hard-to-imagine, distant goal of a good state of health is explained by large discount rates (23). The value of non-smoking, for example, is very small because the benefits are obtained in the remote future. Those who discount most are considered most impulsive. High rates of cigarette consumption have been related to higher rates of delay discounting (24). With a high discount rate this effect would increase and would explain the demonstrated deficient effects of preventive programs.

In an earlier study (25) it was found that smokers were less educated and were more likely to discount future rewards than nonsmokers. Future time perspective has also been found to be a predictor of cannabis use (26). In another study (27) nicotine deprivation was found to increase impulsive choices for both cigarette and monetary rewards in a delay-discounting task. The situation could be described as a choice between the immediate pleasure of having a cigarette and having good health, or avoiding illnesses related to smoking, in the remote future. If a deferred gratification pattern is adopted, sound health could be an alternative future reward. The perspective of rational decision making in economics could be applied to cases of addictive behavior (28), regarding inter-temporal decisions as an investment decision (21). In many inter-temporal situations involving self-control, humans are uncertain whether they could manage this rational long-term choice.

The effect of uncertainty in decision making related to the future has been investigated. A study by Patak and Reynolds (29) sought to determine whether adolescent participants incorporated uncertainty into their valuations for delayed rewards. It was found that delayed rewards were rated as increasingly uncertain with longer delays. Also, ratings of uncertainty were correlated with rate of delay discounting. Another study, by Yi, et al (30), combined delay and probability to explain discounting effects. Some people prefer the proximal addictive reward; that, however, is often followed by a period of remorse. The reverse is also possible, in which case addiction provides a shortsighted relief from discontentment rather than obtaining a long-term state of well-being. The question can also be raised whether a high time-preference rate leads to addiction or whether the onset of addiction itself alters people's inter-temporal equilibrium (28).

Smoking and Pregnancy

Although maintaining abstinence from cigarettes during pregnancy yields important benefits for women and children, only 20-30% of pregnancy cessation lasts one year postpartum (31). Delay discounting has been found to predict postpartum relapse to smoking among pregnant women (32). Discounting has also been found to be related to different stages of smoking and non-smoking (22). As smokers have displayed rapid loss of value for delayed health outcomes (33), the need for smoking-cessation treatments that provide relatively immediate positive consequences for abstinence has been stressed.

Although evidence indicates that individual smoking cessation counseling does not increase quitting rates during pregnancy, the method may have long-term effects (34). It is important to understand the larger process of change in which addict and treatment provider meet, and the possibility of counseling especially tailored to the motivational stage of pregnant women has been explored (35).

In the transtheoretical model (36) five groups have been formed representing stages of readiness for behavior change (i.e., quitting smoking), consisting of relapsers, persons in the precontemplation stage, persons in the contemplation stage, actors and maintainers. Precontemplators (contemplators being persons considering quitting) were found to have a more negative attitude toward quitting than the other groups. General motivation to change smoking behavior and confidence in one's ability to succeed have been found to vary across these five groups representing stages of readiness (37).

Decisional balance and the stage of change have been used to understand the motivation for giving up the habit of smoking (37). An interaction between the motivational stage of attempting to quit smoking and the process it creates has been reported , with smoking cessation related to perceptions of pros and cons of smoking that constitute a decisional balance (38). These pros and cons of smoking have also been related to pregnancy (38). More specifically, pregnant women have a less negative attitude toward their smoking (39). It has also been found that differing predictors may contribute to the different transitional stages of smoking cessation (40).

In a study by Näsman and Ortendahl (41) a decision-analytic model based on the product of values and beliefs (expected utility) related to smoking provided a good description of judgments over a period of time. Four groups of women were investigated formed by the two variables of pregnancy/non-pregnancy and intending/not intending to quit smoking. No difference was found between pregnant and non-pregnant women in expected utility of consequences related to smoking, indicating that pregnancy did not influence judgments performed. Expected utility was negative for pregnant as well as non-pregnant women for both smoking and non-smoking conditions. The result obtained in the study was in accord with earlier findings (39) where, testing the trans-theoretical model, pregnant and non-pregnant smokers were found to be similar in their readiness for quitting smoking. This suggests that psychological aspects like motivational stage rather than physical variables like being pregnant or not have an impact on values and beliefs.

Another important finding in the same study by Näsman and Ortendahl (41) was that for all the consequences of smoking, which included health consequences, consequences related to pregnancy, and consequences related to mood and social relations, expected utility of quitting smoking and of not quitting smoking were both negative. It is reasonable to assume that smokers will find both smoking and not smoking to be negative, but for quite different reasons. One explanation presented earlier (42) implies that the constellation of two negative options generates an avoidance-avoidance conflict, which is a conflict between two equally negative and undesirable goals or alternatives, in which avoiding one requires choosing the other.

For the condition of smoking, the expected utilities for health consequences and consequences related to pregnancy were evaluated as more negative than the psychological and social consequences in the same study (41). Assuming that smoking-related consequences for the body are perceived as somehow more fundamental than psychological and social consequences, the expected utility of smoking could be expected to be most negative for health consequences and consequences related to pregnancy.

Another result obtained in the same study was that the expected utility of not quitting was judged to be more negative than the quitting condition, and the utility difference was largest for health consequences. One conclusion in the study was that outcome in health should be stressed in messages for non-pregnant as well as pregnant women when quitting smoking. Another conclusion was that this consequence should be emphasized, as effects on health are more likely to be irreversible than psychological and social consequences.

Most persons are informed about the hazards connected to smoking during pregnancy not only for the mother but also for the fetus and the infant. It is an important task for health professionals to dispense information about the negative consequences of smoking on health (43). One reason for the lack of conclusive data on behaviors in this field of research may be that models used in explaining addictive behavior assume that people behave rationally once they have obtained reliable factual information. For instance, many smokers make the decision to quit smoking and attempt to do so. Although individuals set up goals, such as to discontinue smoking, it seems that people lack the ability to reach these goals (44).

Cessation interventions may increase success rates by being sensitive to motivational and psychological stage and by shifting strategies depending on stages of readiness (45). Repeated contacts are likely an essential factor for early-stage smokers because feedback provides useful information when it focuses on stage-specific goals and strategies. The greatest benefit, however, might come from maintaining contact with the individuals as they move through the cycle of change over time. Paying careful attention to the stages of motivational change could increase the effectiveness and efficiency of interventions.

Another study of women smokers in the same project (46) found that the non-pregnant women gave smoking-related consequences the least positive ratings across time and intent to quit. Throughout the two-week study the determining variable accounting for the difference in rated values of smoking was pregnancy and non-pregnancy; no difference was noted between women who intended to quit and those who did not. The difference in ratings between pregnant and non-pregnant women was largest for health consequences, while there was no difference in ratings of consequences related to mood and social relations.

Pregnant women have been found in earlier studies (47) to have no significantly increased intention to quit smoking, despite the health risk to the fetus and the newborn child. The study by Ortendahl and Näsman (46) showed no impact on judgments of smoking-related consequences from motivational and psychological aspects like the intent to quit smoking. Instead, in the same study (46) it was the pregnant smokers who gave smoking-related consequences the least negative rated values. This accords with earlier results in which pregnant women have been found to have a less negative perception of their smoking compared to non-pregnant smokers (31). It might be expected that pregnant women would give smoking a more negative value than non-pregnant women. However, the opposite result was obtained in the study by Ortendahl and Näsman (46).

Many smokers worry about their health, and the results of the study indicated that for many women, smoking during pregnancy is a complex and variable behavior. It appears to be accepted knowledge among the general population that, from a health perspective, smoking is a precarious and self-destructive behavior. Dynamic models of smoking incorporating future uncertainty have been proposed (48), where smokers were found to react to personalized health information but not necessarily to general information.

Misconceptions about risk and values may help to rationalize continued smoking (49). One speculative conclusion of the Ortendahl and Näsman study under discussion (46) was that smokers intent on quitting smoking, especially during pregnancy, should be given personalized information concerning values related to smoking in order to increase success rates. Results indicate that incentives for smoking cessation should incorporate varying patterns of presentation of information, including values of smoking and smoking cessation.

Given that the pregnant smokers were found to exhibit a less negative judgment of health consequences related to smoking than the non-pregnant smokers, another of the study's conclusions was that additional strategies are needed to achieve reductions in smoking, especially during pregnancy. It has earlier been found (50) that worry about health led to more quitting activity. One explanation presented for this result was that worry kept attention focused on the treatment. It has also been found (2) that behavioral risk profiles of those who reduce smoking are closer to those of smokers than of non-smokers, and that repeated information and contacts during pregnancy may increase success rates.

A further study by Ortendahl and Näsman (51) investigated perception of smoking-related health consequences. The perceived probability that the smoking-related health consequences would occur if smoking continued was estimated as somewhat unlikely to somewhat likely. The highest mean estimated probability if smoking continued was for losing some physical strength, physical condition becoming worse, getting a heart disease, and getting lung cancer. For the condition of continuing to smoke, the mean estimated probability was low in general for pregnant women who did not intend to quit smoking.

Data from the same study indicated that there are misconceptions among pregnant women, especially among those who do not intend to quit, about the risks related to smoking. This result accorded with the result of an earlier study on pregnant and postpartum women (49). While, as already noted, an increasing number of health care professionals have recognized the problem of smoking during pregnancy (52,53) and several smoking cessation programs have been developed for pregnant women (54), many smokers continue to smoke throughout their pregnancy (55), and those who quit often relapse postpartum (56). One explanation presented in these studies was that pregnant women underestimate smoking-related health consequences; this is supported by the results obtained in the study under discussion. It should be noted that the perceptions applied to smoking-related health consequences are not specifically related to pregnancy but are valid for all smokers.

Most studies on risk perceptions have been performed on non-pregnant women. In one of these studies smokers in general were found not to view themselves at increased risk of heart disease or cancer (57). In our study (51) the mean estimated probability of suffering negative health effects for women intending to quit smoking was found to be somewhat lower compared to the women not intending to quit smoking. This means that women who intended to quit considered the positive consequences of quitting as greater than did those who did not intend to quit. This applied to both pregnant and non-pregnant women and to all smoking-related health consequences except for the consequence of getting fat.

The same study found that the condition of quitting smoking showed an effect in the estimates made by all groups for all smoking-related health consequences except for estimated probability of "your life expectancy becomes shorter" made by pregnant women intending to quit smoking. The difference between the conditions of continuing and quitting smoking was negative for getting fat, meaning that the estimated probability of getting fat is greater for quitting smoking.

The largest difference between the conditions of continuing and quitting smoking was for "physical condition becoming worse", "getting a heart disease", "getting lung cancer", and "losing some physical strength". These smoking-related health consequences were estimated as most probable to occur for the condition of continuing to smoke. For all four of these smoking-related health consequences, pregnant women who did not intend to quit smoking showed the smallest difference, compared to the other groups, between the conditions of continuing and quitting smoking. These women also estimated that the probability for these health consequences to occur if they continued smoking was low.

One tentative explanation of the result presented was that the pregnant women who are not intending to quit smoking continue because they do not consider smoking to be dangerous. Smokers and non-smokers have earlier been found to differ markedly in their perception of health (58), and the smokers did not fully comprehend the harm related to smoking. Another explanation presented was that for pregnant women it is most important to quit the habit of smoking, and that these women may have the greatest denial of the harm, with different excuses for continuing to smoke in order to feel more comfortable about continuing (59). Pregnant women who do not intend to quit might rationalize and have self-exempting beliefs that reduce cognitive dissonance, inhibiting their willingness to quit (60).

Yet it seems likely that many pregnant women are already predisposed to quit smoking because of pregnancy-related physiological changes that make smoking less appealing and/or because they wish to prevent complications of pregnancy. In this case, for them, compared to non-pregnant women, perceptions of future smoking-related health consequences would not have to be as strong to persuade them to quit, and they would have to be weak indeed if the combination of pregnancy and perceived future health consequences of smoking were not enough to motivate them to quit smoking. In either event, it makes sense to take advantage of pregnancy to encourage women to stop smoking and not to start again after delivery.

In another study by the same authors (61) the intent to quit affected the estimated probabilities for the occurrence of smoking-related psychological and social consequences for both the conditions of continuing and of quitting smoking, whereas pregnancy did not affect the estimation of probabilities. The motivational and psychological variable of intent to quit seemed to have a larger impact on risk perceptions than did the physical variable of being pregnant or not. The study confirmed, in general, the findings of other studies of perceptions of health risks (62). In these earlier studies smoking was also associated with risk assessment. Smokers and non-smokers differed markedly in their perceptions of health risks. Smokers were found to be less likely to agree with health risks than their non-smoking counterparts and did not fully comprehend the risks associated with smoking.

Psychological and social health risks do not seem to have been studied to the same extent as somatic health risks. An earlier study by Hampson, et al (63) focused on smoking as a behavior that affects others as well as oneself. Oncken, et al (64) and Carbone, et al (65) have considered the role of perception in quality-of-life effects of smoking in connection with immediate concerns and feelings, and in future risk of mortality.

An important finding in the study was that for all women, the estimated effect of quitting smoking for psychological and social consequences was statistically significant. The effect of quitting smoking was estimated to be largest for the consequences involving a social relationship, with an estimated smaller difference for psychological consequences. Many smokers worry about their own health, and it could be expected that this worry would affect risk perceptions of psychological and social consequences.

Conclusion

Smoking during pregnancy is a complex and variable behavior for many women. Many quit attempts are unprepared (66), suggesting that models of smoking cessation should place greater emphasis on the dynamic nature of motivation to quit. Fluctuations in maternal smoking during pregnancy have been found (67), and a substantial proportion of the women exhibited a pattern of repeated cessation and relapse. Moreover, the intent to quit often spontaneously changes over short periods of time (68). Brief smoking cessation interventions early in pregnancy are likely to be inadequate for many smokers during pregnancy.

Our studies in the project confirmed, in general, that the women who were trying to quit smoking had made a larger number of attempts to quit in the past compared to the women who were not trying to quit. This finding is in accord with results earlier obtained in a study by Walsh, et al (14), where many of the persons who had succeeded in quitting smoking had made numerous attempts to quit before finally achieving success. The act of quitting smoking, therefore, seems to be a dynamic process rather than a discrete event, where many people periodically cycle from smoking to not smoking (67).

An earlier study (51) has related the probability of successful quitting attempts to the number of earlier attempts. The finding suggests that women trying to quit smoking are generally more motivated to stop smoking than those not trying to stop. It indicates that succeeding is preceded by a certain number of quitting attempts, and that the chances are improved by every attempt. Of course, there is an increased statistical probability, but there is also an increased psychological probability. In the same study by Ortendahl and Näsman (51), non-pregnant women who were trying to quit and who had smoked the longest also exhibited the highest number of previous attempts to quit. Longer duration of smoking has been associated in another study (69) with lower likelihood of attempting to quit and of quitting successfully.

Health and addictive behavior is a problem and a focus of interest in much current research. The impact of programs on changing and maintaining positive health habits can only be assessed over time, and it may be that the strategy will change in the future, preferably toward projects that focus on the time aspects of individual behavior. One reason for the inconclusive nature of current research findings may be that if we are to understand health-related behavior and learn to relate to it with greater effectiveness we need to engage in an interdisciplinary approach. Such an approach should include such fields as social psychology, personality psychology, health education, preventive medicine, public health, epidemiology, sociology and economics. By promoting close collaboration among specialists in different disciplines, we might able to make new advances toward understanding the results of preventive efforts. Further, the importance of time for the value of remote outcomes should be considered more than it has been in explaining addictive behavior, since it is evident that such behavior is the result not of a single action but a long series of actions that have been taken.

References

[1]   Reichert VC, Seltzer V, Efferen LS, Kohn N. Women and tobacco dependence. *Med. Clin. North Am.* 2004 Nov;88(6):1467-1481.

[2]   Raatikainen K, Huurinainen P, Heinonen S. Smoking in early gestation or through pregnancy: a decision crucial to pregnancy outcome. *Prev. Med.* 2007 Jan;44(1):59-63.

[3] Cowperthwaite B, Hains SM, Kisilevsky BS Fetal behavior in smoking compared to non-smoking pregnant women. *Infant. Behav. Dev.* 2007 Aug;30(3):422-430.

[4] Klesges LM, Johnson KC, Ward KD, Barnard M. Smoking cessation in pregnant women.*Obstet. Gynecol. Clin. North Am.* 2001 Jun;28(2):269-82.

[5] Cnattingius S. The epidemiology of smoking during pregnancy: smoking prevalence, maternal characteristics, and pregnancy outcomes. *Nicotine Tob. Res.* 2004 Apr;6 Suppl 2:S125-140.

[6] Curry SJ, Sporer AK, Pugach O, Campbell RT, Emery S. Use of tobacco cessation treatments among young adult smokers: 2005 National Health Interview Survey. *Am. J. Public Health* 2007 Aug;97(8):1464-1469.

[7] Solomon LJ, Higgins ST, Heil SH, Badger GJ, Thomas CS, Bernstein IM. Predictors of postpartum relapse to smoking. *Drug Alcohol Depend.* 2007 Apr 30.

[8] French GM, Groner JA, Wewers ME, Ahijevych K. Staying smoke free: an intervention to prevent postpartum relapse. *Nicotine Tob. Res.* 2007 Jun;9(6):663-670.

[9] Law M, Tang JL. An analysis of the effectiveness of interventions intended to help people stop smoking. *Arch. Intern. Med.* 1995 Oct 9;155(18):1933-1941.

[10] Droomers M, Schrijvers CT, Mackenbach JP. Educational differences in the intention to stop smoking: explanations based on the Theory of Planned Behaviour. *Eur. J. Public.* Health 2004 Jun;14(2):194-198.

[11] Curry SJ, Orleans CT, Keller P, Fiore M. Promoting smoking cessation in the healthcare environment: 10 years later. *Am. J. Prev. Med.* 2006 Sep;31(3):269-272.

[12] McCaul KD, Hockemeyer JR, Johnson RJ, Zetocha K, Quinlan K, Glasgow RE. Motivation to quit using cigarettes: a review. *Addict Behav.* 2006 Jan;31(1):42-56.

[13] DiClemente CC, Dolan-Mullen P, Windsor RA. The process of pregnancy smoking cessation: implications for interventions. *Tob. Control* 2000;9 Suppl 3:III16-21.

[14] Walsh RA, Lowe JB, Hopkins PJ. Quitting smoking in pregnancy. *Med. J. Aust.* 2001 17;175(6):320-323.

[15] Selby P, Hackman R, Kapur B, Klein J, Koren G. Heavily smoking women who cannot quit in pregnancy: evidence of pharmacokinetic predisposition. *Ther. Drug Monit.* 2001 Jun;23(3):189-191.

[16] Kinzie MB. Instructional design strategies for health behavior change. *Patient Educ. Couns.* 2005 Jan;56(1):3-15.

[17] Chapman GB, Brewer NT, Coups EJ, Brownlee S, Leventhal H, Leventhal EA.Value for the future and preventive health behavior. *J. Exp. Psychol. Appl.* 2001 Sep;7(3):235-250.

[18] Doran N, McChargue D, Cohen L. Impulsivity and the reinforcing value of cigarette smoking. *Addict Behav.* 2007 Jan;32(1):90-8.

[19] Skinner MD, Aubin HJ, Berlin I. Impulsivity in smoking, nonsmoking, and ex-smoking alcoholics. A*ddict Behav.* 2004 Jul;29(5):973-978.

[20] Doran N, Spring B, McChargue D, Pergadia M, Richmond M Impulsivity and smoking relapse. *Nicotine Tob. Res.* 2004 Aug;6(4):641-647.

[21] Ferguson BS. Economic modeling of the rational consumption of addictive substances.*Subst. Use Misuse* 2006;41(4):573-603.

[22] Reynolds B, Richards JB, Horn K, Karraker K. Delay discounting and probability discounting as related to cigarette smoking status in adults. *Behav. Processes* 2004 Jan 30;65(1):35-42.

[23] Baker F, Johnson MW, Bickel WK. Delay discounting in current and never-before cigarette smokers: similarities and differences across commodity, sign, and magnitude. *J. Abnorm. Psychol.* 2003 Aug;112(3):382-392.

[24] Reynolds B. Do high rates of cigarette consumption increase delay discounting? A cross-sectional comparison of adolescent smokers and young-adult smokers and nonsmokers. *Behav. Processes* 2004 Nov 30;67(3):545-549.

[25] Jaroni JL, Wright SM, Lerman C, Epstein LH. Relationship between education and delay discounting in smokers. *Addict Behav.* 2004 Aug;29(6):1171-1175.

[26] Apostolidis T, Fieulaine N, Soule F. Future time perspective as predictor of cannabis use: exploring the role of substance perception among French adolescents. *Addict Behav.* 2006 Dec;31(12):2339-2343.

[27] Field M, Santarcangelo M, Sumnall H, Goudie A, Cole J. Delay discounting and the behavioural economics of cigarette purchases in smokers: the effects of nicotine deprivation. *Psychopharmacology* (Berl). 2006 Jun;186(2):255-263.

[28] Bretteville-Jensen AL. Addiction and discounting. *J. Health Econ.* 1999 Aug;18(4):393-407.

[29] Patak M, Reynolds B. Question-based assessments of delay discounting: do respondents spontaneously incorporate uncertainty into their valuations for delayed rewards? *Addict Behav.* 2007 Feb;32(2):351-357.

[30] Yi R, Gatchalian KM, Bickel WK. Discounting of past outcomes. *Exp. Clin. Psychopharmacol* 2006 Aug;14(3):311-317.

[31] Mullen PD. How can more smoking suspension during pregnancy become lifelong abstinence? Lessons learned about predictors, interventions, and gaps in our accumulated knowledge. *Nicotine Tob. Res.* 2004 Apr;6 Suppl 2:S217-238.

[32] Yoon JH, Higgins ST, Heil SH, Sugarbaker RJ, Thomas CS, Badger GJ. Delay discounting predicts postpartum relapse to cigarette smoking among pregnant women. *Exp. Clin. Psychopharmacol.* 2007 Apr;15(2):176-186.

[33] Odum AL, Madden GJ, Bickel WK. Discounting of delayed health gains and losses by current, never- and ex-smokers of cigarettes. *Nicotine Tob. Res.* 2002 Aug;4(3):295-303.

[34] Lumley J, Oliver SS, Chamberlain C, Oakley L. Interventions for promoting smoking cessation during pregnancy. *Cochrane Database Syst. Rev.* 2004 Oct 18;(4):CD001055.

[35] DiClemente CC, Schlundt D, Gemmell L.Readiness and stages of change in addiction treatment. *Am. J. Addict.* 2004 Mar-Apr;13(2):103-119.

[36] Prochaska JO, DiClemente CC, Velicer WF, Rossi JS. Standardized, individualized, interactive, and personalized self-help programs for smoking cessation. *Health Psychol.* 1993 Sep;12(5):399-405.

[37] Prochaska JO, Velicer WF, Redding C, Rossi JS, Goldstein M, DePue J, Greene GW, Rossi SR, Sun X, Fava JL, Laforge R, Rakowski W, Plummer BA. Stage-based expert systems to guide a population of primary care patients to quit smoking, eat healthier,

prevent skin cancer, and receive regular mammograms. *Prev. Med.* 2005 Aug;41(2):406-416.

[38] Font-Mayolas S, Planes M, Gras MA, Sullman MJ. Motivation for change and the pros and cons of smoking in a Spanish population. *Addict Behav.* 2007 Jan;32(1):175-180.

[39] Ruggiero L, Tsoh JY, Everett K, Fava JL, Guise BJ. The transtheoretical model of smoking: comparison of pregnant and nonpregnant smokers. *Addict Behav.* 2000 Mar-Apr;25(2):239-251.

[40] Abdullah AS, Yam HK. Intention to quit smoking, attempts to quit, and successful quitting among Hong Kong Chinese smokers: population prevalence and predictors. *Am. J. Health Promot.* 2005 May-Jun;19(5):346-354.

[41] Näsman P, Ortendahl M. 2007. Values and beliefs about consequences related to smoking among pregnant and non-pregnant women. In Press. *J. Obstet. Gynaecol.*

[42] Shadel WG, Niaura R, Goldstein MG, Abrams DB. Cognitive avoidance as a method of coping with a provocative smoking cue: the moderating effect of nicotine dependence. *J. Behav. Med.* 2001 Apr;24(2):169-182.

[43] Castrucci BC, Culhane JF, Chung EK, Bennett I, McCollum KF. Smoking in pregnancy: patient and provider risk reduction behavior. *J. Public Health Manag. Pract.* 2006 Jan-Feb;12(1):68-76.

[44] Ebrahim SH, Merritt RK, Floyd RL. Smoking and women's health: opportunities to reduce the burden of smoking during pregnancy. CMAJ 2000 Aug 8;163(3):288-289.

[45] Dijkstra A, Tromp D, Conijn B.Stage-specific psychological determinants of stage transition. *Br .J. Health Psychol.* 2003 Nov;8(Pt 4):423-437.

[46] Ortendahl M, and Näsman P. Somatic, Psychological and Social Judgments Related to Smoking among Pregnant and Non-Pregnant Women. In Press. *J. Addict. Dis.*

[47] Hutchison KE, Stevens VM, Collins FL Jr. Cigarette smoking and the intention to quit among pregnant smokers. *J. Behav. Me* . 1996;19:307-316.

[48] Clark A, Etile F. Health changes and smoking: an economic analysis. *Subst. Use Misuse* 2006;41:427-451.

[49] Dunn CL, Pirie PL, Lando HA. Attitudes and perceptions related to smoking among pregnant and postpartum women in a low-income, multiethnic setting. *Am. J. Health Promot.* 1998;12: 267-274.

[50] Dijkstra A, Brosschot J. Worry about health in smoking behaviour change. *Behav. Res. Ther.* 2003;41:1081-1092.

[51] Ortendahl M, Näsman P. Perception of smoking-related health consequences among pregnant and non-pregnant women. In Press. *Am. J. Addict.*

[52] Kukla L, Hruba D, Tyrlik M. Smoking and damages of reproduction: evidence of ELSPAC. *Cent. Eur. J. Public Health* 2001;9:59-63.

[53] 53. Nordeng H, Eskild A, Nesheim BI, Aursnes I, Jacobsen G. Drug use during early pregnancy. The impact of maternal illness, outcome of prior pregnancies and socio-demographic factors. *Eur. J. Clin. Pharmacol.* 2001;57:259-263.

[54] Pbert L, Ockene JK, Zapka J, et al. A community health center smoking-cessation intervention for pregnant and postpartum women. Am J Prev Med 2004;26:377-385.

[55] Penn G, Owen L. Factors associated with continued smoking during pregnancy: analysis of socio-demographic, pregnancy and smoking-related factors. *Drug Alcohol Rev.* 2002; 21:17-25.

[56] Lawrence T, Aveyard P, Cheng K, Griffin C, Johnson C, Croghan E. Does stage-based smoking cessation advice in pregnancy result in long-term quitters? 18-month postpartum follow-up of a randomized controlled trial. *Addiction* 2005;100:107-116.

[57] Ayanian JZ, Cleary PD. Perceived risks of heart disease and cancer among cigarette smokers. *JAMA* 1999;281:1019-1021.

[58] Haslam C, Draper E. Stage of change is associated with assessment of the health risks of maternal smoking among pregnant women. *Soc. Sci. Med.* 2000;51:1189-1196.

[59] Kleinjan M, van den Eijnden RJ, Dijkstra A, Brug J, Engels RC. Excuses to continue smoking: The role of disengagement beliefs in smoking cessation. *Addict Behav.* 2006;31:2223-2237.

[60] Peretti-Watel P, Halfen S, Gremy I. Risk denial about smoking hazards and readiness to quit among French smokers: An exploratory study. *Addict Behav.* 2007;32:377-383.

[61] Nasman P, Ortendahl M. Perceived consequences among pregnant and non-pregnant women of continuing or ceasing to smoke. *Int. J. Gynaecol. Obstet.* 2007 Jul 3.

[62] Murphy-Hoefer R, Alder S, Higbee C. Perceptions about cigarette smoking and risks among college students. *Nicotine Tob. Res.* 2004;6 Suppl 3: 371-374.

[63] Hampson SE, Andrews JA, Barckley M, Lichtenstein E, Lee ME. Conscientiousness, perceived risk, and risk-reduction behaviors: a preliminary study. *Health Psychol.* 2000; 19: 496-500.

[64] Oncken C, McKee S, Krishnan-Sarin S, O'Malley S, Mazure CM. Knowledge and perceived risk of smoking-related conditions: a survey of cigarette smokers. *Prev. Med.* 2005;40:779-784.

[65] Carbone JC, Kverndokk S, Rogeberg OJ. Smoking, health, risk, and perception. *J. Health Econ.* 2005; 24: 631-653.

[66] Larabie LC. To what extent do smokers plan quit attempts? *Tob. Control.* 2005 Dec;14(6): 425-428.

[67] Pickett KE, Wakschlag LS, Dai L, Leventhal BL. Fluctuations of maternal smoking during pregnancy. *Obstet. Gynecol.* 2003 Jan;101(1):140-147.

[68] Hughes JR, Keely JP, Fagerstrom KO, Callas PW.Intentions to quit smoking change over short periods of time. *Addict Behav.* 2005 May;30(4):653-362.

[69] Yu SM, Park CH, Schwalberg RH. Factors associated with smoking cessation among U.S. pregnant women. *Matern. Child Health J.* 2002 Jun;6(2):89-97.

In: Smoking and Women's Health   ISBN 978-1-60456-148-7
Editors: M.K. Wesley and I.A. Sternbach, pp.121-146   © 2008 Nova Science Publishers, Inc.

Chapter 4

A Review of Behavioral Interventions for Smoking Cessation and Weight Gain Prevention

Darla E. Kendzor[3], Lauren E. Baillie and Amy L. Copeland

University of Texas M.D. Anderson Cancer Center, Houston, Texas, USA
Louisiana State University, Baton Rouge, Louisiana, USA

Abstract

Research studies have consistently shown a relationship between smoking cessation and weight gain. Unfortunately, concern about postcessation weight gain prevents many individuals from attempting to quit smoking and may contribute to treatment attrition and relapse. Postcessation weight gain is currently of particular concern given the rising prevalence of overweight and obesity in the United States. Effective interventions that target both smoking cessation and postcessation weight gain are needed to address the public health concerns associated with smoking and obesity, in addition to the weight concerns that prevent many individuals from successfully quitting smoking. This chapter provides a qualitative review of the research on combined smoking cessation and behavioral weight control interventions. Fourteen studies that included dietary or physical activity components in combination with a smoking cessation intervention met the inclusion criteria for the present review. Overall, findings suggest that adjunctive weight management interventions provide little or no long-term weight control benefits, although such interventions do not generally have a negative impact on cessation outcomes. Future directions for research are discussed.

3 Corresponding Author: Darla E. Kendzor, Ph.D., University of Texas M. D. Anderson Cancer Center, Department of Health Disparities Research, Unit 125, 1515 Holcombe Boulevard, Houston, Texas 77030, Phone: (713) 745-8558, Fax: (713) 792-1152, Email: dkendzor@mdanderson.org.

Introduction

Cigarette smoking continues to be the leading cause of preventable death in the United States, with approximately 438,000 deaths from cancer, cardiovascular disease, and respiratory disease attributable to cigarette smoking annually (CDC, 2005a). Lung cancer is the most frequent cause of cancer death among adults who smoke and 90% of lung cancer cases are attributable to tobacco smoking (Levitz, Bradley, and Golden, 2004). Smoking reduces life expectancy by an average of 14 years, and 167 billion dollars are lost annually in health care costs and job productivity (CDC, 2005a). Although the prevalence of smoking has been declining in recent years, nearly 21% of adults in the United States continue to smoke (CDC, 2005b). Prevalence rates have remained high despite the societal costs and widespread knowledge of the health consequences of smoking. Innovative smoking cessation programs must be developed to address the specific concerns and difficulties of those who have been unable to quit smoking.

Research suggests that fear of postcessation weight gain and the use of smoking as a weight control strategy are frequently cited reasons why some individuals continue to smoke (Copeland, Martin, Geiselman, Rash, and Kendzor, 2006a; Klesges and Klesges, 1988; Namenek Brouwer and Pomerleau, 2000). Individuals who smoke weigh an average of eight lbs. less than non-smokers and additionally tend to gain less weight with age (Klesges, Meyers, Klesges, and La Vasque, 1989). In addition, the differences in weight between smokers and non-smokers are greater among women than men, and moderate smokers (i.e., 10-20 cigarettes per day) obtain greater weight control benefits from smoking than those who smoke more heavily (Klesges et al., 1989).

Across studies, smoking cessation has consistently been shown to result in significant weight gain (Klesges et al., 1989). Those who remain continuously abstinent for one year may expect to gain an average of 13 lbs. or approximately 6 kilograms (kg) of body weight (Klesges et al., 1997), and approximately 10% of males and 13% of females who quit smoking reportedly gain more than 13 kg or 29 lbs. (Williamson et al., 1991). Those who quit smoking are more likely than never-smokers to become and remain overweight or obese (Chiolero, Jacot-Sadowski, Faeh, Paccaud, and Cornuz, 2007; Flegal, Troiano, Pamuk, Kuczmarski, and Campbell, 1995), and an estimated 24% of the increase in the prevalence of overweight among men and 16% among women may be attributed to smoking cessation (Flegal et al., 1995).

Studies have indicated that postcessation weight gain may not be equal across racial/ethnic and gender groups. African Americans often suffer greater postcessation weight gain than Caucasians, and women gain tend to gain more weight postcessation than men (Filozof, Fernandez Pinilla, and Fernandez-Cruz, 2004; Klesges et al., 1989; Pisinger and Jorgensen, 2007; Williamson et al., 1991). Further, African Americans and women are at higher risk than Caucasians or men of gaining greater than 13 kg following smoking cessation (Williamson et al., 1991). Smoking may have a greater impact on body weight among African Americans, given the recent finding that resting energy expenditure among African Americans who smoke heavily may be greater than the resting energy expenditure of Caucasians who smoke heavily (Clemens, Klesges, Slawson, and Bush, 2003). In addition, there is initial evidence that Mexican Americans may be at greater risk than Caucasians of becoming overweight or obese postcessation (Burke, Hazuda, and Stern, 2000). Racial/ethnic differences in weight status may occur as a result of complex interactions among socioeconomic status, education, gender, and other related variables that affect health behaviors and access to health care (Wang and Beydoun, 2007). Such disparities are alarming given the high prevalence of obesity in the United States and the even higher prevalence of overweight and obesity among African Americans and Latinos (Sanchez-Johnson, 2005; Wang and Beydoun, 2007). As a result, researchers have called for the development of interventions that address the needs of specific racial/ethnic and gender groups (Sanchez-Johnson, 2005; Mazas and Wetter, 2003).

The mechanisms of postcessation weight gain likely involve changes in energy balance, including postcessation increases in caloric intake, decreases in resting energy expenditure, and decreases in energy expenditure during physical activity. Some, but not all, studies have demonstrated acute increases in energy intake following smoking cessation (Hall, McGee, Tunstall, Duffy, and Benowitz, 1989; Moffatt and Owens, 1991; Perkins, Epstein, and Pastor, 1990; Rodin, 1987; Stamford, Matter, Fell, and Papenek, 1986). Caloric intake has been found to increase by approximately 250 to 300 calories in the first few weeks following smoking cessation (Perkins, 1993). Some research has indicated that resting energy expenditure may decrease by four to 16 percent following smoking cessation (Dallosso and James, 1984; Filozof et al., 2004; Moffatt and Owens, 1991), although other studies have failed to find similar decreases (Ferrara, Kumar, Nicklas, McCrone, and Goldberg, 2001; Stamford et al., 1986). The findings of several studies suggest that smoking cessation is not associated with decreases in physical activity (Hall et al., 1989; Perkins et al., 1990; Stamford et al., 1986). However, there is evidence that energy expenditure may be greater among individuals who smoke during light physical activity (Perkins, Epstein, Marks, Stiller, and Jacob, 1989; Walker et al., 1999). Unfortunately, the potential metabolic and anorectic effects of smoking may deter many individuals from quitting smoking or lead to relapse related to weight gain during a quit attempt.

Studies have indicated that cessation-related weight concerns may negatively impact smoking cessation treatment outcomes and increase the risk of treatment attrition (Copeland et al., 2006a; Jeffery, Hennrikus, Lando, Murray, and Liu, 2000; Klesges et al., 1988; Meyers et al., 1997; Mizes et al., 1998; Streater, Sargent, and Ward, 1989; Wetter et al., 1999). However, postcessation weight gain (rather than weight concern) has been shown to be associated with continued smoking abstinence in many studies (Hall, Ginsberg, and Jones, 1986; Killen et al., 1996; Streater et al., 1989; Suchanek Hudman, Gritz, Clayton, Nisenbaum, 1999; Twardella et al., 2006). For example, Hall et al. (1986) reported that weight gain at 26 weeks postcessation predicted continued abstinence at one-year postcessation. However, only those who were continuously abstinent at week 26 were included in the analyses. Thus, individuals who may have relapsed due to weight gain or concern about weight gain prior to week 26 were not included in the analyses. Perhaps those who are willing to make smoking cessation their priority and accept some postcessation weight gain are more likely to successfully maintain continuous abstinence. In contrast, Pirie et al. (1992) reported that 51% of weight-concerned quitters who gained more than five lbs. by the end of an eight-week smoking cessation treatment had relapsed by the six-month follow-up visit, compared with a 40% relapse rate among quitters who gained less than five lbs. It is plausible that weight concern moderates the relationship between weight gain and relapse, such that weight gain is a risk factor for relapse and attrition only among those who are weight-concerned.

In summary, many individuals continue to smoke due to concern that they will gain weight following smoking cessation. Research has indicated that cessation of smoking is associated with a weight gain that is substantial for many individuals. The reasons for postcessation weight gain may include acute postcessation increases in caloric intake, decreases in resting metabolic rate, and decreases in energy expenditure during physical activity. Unfortunately, there is evidence that postcessation weight gain and weight gain concerns are associated with smoking relapse and treatment attrition within cessation interventions. It is plausible that changes in energy balance might potentially be attenuated through decreases in caloric intake and increases in physical activity after smoking cessation. Given the rise in overweight and obesity in the United States and the concerns about postcessation weight gain among many, effective interventions that target both smoking cessation and weight gain are needed. The present chapter will review treatment interventions that were developed to address both smoking cessation and weight gain prevention, and will provide directions for future research.

Method

This chapter will qualitatively review interventions that focused on both smoking cessation and weight gain prevention. Interventions that included a pharmacological component (e.g., nicotine replacement therapy) were included in the review only if the intervention incorporated additional dietary or physical activity components. Computerized searches of Medline and PsychInfo were conducted to identify published research studies written in English that examined the impact of smoking cessation and weight control interventions on weight gain and smoking cessation outcomes. Search terms included smoking, tobacco, smoking cessation, tobacco cessation, physical activity, exercise, weight gain prevention, and diet. The reference sections of related articles were examined to identify additional studies relevant to the present review. Treatment studies were excluded from the review if they did not report on both smoking cessation outcomes and postcessation weight gain (e.g., Hill, 1985; Martin et al., 1997; Taylor, Houston-Miller, Haskell, and Debusk, 1988), or did not utilize a comparison group (e.g., Talcott et al., 1995).

Fourteen studies met the inclusion criteria for the present review. Smoking cessation interventions were categorized for discussion by the primary focus of the adjunctive weight control intervention (i.e., physical activity, dietary, or combined diet and physical activity interventions). Studies were categorized as physical activity interventions if the purpose of the intervention was to increase physical activity levels in the absence of other behavioral targets related to weight management. Dietary interventions included those that aimed to decrease caloric intake, but did not target physical activity levels. Combined diet and physical activity interventions included those that targeted both diet and physical activity within the same intervention.

The primary outcome variables in the present review included point prevalence abstinence (PPA) from smoking, continuous abstinence from smoking (CA), and weight change. PPA refers to abstinence from smoking during a brief specified period of time (typically seven days) prior to the follow-up visit, while CA refers to an extended period of uninterrupted smoking abstinence (typically since the initial quit date). Both types of smoking outcomes were reported in the review when they were available. Weight change refers to any change in weight that has occurred over the course of the study. Numerical weight change values are presented in kg or lbs., and may reflect weight loss, weight maintenance, or weight gain. Other weight-related outcomes including BMI (kg/m²) and percent body fat were reported when available.

Results

Summary information for each of the 14 studies included in the review is provided in Table 1. The studies retained in the review had sample sizes ranging from 20 to 417 participants. Ten of the studies included women only, and most of the remaining studies included a primarily female sample. Only four of the studies reported on the racial/ethnic characteristics of their samples, and these studies included primarily Caucasian participants. Seven of the 14 studies yielded statistically significant weight gain prevention outcomes for the weight management intervention (Danielsson, Rossner, and Westin, 1999; Hall, Tunstall, Vila, and Duffy, 1992; Marcus et al., 1999; Marcus, Albrecht, Niaura, Abrams, and Thompson, 1991; Perkins et al., 2001; Prapavessis et al., 2007; Spring et al., 2004). However, only one study demonstrated long-tem weight control benefits for the intervention group relative to a comparison group (Perkins et al., 2001). Five of the studies demonstrated significantly improved cessation outcomes for a weight management intervention relative to a comparison group (Danielsson et al., 1999; Marcus et al., 1999; Marcus et al., 1991; Perkins et al., 2001; Pirie et al., 1992), and the cessation benefits were maintained at the long-term follow-up visit in all studies. It is important to note that most studies reported that the weight gain prevention intervention did not have a detrimental impact on cessation outcomes. In most cases, smoking cessation rates within the weight management intervention were similar to the cessation rates in the comparison group. The research studies included in the review are summarized below by the primary focus of the adjunctive weight management intervention.

Physical Activity Interventions

Eight studies were identified that evaluated the efficacy of interventions that included a physical activity component as an adjunct to a smoking cessation intervention (Jonsdottir and Jonsdottir, 2001; Marcus et al., 1999; Marcus et al., 1995; Marcus et al., 1991; Prapavessis et al., 2007; Russell, Epstein, Johnston, Block and Blair, 1988; Ussher, West, McEwen, Taylor, and Steptoe, 2003; Ussher, West, McEwen, Taylor, and Steptoe, in press). Russell et al. (1988) compared three interventions groups on weight change and smoking cessation rates in a randomized controlled trial. All groups received a one-week behavioral smoking cessation program in addition to 1) a walking and jogging program that met once per week for one hour, 2) group sessions during which general health education was provided on topics including stress management, muscle relaxation, diet and exercise, or 3) contact control who received only the smoking cessation intervention.

No significant differences were found between groups in smoking abstinence rates or weight change at the end of treatment, or at the three and six month follow-up visits.

It is notable that no improvements in fitness level were observed between from the end of treatment to the six month follow-up in the physical activity group, suggesting the possibility that participants did not maintain their physical activity levels post-treatment.

Marcus et al. (1991) compared two interventions groups that received either a four-week behavioral smoking cessation program alone or in combination with a 15-week exercise training program. The exercise training program included three 30 to 45 minute cycle ergometer training sessions each week. No contact control sessions were included for those who received only the smoking cessation intervention. By the 12-month follow-up visit, only the participants randomized to the exercise condition had remained abstinent. Results indicated that PPA rates were significantly greater by the end of treatment among those in the exercise condition. Participants who received the smoking cessation only intervention experienced a significant weight gain, while those receiving the additional exercise training did not (2 kg vs. 0 kg). Given that contact control sessions were not included for those who received only the smoking cessation treatment, it is unclear whether participants in the combined smoking cessation and exercise group simply benefited from the additional contact with treatment staff.

Marcus et al. (1995) later compared two intervention groups who received a 12-week behavioral smoking cessation intervention in addition to either 1) a 15-week cycle ergometer exercise program or 2) a 15-week contact control program. The exercise program was the same as in Marcus et al. (1991), and the contact control group received three health education lectures per week on topics such as nutrition and weight loss. The contact control group and the exercise group did not differ significantly in abstinence rates at 24 hours post-quit (90% vs. 80%), by the end of treatment, or at the one- (30% vs. 10%) and three-month follow-up visits (30% vs. 10%). Differences between groups may have reached significance if the sample size had been larger, thus providing greater power to detect meaningful differences between groups. In addition, no significant between-groups differences in weight change were found at the end of treatment, although it is notable that the contact control group maintained their baseline weight compared with a 2 kg weight loss in the exercise group.

Table 1. Summary of smoking cessation and weight gain prevention interventions

Study	Sample	Design and Intervention	Weight Outcomes	Smoking Outcomes
Russell, Epstein, Johnson, Block, and Blaire (1988)	$N = 42$; 100% female; Mean age = 28 ($\pm$7) years; Mean CPD = 23 ($\pm$7)	Design: RCT Intervention Groups: 1-week behavioral smoking cessation program plus 1) PA, 2) habit change information, or 3) contact control.	3 months: NS between-groups differences in weight gain. 6 months: NS between-groups differences in weight gain. 18 months: NS between-groups differences in weight gain.	3 months: NS between-groups differences 6 months: NS between-groups differences 18 months: NS between-groups differences
Marcus, Albrecht, Niaura, Abrams, and Thompson (1991)	$N=20$; 100% female; Ages 20-50 yrs; Smoked ≥ 10 CPD; Included women who exercised $\leq$ once per week	Design: RCT Intervention Groups: 1) 4-week behavioral smoking cessation program, or 2) 4-week behavioral smoking cessation program + concurrent 15-week exercise training program.	15 weeks: Participants who received smoking cessation treatment only experienced a significant weight gain, while those who received the exercise intervention did not experience a significant weight change (2 kg vs. 0 kg).	15 weeks: PPA was significantly greater among those who received the exercise program than among those who received behavioral smoking cessation treatment only (50% vs. 0%).
Hall, Tunstall, Vila, and Duffy (1992)	$N = 180$; 73% female; Smoked ≥ 10 CPD and/or 10% over ideal weight	Design: RCT Intervention Groups: 2-week group smoking cessation program including aversive smoking and relapse prevention plus 1) innovative diet and exercise intervention, 2) nonspecific weight-gain prevention, or 3) standard control that included an nutrition and exercise information packet.	6 weeks: NS between-groups differences. Innovative Group: NS differences between abstinent and non-abstinent participants. Nonspecific group: Abstinent participants gained more weight than non-abstinent participants (1.2 kg vs. .02 kg). Control Group: NS differences between abstinent and non-abstinent participants. 52 weeks: NS between-groups differences. Innovative Group: NS differences between abstinent and non-abstinent participants. Nonspecific group: Abstinent participants gained more weight than non-abstinent participants (3.35 kg vs. .44 kg). Control Group: Abstinent participants gained marginally more weight than non-abstinent participants (3.61 kg vs. .71 kg).	6 weeks: PPA was lower in the nonspecific group had than the control group (41% vs. 57%). 12 weeks: PPA was lower in the nonspecific group than the control group (25% vs. 44%). 26 weeks: PPA was lower in the innovative group than the control group (21% vs. 35%). 52 weeks: PPA was lower in the nonspecific group than the control group (22% vs. 35%).

Table 1. (Continued)

Study	Sample	Design and Intervention	Weight Outcomes	Smoking Outcomes
Pirie et al. (1992)	$N = 417$; 100% female; Ages 20-64 yrs; Included only women who wanted to maintain pre-cessation weight	Design: Randomized factorial trial Intervention Groups: 1) FFS 8-week group program, 2) FFS + behavioral weight control, 3) FFS + nicotine gum, or 4) FFS + behavioral weight control + nicotine gum	8 weeks: NS between-groups differences in weight gain. 6 months: NS between-groups differences in weight gain. 12 months: NS between-groups differences in weight gain.	8 weeks: Abstinence rates were highest for FFS + nicotine gum (PPA = 70%; CA = 68%), followed by FFS + behavioral weight control + nicotine gum (PPA = 60%; CA = 55%), FFS + behavioral weight control (PPA = 54%; CA = 44%), and FFS (PPA = 46%; CA = 38%). 6 Months: Abstinence rates were highest for FFS + nicotine gum (PPA = 49%; CA = 38%), followed by FFS + behavioral weight control + nicotine gum (PPA = 35%; CA = 24%), FFS + behavioral weight control (PPA = 32%; CA = 30%), and FFS (PPA = 22%; CA = 17%). 12 Months: Abstinence rates were highest for FFS + nicotine gum (PPA = 44%; CA = 32%), followed by FFS + behavioral weight control (PPA = 28%; CA = 23%), FFS + behavioral weight control + nicotine gum (PPA = 28%; CA = 14%), and FFS (PPA = 19%; CA = 15%).
Marcus et al. (1995)	$N = 20$; 100% female; Ages 22-56 yrs; Smoked 8-40 CPD; Included women who exercised vigorously $\leq$ once per week	Design: RCT Intervention Groups: 12-week behavioral smoking cessation program plus 1) 15-week exercise program, or 2) 15-week contact control.	15 weeks: No change in weight observed in either group.	1 month: NS between-groups differences. 3 months: NS between-groups differences. 12 months: NS between-groups differences.

Study	Sample	Design and Intervention	Weight Outcomes	Smoking Outcomes
Danielsson, Rossner, and Westin (1999)	N = 287; 100% female; Ages 30-60 yrs; Smoked ≥ 10 CPD; Included only women who wanted to maintain pre-cessation weight; BMI range 23-31	Design: RCT Intervention Groups: 16-week group behavioral smoking cessation program, nicotine gum, and behavioral weight control program plus 1) very low energy diet, or 2) no-diet control.	16 weeks: Abstinent participants in the low energy diet group lost 2.1 kg compared with a weight gain of 1.6 kg in the control group. 52 wks: NS between-groups differences in weight change.	16 weeks: CA was greater in the low energy diet group (50%) than in the control group (35%). 52 weeks: CA was greater in the low energy diet group (28%) than in the control group (16%).
Marcus et al. (1999)	N = 281; 100% female; Ages 18-65 yrs; Smoked ≥ 10 CPD; Included women who exercised < twice per week	Design: RCT Intervention Groups: 12-week group cognitive-behavioral smoking cessation program plus: 1) vigorous aerobic exercise, or 2) contact control.	8 weeks: Abstinent participants in the exercise group gained less weight than those in the control group (3.03 kg vs. 5.36 kg) 20 weeks: NS between-groups differences in weight gain. 60 weeks: NS between-groups differences in weight gain.	8 weeks: Abstinence rates were higher in the exercise group than the control group (CA = 19% vs. 10%). 20 weeks: Abstinence rates were higher in the exercise group than the control group (PPA = 25% vs. 14%; CA = 16% vs. 8%). 60 weeks: Abstinence rates were higher in the exercise group than the control group (CA = 12% vs. 5%).
Jonsdottir and Jonsdottir (2001)	N = 67; 49% female	Design: Quasi-Experimental Intervention Groups: 1) NRT + health education + group counseling (1 month) + individual counseling (1 year) or 2) NRT + health education + group counseling (2 months) + individual counseling (1 year) + exercise	1 year: NS between-groups differences in weight gain.	1 year: NS between-groups differences.

Table 1. (Continued)

Study	Sample	Design and Intervention	Weight Outcomes	Smoking Outcomes
Perkins et al. (2001)	$N = 219$; 100% female; Ages 18-65 yrs; Included only women who were concerned about postcessation weight gain	Design: RCT Intervention Groups: 7-week cognitive-behavioral group smoking cessation counseling plus 1) behavioral weight control focused on reduction of caloric intake, 2) CBT to reduce weight-concern, or 3) group contact control.	4 weeks: Abstinent participants in the behavioral weight control (.6 kg vs. 2.2 kg) and CBT groups (1.1 kg vs. 2.2 kg) gained less weight than those in the control group. 3 months: NS between-groups differences. 6 months: Abstinent participants in the CBT group gained less weight than those in the control group (2.9 kg vs. 6.4 kg). 12 months: Abstinent participants in the CBT group gained less weight than those in the control group (2.5 kg vs. 7.7 kg).	4 weeks: CA was greater in the CBT group than the control group (56% vs. 31%). 3 months: NS between-groups differences 6 months: CA was greater in the CBT group than the control group (28% vs. 12%). 12 months: CA was greater in the CBT group than the control group (15% vs. 7%).
Ussher, West, McEwen, Taylor, and Steptoe (2003) Ussher, West, McEwen, Taylor, and Steptoe (in press)	$N = 299$; 62.9% female; 87.9% Caucasian; Ages 18-65 years; Smoked ≥ 10 CPD; Included individuals who engaged in < 30 minutes of moderate PA 5 days per week or <20 minutes of vigorous PA 3 days per week	Design: RCT Intervention Groups: 1) 7-week cognitive-behavioral smoking cessation program + NRT + exercise, or 2) 7-week cognitive-behavioral smoking cessation program + NRT + contact control.	6 weeks: NS between-groups differences in weight gain, BMI, and percent body fat. 12 months: Abstinent participants in the exercise group gained marginally less weight than those in the control group (3.9 kg vs. 7.2 kg).	6 weeks: NS between-groups differences in CA. 12 months: NS between-groups differences in CA.

Study	Sample	Design and Intervention	Weight Outcomes	Smoking Outcomes
Spring et al. (2004)	$N = 315$; 100% female; 66% Caucasian, 31% African American; Ages 20-75 years; Smoked $\geq$ 10 CPD	Design: RCT Intervention Groups: 16-week group behavioral smoking cessation program plus 1) early diet/PA group (1st 8 weeks), 2) late diet/PA group (2nd 8 weeks), or 3) control group with weight loss-counseling at the end of treatment (week 16).	7 weeks: The early diet group gained less weight than the control group. 9 months: NS between-groups differences in weight gain. However, weight gain slowed significantly over time for those in the late diet group.	Week 7 to 9 months: NS between-groups differences in PPA over time.
Copeland, Martin, Geiselman, Rash, and Kendzor (2006)	$N = 79$; 100% female; 89.5% Caucasian, 10.5% African American; Mean age 36.5 ($\pm$8.1); Smoked $\geq$ 10 CPD; Included only weight-concerned women	Design: Randomized Trial Intervention Groups: 2-week cognitive-behavioral group smoking cessation treatment + NRT plus 1) individually tailored cessation maintenance and weight control sessions, or 2) group cessation maintenance and weight control sessions.	3 months: NS between-groups differences in weight gain. 6 months: NS between-groups differences in weight gain.	3 months: PPA was greater among participants in the tailored intervention than in the group intervention (24% vs. 14%). 6 months: PPA was greater among participants in the tailored intervention than in the group intervention (21% vs. 8%).

Table 1. (Continued)

Study	Sample	Design and Intervention	Weight Outcomes	Smoking Outcomes
Prapavessis et al. (2007)	$N = 142$; 100% female; Ages 18-62 years; Smoked ≥ 10 CPD; Included only women who exercised < 30 minutes twice per week	Design: Randomized Factorial Trial Intervention Groups: 1) Exercise + nicotine patch, 2) exercise only, 3) CBT + nicotine patch, or 4) CBT only.	12 weeks: Participants in the exercise groups gained less weight than those in the CBT groups. 52 weeks: NS between-groups differences in weight gain.	6 weeks: CBT + nicotine patch group produced greater PPA than the exercise only group (81% vs. 51%). Exercise + nicotine patch group produced greater PPA than the exercise only group (85% vs. 51%). CA was greater in the groups that received patches than those that did not (73% vs. 53%). 18 weeks: NS between-groups differences in PPA or CA. 52 weeks: CBT only group produced greater PPA than the exercise only group (44% vs. 17%). CBT + nicotine patch group produced greater PPA than the exercise only group (42% vs. 17%). Exercise + nicotine patch group produced greater PPA than the exercise only group (36% vs. 17%).

Note: CA = continuous abstinence; CBT = cognitive behavioral therapy; CPD = cigarettes per day; NRT = nicotine replacement therapy; NS = non-significant; PA = physical activity; PPA = point prevalence; RCT = randomized controlled trial.

More recently, Marcus et al. (1999) compared two intervention groups who received a 12-week behavioral smoking cessation intervention in addition to either 1) a 15-week vigorous aerobic exercise program or 2) a 15-week contact control program that included general health-related lectures, films, and handouts. CA rates were greater at the end of treatment among those in the exercise group than in the contact control group (19.4% vs. 10.2%), and the exercise group maintained significantly greater CA rates at the 20- and 60-week follow-up visits (16.4% vs. 8.2%; 11.9% vs. 5.4%). Further, abstinent participants in the exercise group gained significantly less weight at the end of treatment than participants in the control group (3.03 kg vs. 5.36 kg). Unfortunately, the weight-control benefit was not maintained at either the 20- or 60-week follow-up visits. The authors suggested that the weight control effects of the exercise program may have disappeared at the follow-up visits due to low rates of post-treatment physical activity maintenance. In support of this explanation, only 10% of participants randomized to the exercise group reported that had engaged in regular exercise in the 12 months following treatment completion.

Jonsdottir and Jonsdottir (2001) compared the efficacy of two smoking cessation interventions in a quasi-experimental design. Participants enrolled at either of two locations and paid for the intervention that was delivered at the location of their choice. Participants received 1) nicotine replacement therapy, group counseling for two months, individual counseling for one year, and health education or 2) nicotine replacement therapy, group counseling for one month, individual counseling for one year, health education, and a six-month exercise program that involved three 40 to 80 minute sessions per week. The exercise intervention was more expensive for participants than the standard intervention. No between groups differences were observed in CA rates or self-reported weight gain after one year, although 40% of the participants in the study were unwilling to report their weight at the conclusion of the intervention.

Ussher et al. (2003) compared two interventions that each included a seven-week cognitive-behavioral smoking cessation program and the nicotine patch in addition to either 1) brief exercise counseling during each treatment session or 2) a contact control program during which health advice was provided during treatment sessions. During the brief exercise counseling sessions, participants were advised to gradually increase to 30 minutes or more of moderate to vigorous physical activity on five or more days per week. The health advice received by those in the contact control group focused on eating healthfully, alcohol use, and stress management. No significant between groups differences in CA rates, weight change, body mass index (BMI), or percentage of body fat were observed between groups at six weeks post-quit. Similarly, no differences in CA rates were reported at the 12-month follow-up visit, although participants in the exercise intervention gained marginally less weight than those in the control group (3.9 kg vs. 7.2 kg; Ussher et al., in press).

Prapavessis et al. (2007) compared the efficacy of four interventions in a randomized factorial trial. The intervention groups were 1) 12-week cognitive behavioral cessation program, 2) 12-week aerobic exercise training program, 3) 12-week cognitive behavioral cessation program plus a 10-week supply of the nicotine patch, and 4) 12-week aerobic exercise training program exercise plus a 10-week supply of the nicotine patch. Higher PPA rates were found at the end of treatment in the two groups that received the nicotine patch than in the exercise only group. Further, CA was greater in the groups that received the nicotine patch than in those that did not. At the 52-week follow-up visit, PPA rates were greatest among participants in the group that received only the smoking cessation intervention (44%), followed by the smoking cessation intervention in combination with NRT (42%), exercise training in combination with NRT (36%), and exercise training alone (17%). However, participants randomized to the exercise groups gained significantly less weight by the end of treatment than participants in the cognitive behavioral smoking cessation groups. Unfortunately, this weight control effect disappeared by the 12-month follow-up visit. It is possible that participants had difficulty maintaining the exercise routine after the intervention was completed and were therefore unable to maintain the reductions in weight gain.

Overall, the results of these studies provide minimal evidence that adding a physical activity component to a standard smoking cessation treatment may improve smoking abstinence rates. The findings of two studies suggest that abstinence rates may improve within interventions that include an exercise component (Marcus et al., 1991; Marcus et al., 1999), while the remaining six studies failed to find any benefit of including an exercise component (Jonsdottir and Jonsdottir, 2001; Marcus et al., 1995; Prapavessis et al., 2007; Russell et al., 1988; Ussher et al., 2003; Ussher et al., in press). The findings of Prapavessis et al. (2007) indicate that exercise training alone and in combination with nicotine replacement therapy may actually result in poorer cessation outcomes than cognitive behavioral smoking cessation treatment alone or in combination with NRT.

Similarly, research studies have indicated that adding an exercise component to a smoking cessation intervention has a minimal effect on postcessation weight gain. Four of the studies reviewed found no differences in weight gain between groups receiving a physical activity intervention and those that did not include a physical activity component (Russell et al., 1988; Marcus et al., 1995; Ussher et al., 2003, Jonsdottir and Jonsdottir, 2001). Marcus et al. (1999) and Prapavessis et al. (2007) reported that participants who received exercise training in addition to smoking cessation treatment gained significantly less weight than those who did not receive a physical activity intervention, although the weight gain prevention effect reported in these studies did not persist beyond the end of treatment. Ussher et al. (in press) reported that individuals who participated in an exercise intervention gained marginally less weight than those in the control group after one year. Finally, Marcus et al. (1991) reported that individuals who participated in a smoking cessation intervention experienced significant weight gain, while those in the physical activity intervention did not. In the studies which found a significant effect of physical activity on weight gain, the interventions seemed only to delay postcessation weight gain until the end of treatment. It is possible that post-treatment weight gain may occur as a result of poor maintenance of regular physical activity after the treatment has concluded.

Dietary Interventions

Two studies were identified that evaluated the efficacy of interventions that included a dietary component as an adjunct to a smoking cessation intervention (Danielsson et al., 1999; Perkins et al., 2001). Danielsson et al. (1999) compared two intervention groups that each included a 16-week group behavioral smoking cessation program, a minimum three-month supply of nicotine gum, and a behavioral weight management program in addition to either 1) intermittent very low energy diet (1.76 MJ/day) or 2) a no-diet control group. Weight-concerned females randomized to the intermittent very low energy diet group were placed on the diet for three separate two- week periods during the 16-week cessation program.

Results indicated that CA rates were significantly greater among those who received the intermittent low energy diet than among those in the control group at the end of treatment (50% vs. 35%). CA rates remained greater among those in the low energy diet group than in the control group after 52 weeks (28% vs. 16%). Among those who successfully quit smoking, participants who received the dietary intervention gained significantly less weight than their control group counterparts at the end of treatment (-2.1 kg vs. +1.6 kg). However, this effect was not maintained at the 52-week follow-up visit. These findings suggest that a low energy diet may be a useful means by which to delay postcessation weight gain within smoking cessation treatment interventions.

Perkins et al. (2001) compared participants randomized to three interventions that each included seven weeks of cognitive behavioral smoking cessation counseling in addition to 1) behavioral weight control focused on reducing snacking and total caloric intake, 2) cognitive-behavioral treatment to reduce weight concerns and to help participants accept modest weight gain, or 3) contact control involving cessation-related discussion groups. At the end of treatment, CA rates were significantly greater among participants who received the cognitive-behavioral treatment to reduce weight concerns than the control group (56% vs. 31%). CA rates remained higher among those who received the cognitive-behavioral treatment than among those in the control group at the six and 12-month follow-up visits (28% vs. 12%; 15% vs. 7%). Interestingly, no differences in continuous abstinence rates were found between the cognitive-behavioral treatment and behavioral weight control groups.

Participants in the cognitive-behavioral and behavioral weight control groups showed significantly less weight gain at the end of treatment (1.1 kg and .6 kg) than participants the control group (2.2 kg). Weight gain remained significantly lower in the cognitive-behavioral treatment group than in the control group at the six- (2.9 kg vs. 6.4 kg) and 12-month follow-up visits (2.5 kg vs. 7.7 kg). No differences in weight gain were found between the behavioral weight control and control group at any follow-up visit. Findings suggest that cognitive-behavioral treatment to reduce weight concerns may be more helpful than behavioral weight control interventions aimed at reducing postcessation weight gain.

In summary, only two studies included an adjunctive weight management intervention that focused primarily on reducing caloric intake. Danielsson et al. (1999) reported that an intermittent low-energy diet resulted in weight loss at the end of treatment, while participants in the control group gained weight. However, this effect did not persist to the 52-week follow-up visit. Perkins et al. (2001) reported that participants randomized to a cognitive-behavioral intervention aimed at reducing weight concerns or a behavioral weight control intervention experienced less weight gain than a contact control group at the end of treatment. This effect persisted at the six and 12-month follow-up visits among those randomized to the cognitive-behavioral intervention, but not among those randomized to the behavioral weight control intervention.

Overall, the two studies that included a dietary weight management intervention showed improved smoking cessation rates relative to a comparison group. Danielsson et al. (1999) reported that CA rates were greater among those randomized to the intermittent low energy diet condition than those in the control group, both at the end of treatment and at the 52 week follow-up visit. Perkins et al. (2001) reported improved CA rates among those randomized to a cognitive-behavioral treatment aimed at reducing weight concerns (rather that body weight) relative to a control group at the end of treatment, and at the six and 12-month follow-up visits. Conversely, the behavioral weight control intervention produced cessation outcomes that were similar to the control group.

Combined Physical Activity and Dietary Interventions

Four studies were identified that evaluated the efficacy of interventions that included dietary and physical activity components as adjuncts to a smoking cessation intervention (Copeland, Martin, Geiselman, Rash, and Kendzor, 2006b; Hall et al., 1992; Pirie et al., 1992; Spring et al., 2004). Hall et al. (1992) compared three interventions that each included a two-week group smoking cessation program involving aversive smoking and relapse prevention skills training. Participants were randomized to either 1) a control group that received a nutrition and exercise packet, 2) an innovative weight gain prevention program, or 3) a non-specific weight gain prevention intervention. The control group did not meet during the four weeks when the weight gain prevention components of the innovative and non-specific treatment groups were administered. The four-week innovative weight gain prevention intervention included daily monitoring of weight, caloric reduction contingent on a weight gain of two lbs., an exercise plan in which the participant was encouraged to engage in an activity of their own choosing on three or more days per week, and behavioral self-management training (e.g., identifying antecedents to overeating, eating more slowly, limiting eating to specific locations in the home). The four-week nonspecific weight gain prevention intervention was based on an insight-oriented rationale and involved discussion of eating habits, the provision of information about nutrition and exercise, group support, and therapy.

No significant differences in weight change were found between the intervention groups at six or 52 weeks. However, weight change did not differ between those who abstained from smoking and those who had resumed smoking at six and 52 weeks in the innovative intervention. These findings suggest that the innovative intervention was successful at preventing postcessation weight gain. Conversely, abstinent participants in the non-specific intervention group gained more weight than those who were not abstinent at six and 52 weeks. No differences in weight change were found between abstainers and non-abstainers in the control group after six weeks, although abstinent participants gained marginally more weight after 52 weeks than the non-abstinent participants (3.61 kg vs. .71 kg). Findings suggest that the innovative weight gain prevention intervention may have reduced postcessation weight gain among abstainers relative to the control and non-specific treatment groups.

PPA rates were significantly lower in the non-specific weight gain prevention intervention than in the standard treatment group at six, 12, and 52 weeks. The odds of relapse were significantly greater in the innovative weight gain prevention intervention than in the control group at 26 weeks and marginally greater at 12 and 52 weeks. Further, the risk of relapse was greater in the combined non-specific and innovative interventions than in the standard treatment intervention at weeks six, 12, 26, and 52 weeks. Although findings suggest that the innovative weight gain prevention program may have prevented some weight gain among abstinent participants, the odds of relapse appeared to increase in both of the weight gain prevention groups (i.e., innovative and non-specific) relative to the control group.

Pirie et al. (1992) compared four intervention groups using a randomized factorial design. All groups participated in the eight week Freedom from Smoking (FFS) program developed by the American Lung Association. The intervention groups were as follows: 1) FFS alone, 2) FFS and a behavioral weight control intervention, FFS and nicotine gum, and 4) FFS, the behavioral weight control intervention, and nicotine gum. The FFS program focused on cognitive-behavioral skills training and social support. In the groups that received the behavioral weight control intervention, participants were encouraged to decrease their caloric intake by 100 to 300 calories per day and walk for one hour on three days each week. In the two groups that received nicotine gum, a supply of gum was provided throughout treatment and for the three months following completion of the treatment.

No significant differences in weight change between groups were found among participants who were continuously abstinent for 12 months. PPA and CA rates were greatest at eight weeks (end of treatment) and at the six and 12-month follow-up visits among participants who received the FFS program in combination with nicotine gum. Conversely, participants who received only the FFS program had the lowest PPA and CA rates at eight weeks and the six and 12-month follow up visits. Participants who received the behavioral weight control program in combination with either FFS alone or FFS and nicotine gum had PPA and CA rates that fell between the other two interventions. Findings suggest that adding a weight control component to a standard smoking cessation intervention does not necessarily have a detrimental impact on abstinence rates. Participants in the groups that received the weight control intervention did at least as well as those who received only the FFS intervention. It is notable that the weight control component did not produce significant differences in weight change between the intervention groups. However, abstainers and those who returned to smoking were not compared within each condition to determine whether similar weight gain had occurred.

Spring et al. (2004) compared three intervention groups in a randomized controlled trial. Each of the three groups received a 16-week cognitive-behavioral group smoking cessation intervention in combination with 1) an early weight management intervention delivered during the first eight weeks of smoking cessation treatment, 2) a late weight management intervention delivered during the last eight weeks of the smoking cessation treatment, or 3) a control group. The dietary component of the early and late diet interventions involved a prepackaged meal plan that provided a high-carbohydrate and low-fat diet containing 150 fewer calories than the typical daily intake of each participant. Participants were encouraged to engage in 30 minutes of moderate physical activity on at least five days per week, and participants walked for 30 minutes with the group after each treatment session during the weight management module. The control group received weight loss counseling during week 16 of the smoking cessation intervention.

Participants in the early diet group experienced significantly less weight gain than those in the control group at week seven, although no differences were found in weight gain after nine months post-quit. However, analysis indicated that the weight gain had slowed significantly over time for those in the late diet group. At nine months post-quit, participants had gained 6.20 lbs. in the control group, 7.57 lbs. in the early diet group, and 4.88 lbs. in the late diet group. No significant differences in PPA rates were found between groups over time (i.e., visit seven through nine months post-quit). At nine-months post-quit, PPA rates were 18.2% for those in the control group, 21.4% for those in the early diet group, and 19.5% for those in the late diet group. Overall, findings suggest that adding a weight management component to smoking cessation treatment does not negatively impact cessation outcomes, and that weight management interventions delivered later in smoking cessation treatment may slow postcessation weight gain.

Recently, Copeland et al. (2006b) compared the efficacy of two intervention groups for weight-concerned females that each received a two-week cognitive-behavioral group smoking cessation intervention and an eight-week supply of the nicotine patch in addition to either 1) individual tailored smoking cessation maintenance and weight gain prevention follow-up sessions or 2) group smoking cessation maintenance and weight gain prevention follow-up sessions. Participants in both intervention groups met with clinical psychologists, registered dieticians, and exercise physiologists in either an individual or group format. Individual and group follow-up sessions focused on relapse prevention as well as dietary and exercise strategies for weight management.

No differences in weight gain were found between the treatment interventions. However, PPA rates were greater among participants in the individually tailored intervention than in the group intervention at the three and six month follow-up visits (23.7% vs. 13.9% and 21.1% vs. 8.3% respectively). Further, participants in the individual, tailored intervention had marginally higher CA rates after three and six months (20% vs. 13.9% and 17.5% vs. 8.3% respectively). Interestingly, treatment type (individual vs. group) moderated the relationship between weight gain and smoking relapse, such that weight gain was more strongly associated with relapse among participants in the group intervention than among those assigned to the individual intervention.

In summary, smoking cessation outcomes have been mixed within smoking cessation interventions that have included both dietary and physical activity components. Two studies have indicated that adding a combination of dietary and physical activity components to a smoking cessation intervention does not negatively impact cessation outcomes (Pirie et al., 1992; Spring et al., 2004), while the findings of another study have suggested that adding these components may have a detrimental effect on smoking cessation (Hall et al., 1992). The study conducted by Hall et al. (1992) was different from the other two studies in at least two potentially important ways: 1) males were included in the intervention and 2) participants were instructed to initiate caloric reduction following a two pound weight gain rather than advising more permanent changes in their eating habits regardless of their weight. It is possible that males may have responded less favorably to the weight control intervention than females, and daily weighing and weight gain contingent caloric reduction may have been too complex or effortful for participants who were also attempting to quit smoking. Establishing a consistently healthful and reduced calorie diet may help individuals to develop new habits that require less effort over time with practice. Finally, the findings of Copeland et al. (2006b) suggest that utilizing an individualized format for delivering dietary and physical activity components within cessation interventions may produce better smoking cessation outcomes than interventions delivered in a group format.

Weight outcomes have also been mixed across studies of combined physical activity and dietary interventions. The findings of two studies have suggested the possibility that combined dietary and physical activity interventions may reduce postcessation weight gain (Hall et al., 1992; Spring et al., 2004), while other research suggests that such interventions have failed to prevent weight gain (Pirie et al., 1992). Hall et al. (1992) found no differences in weight gain at 52 weeks between abstinent and non-abstinent participants receiving the innovative weight control intervention, although abstinent participants gained marginally more weight than the non-abstinent participants in the control group. Spring et al. (2004) reported that participants who received the dietary and physical activity intervention during the first eight weeks of smoking cessation treatment gained less weight by the end of treatment than the control group. However, the weight control effects of the early diet intervention did not endure. Participants who received the dietary and physical activity intervention during the last eight weeks of the smoking cessation intervention experienced slowed weight gain over time relative to the early diet intervention and the control group. Finally, Copeland et al. (2006b) found that individual and group sessions produced similar weight outcomes suggesting that the format for delivery of weight management information may not be as important as it is for smoking cessation.

Conclusion

In summary, combined smoking cessation and weight management interventions have not been particularly effective at preventing postcessation weight gain in the long-term. There is some evidence that adjunctive weight management interventions focused primarily on increasing physical activity may offer modest short-term weight gain prevention benefits (Marcus et al., 1999; Marcus et al., 1991; Prapavessis et al., 2007), although not all studies agree (Marcus et al., 1995; Ussher et al., 2003). Similarly, adjunctive weight control interventions that focus primarily on reducing caloric intake may have a short-term weight gain prevention effect (Danielsson et al., 1999; Perkins et al., 2001). One study showed that the use of an intermittent very low energy diet produced initial weight loss among individuals participating in a smoking cessation program, although there was no long-term weight gain prevention relative to the control group. Interestingly, cognitive-behavioral therapy to reduce weight concerns (rather than weight gain) was associated with reduced weight gain relative to a control group at the 12-month follow-up visit (Perkins et al., 2001). The few smoking cessation interventions that have included both dietary and exercise components have produced modest, if any, weight control benefit (Hall et al., 1992; Pirie et al., 1992; Spring et al., 2004), although the findings of one study suggests that weight control interventions delivered later in treatment may slow the rate of postcessation weight gain (Spring et al., 2004).

It is important to note that most studies that included an adjunctive weight management intervention did not have a detrimental impact on smoking cessation outcomes (Jonsdottir and Jonsdottir, 2001; Marcus et al., 1995; Perkins et al., 2001; Russell et al, 1988; Spring et al., 2004; Ussher et al., 2003; Ussher et al., in press), and in several studies the addition of a weight management component was associated with improved cessation outcomes relative to a comparison group (Danielsson et al., 1999; Marcus et al., 1991; Marcus et al., 1999; Pirie et al., 1992). With regard to physical activity interventions, the majority of studies reported that cessation outcomes did not improve relative to a comparison group (Jonsdottir and Jonsdottir, 2001; Marcus et al., 1995; Prapavessis et al., 2007; Russell et al., 1988; Ussher et al., 2003, Ussher et al., in press), although two studies noted greater cessation rates within the physical activity intervention (Marcus et al., 1991; Marcus et al., 1999). Studies of dietary interventions have indicated that the inclusion of an intermittent very low energy diet may be associated with increased abstinence rates after one year (Danielsson et al., 1999). Interestingly, a cognitive-behavioral therapy to reduce weight concerns, but not a dietary weight control intervention, was associated with increased abstinence rates after 12 months (Perkins et al., 2001). Only one cessation intervention that included both dietary and physical activity components has produced superior abstinence rates relative to a comparison group (Pirie et al., 1992). No differences between groups were found in another study that tested a combined dietary, physical, activity, and smoking cessation intervention (Spring et al., 2004), and the remaining study reported a marginally significant negative impact of the combined dietary and physical activity intervention on cessation outcomes (Hall et al., 1992). Finally, the findings of one study has indicated that smoking cessation interventions which include a weight control component may be more effective at improving outcomes cessation when delivered in an individualized rather than a group format (Copeland et al., 2006b).

Researchers should consider utilizing larger sample sizes and factorial designs in order to determine the relative efficacy of specific treatment components for smoking cessation and/or weight gain prevention. The individual and combined benefits of specific weight management components such as vigorous exercise, moderate physical activity, low energy diet, and moderate caloric restriction within smoking cessation interventions remain unclear. In addition, more research is needed to determine the optimal timing of the weight management intervention relative to the quit date. The findings of Spring et al. (2004) suggest that the weight management component may have a more beneficial effect on weight outcomes if the intervention begins a few weeks after the quit date. However, the minimum duration of the weight control intervention that would be required in order to improve abstinence rates and/or prevent weight gain remains to be determined. It may be beneficial to monitor post-treatment diet and exercise habits to verify continued adherence with the weight management components of the treatment. Periodic follow-up sessions that involve supervised physical activity, informational review sessions, or goal-setting may help to facilitate the maintenance of post-treatment diet and physical activity habits.

Combined behavioral and pharmacological interventions for weight gain may provide weight gain prevention benefits in excess of either treatment alone. Pharmacological interventions such as nicotine gum and naltrexone have demonstrated some weight control benefits among those attempting smoking cessation (e.g., Doherty, Militello, Kinnunen, and Garvey, 1996; King et al., 2006; Nordstrom, Kinnunen, Utman, and Garvey, 1999; O'Malley et al., 2006). However, it is unclear whether the weight control effects of pharmacological interventions persist beyond the discontinuation of the medications. Thus, behavioral interventions in combination with pharmacological interventions may facilitate both initial and prolonged weight gain prevention for those who are concerned about postcessation weight gain.

Effective smoking cessation and weight management interventions that specifically target overweight and obese individuals must be developed in order to prevent or limit additional weight gain. Recent research suggests that nearly five percent of adults in the United Status are currently smoking and are also obese, and the prevalence of comorbid smoking and obesity among African Americans is even higher at approximately seven percent (Healton, Vallone, McCausland, Xiao, and Green, 2006). This is of particular importance given the potentially synergistic contribution of obesity and cigarette smoking to the development of cardiovascular disease (Van Gaal, Mertens, and De Block, 2006), and the increased risk of circulatory disease mortality among obese individuals who smoke (Freedman et al., 2006). Multiple behavior change interventions that address cigarette smoking, overweight/obesity, and sedentary lifestyles may be particularly useful in medical settings where the prevalence of chronic health problems related to these behaviors is greater.

Other medical populations, such as individuals seeking weight loss surgery, may also benefit from multiple behavior change interventions. It is relatively common for obese individuals who are candidates for weight loss surgery to be advised that they must simultaneously quit smoking, engage in more physical activity, and eat more healthfully prior to surgery. Such behavioral changes are particularly important given that greater pre-surgery weight and current smoking are associated with greater risk of postoperative complications (Livingston, Arterburn, Schifftner, Henderson and De Palma, 2006). A recent study indicated that nearly 27% of weight loss surgery candidates were current smokers, and that the average self-reported postcessation weight gain during previous quit attempts within this population was greater than 28 lbs. (Levine, Kalarchian, Courcoulas, Wisinski, and Marcus, 2007). Thus, individuals seeking weight loss surgery may be at increased risk of suffering greater postcessation weight gain and may find interventions that address both smoking cessation and weight management to be of benefit prior to surgery.

Finally, the efficacy of combined smoking cessation and weight management interventions within specific racial/ethnic and gender groups is not clear. Ten of the 14 studies reviewed in the present chapter included women only, and most of the remaining studies utilized primarily female samples. It is likely that men who are concerned about postcessation weight gain or who have obesity-related health problems would also benefit from interventions targeting postcessation weight gain and smoking cessation. Most of the studies reviewed failed to describe the demographic characteristics of their samples, and none of the studies compared the efficacy of the interventions among racial/ethnic groups. As a result, it is unclear for which racial/ethnic groups such interventions may be beneficial. Research is needed to determine which racial/ethnic groups may benefit from combined smoking cessation and weight gain prevention programs. Further, interventions that address the needs of specific populations must be developed.

Several limitations of the present review should be noted. The search strategy utilized in the present review could be considered narrow, given that only studies which included both weight and smoking cessation outcomes were included. Thus, cessation interventions that included components known to affect weight were excluded if they did not measure postcessation weight change. The qualitative nature of the review and the inclusion of studies with a wide variety of study designs, methodology, sample characteristics, and follow-up lengths limited the ability to directly compare the efficacy of specific intervention components and to draw conclusions. None of the studies included in the review reported on follow-up visits beyond 18 months, thus limiting the ability to draw conclusions about the long-term benefits of smoking cessation and weight management interventions. Nevertheless, the present review summarizes the current literature and provides direction for future research. Researchers are encouraged to utilize the information presented in the review in order to develop innovative interventions or improve existing interventions for individuals who would like to quit smoking and are also concerned about postcessation weight gain.

References

Burke, J. P., Hazuda, H. P., and Stern, M. P. (2000). Rising trend in obesity in Mexicans Americans and non-Hispanic whites: Is it due to cigarette smoking cessation. *International Journal of Obesity, 24,* 1689-1694.

Centers for Disease Control and Prevention (CDC). (2005a). Annual smoking-attributable mortality, years of potential life lost, and productivity losses - United States, 1997–2001. *Morbidity and Mortality Weekly Report, 54,* 625-628.

Centers for Disease Control and Prevention (CDC). (2005b). Cigarette Smoking Among Adults – United States, 2004. *Morbidity and Mortality Weekly Report, 54,* 1121-1124.

Chiolero, A., Jacot-Sadowski, I., Faeh, D., Paccaud, F., and Cornuz, J. (2007). Association of cigarettes smoked daily with obesity in a general population. *Obesity, 15,* 1311-1318.

Clemens, L. H., Klesges, R. C., Slawson, D. L., and Bush, A. J. (2003). Cigarette smoking is associated with energy balance in premenopausal African-American adult women differently than in similarly aged white women. *International Journal of Obesity, 27,* 1219-1226.

Copeland, A. L., Martin, P. D., Geiselman, P. J., Rash, C. J., and Kendzor, D. E. (2006a). Predictors of pretreatment attrition from smoking cessation among pre- and post-menopausal, weight-concerned women. *Eating Behaviors, 7,* 243-251.

Copeland, A. L., Martin, P. D., Geiselman, P. J., Rash, C. J., and Kendzor, D. E. (2006b). Smoking cessation for weight-concerned women: Group vs. individually tailored, dietary, and weight-control follow-up sessions. *Addictive Behaviors, 31,* 115-127.

Dallosso, H. M., and James, W. P. (1984). The role of smoking in the regulation of energy balance. *International Journal of Obesity, 8,* 365-375.

Danielsson, T., Rossner, S., and Westin, A. (1999). Open randomized trial of intermittent very low energy diet together with nicotine gum for stopping smoking in women who gained weight in previous attempts to quit. *British Medical Journal, 319,* 490-494.

Doherty, K., Militello, F. S., Kinnunen, T., and Garvey, A. J. (1996). Nicotine gum dose and weight gain after smoking cessation. *Journal of Consulting and Clinical Psychology, 64,* 799-807.

Ferrara, C. M., Kumar, M., Nicklas, B., McCrone, S., and Goldberg, A. P. (2001). Weight gain and adipose tissue metabolism after smoking cessation in women. *International Journal of Obesity, 25,* 1322-1326.

Filozof, C., Fernandez Pinilla, M. C., and Fernandez-Cruz, A. (2004). Smoking cessation and weight gain. *Obesity, 5,* 95-103.

Flegal, K. M., Troiano, R. P., Pamuk, E. R., Kuczmarski, R. J., and Campbell, S. M. (1995). The influence of smoking cessation on the prevalence of overweight in the United States. *New England Journal of Medicine, 333,* 1165-1170.

Freedman, D. M., Sigurdson, A. J., Rajaraman, P., Doody, M. M., Linet, M. S., and Ron, E. (2006). The mortality risk of smoking and obesity combined. *American Journal of Preventive Medicine, 31,* 355-362.

Hall, S. M., Ginsberg, D., and Jones, R. T. (1986). Smoking cessation and weight gain. *Journal of Consulting and Clinical Psychology, 54,* 342-346.

Hall, S. M., McGee, R., Tunstall, C., Duffy, J., and Benowitz, N. (1989). Changes in food intake and activity after quitting smoking. *Journal of Consulting and Clinical Psychology, 57,* 81-86.

Hall, S. M., Tunstall, C. D., Vila, K. L., and Duffy, J. (1992). Weight gain prevention and smoking cessation: Cautionary findings. *American Journal of Public Health, 82,* 799-803.

Healton, C. G., Vallone, D., McCausland, K. L., Xiao, H., and Green, M. P. (2006). Smoking, obesity, and their co-occurrence in the United States: Cross sectional analysis. *British Medical Journal, 333,* 25-26.

Hill, J. S. (1985). Effect of a program of aerobic exercise on the smoking behavior of a group of adult volunteers. *Canadian Journal of Public Health, 76,* 183-186.

Jeffery, R. W., Hennrikus, D. J., Lando, H. A., Murray, D. M., and Liu, J. W. (2000). Reconciling conflicting findings regarding postcessation weight concerns and success in smoking cessation. *Health Psychology, 19,* 242-246.

Jonsdottir, D. and Jonsdottir, H. (2001). Does physical exercise in addition to a multicomponent smoking cessation program increase abstinence rate and suppress weight gain? An intervention study. *Scandinavian Journal of the Caring Sciences, 15,* 275-282.

Killen, J. D., Fortmann, S. P., Kraemer, H. C., Varady, A. N., Davis, L., and Newman, B. (1996). Interactive effects of depression symptoms, nicotine dependence, and weight change on late smoking relapse. *Journal of Consulting and Clinical Psychology, 64,* 1060-1067.

King, A., de Wit, H., Riley, R. C., Cao, D., Niaura, R., and Hatsukami, D. (2006). Efficacy of naltrexone in smoking cessation: A preliminary study and an examination of sex differences. *Nicotine and Tobacco Research, 8,* 671-682.

Klesges, R. C., Brown, K., Pascale, R. W., Murphy, M., Williams, E., and Cigrang, J. A. (1988). Factors associated with participation, attrition, and outcome in a smoking cessation program at the workplace. *Health Psychology, 7,* 575-589.

Klesges, R. C., and Klesges, L. M. (1988). Cigarette smoking as a dieting strategy in a university population. *International Journal of Eating Disorders, 7,* 413-419.

Klesges, R. C., Meyers, A. W., Klesges, L. M., and LaVasque, M. E. (1989). Smoking, body weight, and their effects on smoking behavior: A comprehensive review of the literature. *Psychological Bulletin, 106,* 204-230.

Klesges, R. C., Winders, S. E., Meyers, A. W., Eck, L. H., Ward, K. D., Hultquist, C. M. et al. (1997). How much weight gain occurs following smoking cessation? A comparison of weight gain using both continuous and point prevalence abstinence. *Journal of Consulting and Clinical Psychology, 65,* 286-291.

Levine, M. D., Kalarchian, M. A., Courcoulas, A. P., Wisinski, M. S., and Marcus, M. D. (2007). History of smoking and postcessation weight gain among weight loss surgery candidates. *Addictive Behaviors, 32,* 2365-2371.

Levitz, J. S., Bradley, T. P., and Golden, A. L. (2004). Overview of smoking and all cancers. *Medical Clinics of North America, 88,* 1655-1675.

Livingston, E. H., Arterburn, D., Schifftner, T. L., Henderson, W. G., and De Palma, R. G. (2006). National Surgical Quality Improvement Program analysis of bariatric operations: modifiable risk factors contribute to bariatric surgical adverse outcomes. *Journal of the American College of Surgeons, 203,* 625-633.

Marcus, B. H., Albrecht, A. E., King, T. K., Parisi, A. F., Pinto, B. M., Roberts, M., et al. (1999). The efficacy of exercise as an aid for smoking cessation in women. *Archives of Internal Medicine, 159,* 1229-1234.

Marcus, B. H., Albrecht, A. E., Niaura, R. S., Abrams, D. B., and Thompson, P.D. (1991). Usefulness of physical exercise for maintaining smoking cessation in women. *American Journal of Cardiology, 68,* 406-407.

Marcus, B. H., Albrecht, A. E., Niaura, R. S., Taylor, E. R., Simkin, L. R., Feder, S. I., et al. (1995). Exercise enhances the maintenance of smoking cessation in women, *Addictive Behaviors, 20,* 87-92.

Martin, J. E., Calfas, K. J., Patten, C. A., Polarek, M., Hofstetter, C. R., Noto, J., et al. (1997). Prospective evaluation of three smoking interventions in 205 recovering alcoholics: One-year results of project SCRAP-Tobacco. *Journal of Consulting and Clinical Psychology, 65,* 190-194.

Mazas, C. A. and Wetter, D. W. (2003). Smoking cessation interventions among African Americans: Research needs. *Cancer Control, 10,* 87-89.

Meyers, A. W., Klesges, R. C., Winders, S. E., Ward, K. E., Peterson, B. A., and Eck, L. H. (1997). Are weight concerns predictive of smoking cessation? A prospective analysis. *Journal of Consulting and Clinical Psychology, 65,* 448-452.

Mizes, J. S., Sloan, D. M., Segraves, K., Spring, B., Pingitore, R., and Kristeller, J. (1998). The influence of weight-related variables on smoking cessation. *Behavior Therapy, 29,* 371-385.

Moffatt, R. J., and Owens, S. G. (1991). Cessation from cigarette smoking: Changes in body weight, body composition, resting metabolism, and energy consumption. *Metabolism, 40,* 465-470.

Namenek Brouwer, R. J. and Pomerleau, C. S. (2000). "Prequit attrition" among weight-concerned women smokers. *Eating Behaviors, 1,* 145-151.

Nordstrom, B. L., Kinnunen, T., Utman, C. H., and Garvey, A. J. (1999). Long-term effects of nicotine gum on weight gain after smoking cessation. *Nicotine and Tobacco Research, 1,* 259-268.

O'Malley, S. S., Cooney, J. L., Krishnan-Sarin, S., Dubin, J. A., McKee, S. A., Cooney, N. L., et al. (2006). A controlled trial of naltrexone augmentation of nicotine replacement therapy for smoking cessation. *Archives of Internal Medicine, 166,* 667-674.

Perkins, K. A. (1993). Weight gain following smoking cessation. *Journal of Consulting and Clinical Psychology, 61,* 768-777.

Perkins, K. A., Epstein, L. H., Marks, B. L., Stiller, R. L., and Jacob, R. G. (1989). The effect of nicotine on energy expenditure during light physical activity. *New England Journal of Medicine, 320,* 898-903.

Perkins, K. A., Epstein, L. H., and Pastor, S. (1990). Changes in energy balance following smoking cessation and resumption of smoking in women. *Journal of Consulting and Clinical Psychology, 58,* 121-125.

Perkins, K. A., Marcus, M .D., Levine, M. D., D'Amico, D., Miller, A., Broge, M., et al. (2001). Cognitive-behavioral therapy to reduce weight concerns improves smoking cessation outcome in weight-concerned women. *Journal of Consulting and Clinical Psychology, 69,* 604-613.

Pirie, P. L., McBride, C. M., Hellerstedt, W., Jeffery, R. W., Hatsukami, D., Allen, S., et al. (1992). Smoking cessation in women concerned about weight. *American Journal of Public Health, 82,* 1238-1243.

Pisinger, C. and Jorgensen, T. (2007). Waist circumference and weight following smoking cessation in a general population: The Inter99 study. *Preventive Medicine, 44,* 290-295.

Prapavessis, H., Cameron, L., Baldi, J. C., Robinson, S., Borrie, K., Harper, T., et al. (2007). The effects of exercise and nicotine replacement therapy on smoking rates in women. *Addictive Behaviors, 32,* 1416-1432.

Rodin, J. (1987). Weight change following smoking cessation: The role of food intake and exercise. *Addictive Behaviors, 12,* 303-317.

Russell, P. O., Epstein, L. H., Johnson, J. J., Block, D. R., and Blaire, E. (1988). The effects of physical activity as maintenance for smoking cessation. *Addictive Behaviors, 13,* 215-218.

Sanchez-Johnson, L. A. P. (2005). Smoking cessation, obesity and weight concerns in black women: A call to action for culturally competent interventions. *Journal of the National Medical Association, 97,* 1630-1638.

Spring, B., Doran, N., Pagoto, S., Schneider, K., Pingitore, R., and Hedeker, D. (2004). Randomized controlled trial for behavioral smoking and weight control treatment: Effect of concurrent versus sequential intervention. *Journal of Consulting and Clinical Psychology, 72,* 785-796.

Stamford, B. A., Matter, S., Fell, R. D., and Papenek, P. (1986). Effects of smoking cessation on weight gain, metabolic rate, caloric consumption and blood lipids. *American Journal of Clinical Nutrition, 43,* 486-494.

Streater, J. A., Sargent, R. G., and Ward, D. S. (1989). A study of the factors associated with weight change in women who attempt smoking cessation. *Addictive Behaviors, 14,* 523-530.

Suchanek Hudman, K., Gritz, E. R., Clayton, S., and Nisenbaum, R. (1999). Eating orientation, postcessation weight gain, and continued abstinence among female smokers receiving an unsolicited smoking cessation intervention. *Health Psychology, 18,* 29-36.

Talcott, G. W., Fiedler, E. R., Pascale, R. W., Klesges, R. C., Peterson, A. L., and Johnson, R. S. (1995). Is weight gain after smoking cessation inevitable? *Journal of Consulting and Clinical Psychology, 63,* 313-316.

Taylor, C. B., Houston-Miller, N., Haskell, W. L., and Debusk, R. F. (1988). Smoking cessation after acute myocardial infarction: The effects of exercise training. *Addictive Behaviors, 13,* 331-335.

Twardella, D., Loew, M., Rothenbacher, D., Stegmaier, C., Ziegler, H., and Brenner, H. (2006). The impact of body weight on smoking cessation in German adults. *Preventive Medicine, 42,* 109-113.

Ussher, M., West, R., McEwen, A., Taylor, A., and Steptoe, A. (2003). Efficacy of exercise counseling as an aid for smoking cessation: A randomized controlled trial. *Addiction, 98,* 523-532.

Ussher, M., West, R., McEwen, A., Taylor, A., and Steptoe, A. (in press). Randomized controlled trial of physical activity counseling as an aid to smoking cessation: 12 month follow-up. *Addictive Behaviors.*

Van Gaal, L. F., Mertens, I. L., and De Block, C. E. (2006). Mechanisms linking obesity with cardiovascular disease. *Nature, 444,* 875-880.

Walker, J. F., Collins, L. C., Rowell, P. P., Goldsmith, J., Moffatt, R. J., and Stamford, B. A. (1999). The effect of smoking on energy expenditure and plasma catecholamine and nicotine levels during light physical activity. *Nicotine and Tobacco Research, 1,* 365-370.

Wang, Y. and Beydoun, M. A. (2007). The Obesity Epidemic in the United States – Gender, Age, Socioeconomic, Racial/Ethnic, and Geographic Characteristics: A Systematic Review and Meta-Regression Analysis. *Epidemiologic Reviews, 29,* 6-28.

Wetter, D. W., Kenford, S. L., Smith, S. S., Fiore, M. C., Jorenby, D. E., and Baker, T. B. (1999). Gender differences in smoking cessation. *Journal of Consulting and Clinical Psychology, 67,* 555-562.

Williamson, D. F., Madans, J., Anda, R. F., Kleinman, J. C., Giovino, G. A., and Byers, T. (1991). Smoking cessation and severity of weight gain in a national cohort. *New England Journal of Medicine, 324,* 739-745.

In: Smoking and Women's Health

ISBN 978-1-60456-148-7

Editors: M.K. Wesley and I.A. Sternbach, pp.147-163 © 2008 Nova Science Publishers, Inc.

Chapter 5

Gender Differences in Nicotine Research: Implications for Smoking Cessation Programs

Dmitri Poltavski

School of Medicine and Health Sciences, Center for Health Promotion
and Translation Research, North Dakota, USA

Abstract

There is some growing empirical evidence suggesting significantly lower success rates of Nicotine Replacement Therapies (NRTs) in women than in men despite a generally lower self-reported nicotine dependence in women, fewer number of cigarettes smoked per day and lower nicotine exposure. Nevertheless, some more recent reviews question the significance of such findings suggesting that the observed trends may be of little clinical significance. At the same time several lines of basic nicotine research provide converging evidence that men and women respond to nicotine treatment differently in a variety of domains: physiological, affective and cognitive. Moreover, such response differences may be further accentuated by underlying genetic differences in a particular type of dopamine receptor. Overall these findings seem to add empirical support to conclusions that gender differences observed in smoking cessation trials are real and may be clinically important. Yet, experimental nicotine studies have often been plagued by methodological shortcoming related to nicotine dose used, types of cognitive and affective tasks, types of nicotine replacement, duration of nicotine deprivation, lack of control for the stages of the menstrual cycle and use of oral contraceptives in women. Therefore, evaluation of available evidence and interpretation of emerging findings becomes increasingly challenging when one considers the above confounding factors. The present review is thus aimed at a systematic critical scrutiny of extant research on gender differences in response to nicotine and suggests most promising avenues for future investigations in this area.

Introduction

Rationale for Studying Gender Differences in Nicotine Addiction

Nicotine replacement therapy (NRT) is one of the most commonly used components of smoking cessation programs. It is aimed at alleviation of many of the physiological and psychomotor withdrawal symptoms usually experienced following smoking cessation and may therefore increase the likelihood of remaining abstinent (Gourlay 1990). All of the commercially available forms of NRT (gum, transdermal patch, nasal spray, inhaler and sublingual lozenge) have been found effective as part of a program to counteract tobacco addiction. They increase the odds of long-term abstinence 1.5 to 2 times regardless of setting (Silagy et al., 2004). Nevertheless, some forms of NRT may be more effective than others. Specifically, nicotine patches that are the most popular form of nicotine replacement, may at the same time be the least effective especially in the long run (13.7% quit rate at 12 months follow-up), when compared to nicotine gum (17.4% quit rate), nicotine inhaler (17% quit rate) and intranasal spray (24% quit rate; Silagy et al., 2004). Additionally, despite the well-supported efficacy of NRTs, the best available quit rates do not exceed 25% even when pharmacological treatments are complimented with behavioral counseling and follow-up support (Silagy et al., 2004).

Furthermore, some studies (e.g. Davis et al., 1994; Swan, Jack, and Ward, 1997; Perkins, 1996; Gourlay et al., 1994; Wetter et al., 1999; West et al., 2001) suggested a significantly lower success rate of NRTs in women than in men despite a generally lower self-reported nicotine dependence in women, fewer number of cigarettes smoked per day and lower nicotine exposure (verified by biochemical analyses of blood and salivary cotinine and expired CO) than in men. Lower success rates for women, however, have not been universally observed. Some more recent reviews (e.g. Killen et al, 2002; Shiffman et al., 2005; Munafo et al., 2004) suggest that despite a consistently demonstrated trend favoring men in treatment outcomes with NRTs, these gender differences may be too small to be clinically significant. A closer look at such conclusions reveals that they are often based on aggregated data from a variety of studies that used combination treatments with pharmacotherapy, self-help videos and behavioral counseling (e.g. Killen et al., 2002; Munafo et al., 2004) or several nicotine doses both within and across studies (e.g. Killen et al., 2002; Munafo et al., 2004), which may influence gender differences in treatment outcomes with NRT.

Specifically, the effectiveness of combination treatments in which NRT was paired with behavioral counseling has been shown to be gender-dependent with women benefiting better from the combination therapy compared to NRT alone, while no such differences have been observed for men (Cepeta-Benito, Reynoso and Erath, 2004). Treatment outcomes in clinical cessation trials have also been influenced by the dose of NRT. In these studies no significant differences in outcome rates were observed for men over a variety of doses, but women showed dose-dependent differences in abstinence rates at various follow-up intervals (e.g. Swan, Jack, and Ward, 1997; Evans et al., 2006).

Not surprisingly, when odds ratios for the likelihood of quitting are considered only for those studies in which a single treatment dose was used or when higher multiple nicotine doses were used but patch treatment was not combined with other forms of therapy, greater advantage was consistently found for men. Specifically, with a 21mg patch used in a study by Killen et al., (1997) the odds ratio at 6 months abstinence was 2.37 for males and 1.01 for females; with 21mg, 35mg and 42mg of nicotine patches used in the study by Hughes et al. (1999) the odds ratios were 3.22 for men and 1.06 for women, respectively. Finally with 15mg and 25 mg patches used in the study by Paoletti et al. (1996) the corresponding odds ratios at six months were 2.02 for men and .97 for women.

Similarly, in the review of smoking cessation trials by Killen et al. (2002) the only experimental condition in which gender differences did reach statistical significance involved a pure treatment with 15 mg transdermal nicotine patches at 6 months follow-up. In this condition the abstinence rate for men was 20% vs. 7% rate for women. A similar trend was observed in the same condition immediately following the treatment period with 29% abstinence rate for men and 22% for women. In the 21mg of nicotine condition the NRT was again more effective for men than for women both immediately after the end of the treatment period (46% vs. 35%) and at six months follow-up (29% vs. 22%). In line with this evidence, Shiffman et al. (2005) reported a non-significant trend towards better abstinence rates for men after considering trials using only a 21mg nicotine- patch- treatment regimen and noted that this gender advantage reached statistical significance in the 14mg- of- nicotine patch condition both at 6 and 12-month follow-ups. Additionally, the researchers also reported that among women heavier smokers (15 + cig/day) show significantly lower quit rates following NRT than lighter smokers with no such difference reported for men. These findings again suggest better outcomes for men following transdermal NRT and that the magnitude of this gender difference may be dose-dependent.

In a meta- analysis of 21 randomized smoking cessation trials using NRTs Cepeta-Benito et al. (2004) evaluated gender differences in NRT efficacy at 3 months 6 months and 12 months while controlling for the NRT intensity (combination with pharmacotherapy and counseling). The researchers concluded that the efficacy of NRT was significantly greater in men than in women at 12 months follow-up regardless of the NRT type or intensity. At the same time NRT was efficacious for women at 6 months follow-up only in conjunction with an intensive treatment approach (behavioral counseling). Furthermore, the researchers suggested greater relative efficacy of bupropion treatment by itself and/or in combination with NRT for women compared with men.

Genetic Evidence Supporting Sexual Dimorphism in Smoking Cessation Rates:

Recent genetic evidence involving a particular dopamine receptor subtype also indicates some intra-gender variability among women in relation to NRT efficacy, which may further contribute to the list of factors, shown to affect gender differences in smoking cessation trials. The role of dopamine in the rewarding effects of nicotine has been supported by abundant empirical evidence (e.g. Balfour, 2004; Pontieri, Tanda, Orzi, and Di Chiara, 1996). Nicotine binds to cholinergic receptors in the ventral tegmental area in the brain which stimulates the nucleus accumbens (NAC) to release dopamine from its nerve terminals (Nisell, Nomikos, and Svensson, 1994). This results in activation of post-synaptic dopamine receptors including the D_2 subtype. Some researchers believe that stimulation of these receptors results in perception of pleasure (Koob and Le Moal, 1997). Genetic variations affecting the dopamine D_2 receptor have been suggested to predispose to the development and maintenance of tobacco addiction (Johnstone et al., 2004). A particular genotype for the D_2 receptor (i.e. CC) has been shown to have a higher transcriptional efficiency which results in a greater number of D_2 receptors available to bind dopamine, thus making cigarette smoking possibly more rewarding (Lerman et al., 2006). Women with the CC genotype for the dopamine D_2 receptor subtype, however, may be more sensitive to the rewarding effects of nicotine than men. Specifically, Yudkin et al. (2004) found that women with this genotype benefited significantly less than women with the TT genotype from an NRT using transdermal nicotine patches at all follow-up points (i.e. 3, 6, and 12 months). The differences in the effectiveness of the patch across the same genotypes in men were not significant.

Furthermore, according to the recent imaging data the same dopamine receptor subtype, D_2, may also be implicated in a number of cognitive functions including executive function, memory and verbal fluency. Specifically, Takahashi et al. (2007) reported that dopamine D_2 receptor binding in the hippocampus was not only associated with performance on working memory tests which are typically considered to be within the hippocampal purview but also on tests of frontal lobe function and verbal fluency, on which the role of the hippocampus had hitherto been downplayed. Additionally, administration of D_2 receptor agonists in humans has been reported to improve the above cognitive faculties (Berthier, 2005; McDowell et al., 1998). Interestingly, among other brain regions the hippocampus has been implicated not only in anatomical sex differences but also in functional sexual dimorphism. Juraska (1998), for instance, reported increased dendritic arborization in the hippocampus of female rats placed in an' enriched environment' with opportunities to socialize with fellow rodents and play with toys. Such branching of dendritic trees is presumed to reflect an increase in neuronal connections and consequently, improvement in such cognitive functions as memory consolidation. Exposure to the same type of environment, however, had no effect on dendritic trees of male rodents albeit pruning them slightly. At the same-time drug-seeking behavior induced by exposure to environmental cues associated with drug use has been shown in numerous animal studies to be mediated by the D_2 and D_3 dopamine receptor subtypes (e.g. Crombag, Grimm, Shaham, 2002; Cervo et al., 2003; Kroyan et al., 2000; Gal and Gyertyan, 2006). Coupled with the evidence of a possible greater role of the CC genotype for the D_2 receptors in the efficacy of smoking cessation trials for women as well as a potentially greater effect of the environment on the woman's brain, this research suggests that female smokers may be more sensitive to environmental variables associated with smoking (e.g. smoking- related cues, social stress) than men.

Smoking Cues Vs. Stress-Related Cues

Some available behavioral evidence is consistent with this suggestion. For instance, Perkins (1996; 2001) reported that women depend to a greater extend on sensory cues for maintenance of cigarette smoking than men. Sayette and Hufford (1995) has also found greater facial responses of female smokers to presentation of smoking cues. This finding has been further generalized to non-specific mood-inducing stimuli (Mirowsky and Ross, 1995). Nevertheless, in a recent study in which smoking-related and stress-related cues were directly juxtaposed, female smokers reported significantly greater cigarette cravings than male smokers only in the stress-cue but not in the smoking-cue condition (Colamussi, Bovbjerg and Erblich, 2007). Specifically, the researchers measured self-reported anxiety levels and cigarette cravings of male and female smokers after listening to three types of scripts (neutral, stress and smoking-related). The neutral script described somebody changing a light-bulb, the stress script described a trip to a dentist, while the smoking-related script involved lighting-up a cigarette after a meal. Throughout each script the participants were instructed to imagine the scene in as much detail as possible drawing from personal experience where appropriate. The authors, however, drew their conclusions on the basis of only subjective self-reports of cigarette cravings and perceived nicotine withdrawal, and admitted that they did not control for phases of the menstrual cycle and use of oral contraceptives.

Failure to control for these variables may influence the validity of the findings. Specifically, using only self-report measures the researchers may have obtained more accurate data from men than from women, since women may be less sensitive to pharmacological effects of nicotine and consequently, less accurate in reporting such effects on their cigarette cravings and tobacco withdrawal. Support for this hypothesis comes from a study by Perkins et al. (2006) who administered self-report measures of smoking reward and reinforcement to four groups of male and female smokers who were either given nicotine-containing cigarettes or denicotinized cigarettes, and were either explicitly told what cigarette dose they received or were given no such explanation. The researchers found that dose instructions enhanced the effects of nicotine on smoking reward and reinforcement in women and tended to diminish or reverse these effects in men, suggesting that women may be more sensitive to non-pharmacological factors such as smoking cues rather than the actual nicotine dose.

Likewise, controlling for stages of the menstrual cycle in studies of female tobacco addiction may be of significance, as cigarette-related cues have been shown to increase the intensity of cigarette cravings in women in the luteal phase of the menstrual cycle compared to the follicular phase (Franklin et al., 2004). Abstaining female smokers have also been reported to have greater cigarette cravings and negative affect in the luteal phase of the menstrual cycle compared to the follicular phase with transdermal nicotine treatment (21mg) minimizing the difference (Allen, Hatsukami and Christianson, 2000). These differences have been explained on the basis of a strong correlation between peak plasma estradiol and progesterone concentrations in the late luteal phase and changes in the dopaminergic system including receptors, transporters and levels of dopamine itself, which have been strongly implicated in mediating maintenance of cigarette smoking in women (Morrissette and Di Paolo, 1993). Similarly, the use of oral contraceptives has been shown to intensify cigarette craving in abstaining women in comparison to non-OC-users and to be associated with diminished attenuation of anxiety following cigarette smoking, while no significant differences on those measures were observed in non-OC-users in different phases of the menstrual cycle phases (Masson and Gilbert, 1999).

Nevertheless, despite the methodological shortcomings of the Colamussi et al. (2007) experiment, those studies that supplemented their self-report instruments with physiological measures lend further support to the hypothesis that stress-related stimuli and negative affect may play a particularly prominent role in female nicotine addiction. For instance, Hogle and Curtin (2006) measured the eye-blink component of the startle reflex and salivary cortisol in nicotine-deprived (24 hours) and non-deprived smokers using a fear-conditioning paradigm. The researchers found that nicotine-deprived female smokers displayed increased fear-potentiated startle during the recovery period after the fear cue had been terminated. They also showed a greater cortisol response to the stress-cue (presentation of a color square that had been previously paired with electric shock) than non-nicotine-deprived female smokers. No such differences were observed in men. Nicotine-deprived women also reported greater negative affect associated with nicotine withdrawal at the beginning of the experiment (before the presentation of the stressor), suggesting that they were reporting on their poor overall ability to effectively regulate their negative affective response rather than on their direct experiences of immediate stressors. Nicotine-deprived male smokers, however, reported significantly lower positive affect at baseline than non-deprived men. No such differences in positive affect were observed among women. Thus, withdrawn male smokers may experience decreased positive reinforcement from natural and conditioned reinforces in their environment, while withdrawn female smokers experience increased negative affective symptoms.

Although the study did not test the smoking cue hypothesis, it yielded strong evidence supporting the hypothesis of increased sensitivity of women to stress cues and impaired recovery from negative affect. The findings also suggest that nicotine use may be particularly important to overcome deficits in emotional regulation that occur during acute nicotine withdrawal, at least for women. This finding partially discredits the hypothesis that women are less sensitive to the pharmacological effects of nicotine than men.

Exposure to both types of cues has been directly tested in a study by Robinson et al. (2007) who also supplemented self-report instruments of cigarette cravings and nicotine withdrawal with measures of physiological response to stimuli. Specifically, the researchers measured startle eyeblink responses in nicotine deprived (12 h deprivation) and non-deprived smokers treated with either a placebo or a nicotine-containing nasal spray during a task that combined smoking- related and stress-related cues. V-olunteers were presented with color-slides that contained images from 4 categories: positive affect, neutral, negative affect and smoking-related. Smoking-related slides consisted of images of burning cigarettes and people smoking in a social context. The researchers also utilized self-report measures of in-session mood and cigarette cravings. The results did not show any gender differences for different types of slides, but the researchers did find that although nicotine treatment of nicotine-deprived female smokers resulted in expected attenuation of the startle eyeblink response (pharmacological effect), this reduction was not accompanied by a corresponding decrease in self-reported negative affect. Since the route of nicotine administration involved nasal spray it may thus have affected the way female smokers assessed subtle changes in their negative mood brought on by nicotine. Thus, although the findings did not provide any direct evidence of greater significance of either stress-related or smoking-related cues for women, it did corroborate the observation that women may not be as accurate as men is judging their internal states. A study by Furedy et al. (1999) further confirms this notion. In their experiment the investigators found that despite the fact that many women reported "relaxation" as the primary reason for cigarette smoking, smoking a cigarette of preferred brand and yield resulted in greater skin resistance level (SRL) in men in response to a verbal task challenge and lower SRL in women. These findings indicate greater relaxation in men and greater arousal in women.

If female smokers do, indeed, react to a greater extend to stress-related cues than male smokers, this gender difference may not generalize to non-smokers. Generally greater increases in epinephrine, norepinephrine and salivary cortisol levels in response to psychological stress (e.g. public speech anticipation and delivery, mental arithmetic) have been observed in men with no gender differences found on the above biochemical measures in response to either physical stress (e.g. bicycle ergometry) or CRH challenge (Biondi and Picardi, 1999). Additionally, chronic nicotine administration has been associated with higher tonic cortisol levels in smokers than in non-smokers with male smokers also showing greater cortisol awakening response (CAR) than male non-smokers, while no such difference has been reported for women (Steptoe and Ussher, 2006). Since CAR is thought to represent an anticipatory response to the stress of the day (Kunz-Ebrecht et al., 2004), it adds further evidence that males may be more sensitive to general stressors than females. At the same time phasic cortisol responses in female smokers to psychological stressors (e.g. fear conditioning paradigm) are significantly greater than in female non-smokers (Hogle and Curtin, 2006).

Findings of cardiovascular reactivity (heart rate and mean arterial blood pressure) in abstaining male and female smokers in response to various types of situational manipulation of smoking-related cues have been mixed, with male abstaining smokers showing greater reactivity to in-vivo exposure and females being more reactive in abstract smoking situations (Niaura et al., 1998). Additionally, it's been suggested that women have greater concern about post-cessation weight gain than men, and greater difficulty with negative mood associated with quitting as well as greater need for social support to quit smoking (Jensvold, Hamilton, and Halbreich, 1996). In aggregate all these factors may contribute to the gender disparities in abstinence rates observed in smoking cessation trials.

One additional factor that hasn't been explored in nicotine gender research but which may, nevertheless, be of importance for women undergoing nicotine replacement therapy are cognitive effects of nicotine, their relation to NRT dose and how these possible cognitive dose effects may correspond to dose effects seen in the affective domain (cravings, negative affect, withdrawal).

When the latter area is considered women have been reported to have less attenuated withdrawal relief and poorer outcome with lower doses of nicotine replacement (e.g. 15 microgram/kg of nicotine vs. 30 micrograms/kg by way of nasal spay; Perkins et al., 1992). Higher doses of nicotine delivered either with a transdermal patch (e.g. 21 mg) or nasal spray (e.g. 30 microgram/kg), however, resulted in similar ameliorating effects on negative affect and withdrawal in both abstaining male and female smokers (VanderKaay and Patterson, 2006; Perkins et al., 1992).

Effects of nicotine on anxiety also show a dose-dependent pattern. Nicotine has been found to be both anxiolytic and anxiogenic in human and animal studies (see Cheeta, Kenny, and File, 2000 for a review). Some studies in humans reported that smokers became more anxious after smoking a cigarette (Parrot and Garnham, 1998; Netter et al., 1998) and Newhouse et al. (1990) reported that nicotine increased anxiety in non-smokers. In the social interaction test it has been showed that low doses of nicotine have anxiolytic effects, whereas higher doses have anxiogenic effects (File et al., 1999). Animal studies further revealed that anxiolytic effects of nicotine are primarily mediated by increased production of serotonin in the dorsal hippocampus at low doses, while the anxiogenic effect is reached at higher doses of nicotine when in addition to 5-HT noradrenaline is also released in the lateral septum (see Cheeta et al., 2000, for a review).

Cognitive Effects of Nicotine and Gender:

Besides its effects on mood, affect and reward in smokers, there is also some evidence to suggest that cigarette smoking may affect cognitive functions of men and women in different ways. For example, unlike men women have been reported to experience greater physiological arousal during completion of a cognitive task immediately after smoking a cigarette (Furedy et. al., 1999). Women were also found to be more alert and less physically tired then men after completing a stressful cognitive battery if they had smoked a cigarette of their preferred brand and yield prior to cognitive testing (File et al., 2002). These findings are consistent with the previously discussed psychophysiological data reported by Furedy et al. (1999) that female smokers demonstrate lower skin resistance levels in response to a verbal task challenge and after smoking a cigarette of preferred brand and yield suggesting improved arousal.

As a cholinergic agonist nicotine has been generally found to improve cognitive function, particularly performance on attentional measures as indexed by the Continuous Performance Task (CPT) and memory tasks involving explicit effortful processing such as recall of semantically related material. These effects were observed not only in abstaining smokers but also in non-smokers following an acute nicotine challenge (see Rezvani and Levin 2001, for a review). These improvements in working memory function and attention have been correlated in imaging studies with activation of the prefrontal cortex (Domino et al., 2000a,b,), orbitofrontal cortex (Stein et al., 1998) and anterior cingulated cortex (Kumari et al., 2003).

These ameliorating effects of acute nicotine on cognitive performance have been explained on the basis of upregulation of high-affinity nicotinic receptors (nAChRs) in the smoker's brain following chronic nicotine exposure, particularly $\alpha4\beta2$ and $\alpha7$ sub-types in the hippocampus (see Levin 2002, for a review). Upregulation of nACh receptors has been associated with receptor sensitization to nicotine and potentiation of nicotine response (Sallette et al., 2005). While both $\alpha4\beta2$ and $\alpha7$ nicotinic receptor subtypes have been found important for working memory, $\alpha7$ receptors are thought to be more essential for the expression of the actions of chronic nicotine on working memory function (Levin et al., 2002).

At the same time chronic long-term exposure to nicotine in humans is associated with impairments of executive function and working memory (Razani et al., 2004) that may persist for many years after smoking cessation (Neuhaus et al., 2006). Anatomical correlates of these deficits have been observed in reduced gray matter volumes and densities of prefrontal cortex, anterior cingulate, and the occipital cortex in smokers compared to non-smokers (Brody et al., 2004). Furthermore, during the completion of a standard odd-ball task, minimally deprived smokers (1 hour) have been found to show decreased P300 amplitude in the dorsolateral prefrontal and orbitofrontal cortical areas as well as in the posterior cingulated cortex (Neuhaus et al., 2006). Additionally, parietal P300 amplitude (Pz) was negatively correlated with the length of smoking history and the number of daily cigarettes, suggesting greater cognitive impairments in 'veteran' smokers. These deficits in heavy smokers with a long history of nicotine exposure have been explained more on the basis of mild chronic hypoxia due to vasoconstrictive properties of nicotine rather than its neuronal effects (Razani et al., 2004).

Thus, long smoking histories in humans are associated with cognitive detriments, while shorter periods of chronic exposure to nicotine (yet to be empirically defined) in human and animal studies produce facilitation of certain brain functions. For instance, Fujii et al. (1999) found that acute nicotine administration to chronically nicotine- treated rats (2 week exposure) produces a synergistic effect on long-term potentiation (LTP) in the rat hippocampus, which is important for memory consolidation. This effect was expressed in lowering of the LTP threshold in comparison to acute treatment alone when the same nicotine dose was used. These findings suggest a dose-related mechanism of nicotine-induced cognitive facilitation.

Such an assumption wouldn't be inconsistent with the conclusions of Newhouse et al. (2004) who pointed out in their meta-analysis of cognitive effects of nicotine that nicotine stimulation tends to conform to the Yerkes–Dodson principle with intermediate levels of stimulation-producing optimal performance and high levels of stimulation-impairing performance. Indeed, some studies in humans (using male smokers as subjects) showed impairment in prose recall following administration of higher nicotine doses (e.g. 1.5mg of nicotine cigarette: Krebs, Petros, and Beckwith, 1994; or 21mg of nicotine patch: Poltavski and Petros, 2005).

Nicotine dose response in the brain shows sexual dimorphism as well. Specifically, female rats have been found to have higher densities of nAChRs and chronic nicotine treatment of 0.6mg/kg has been shown to produce an upregulation of nACHRs in male rats but not in females (Koylu et al., 1997). Greater treatment doses, however, (>0.8mg/kg) also resulted in nAChR upregulation in females (Collins et al., 1990). Effects of different nicotine doses on cognitive performance further show sex-dependent differences. Namely, male rats seem to benefit in active avoidance learning at all doses of nicotine tested, while performance of female rats deteriorates at higher doses [>0.6mg/kg] (Yilmaz et al., 1997). To the knowledge of the author, there have not yet been any studies to date that directly compared cognitive effects of different doses of acute nicotine in men and women.

In the very few studies, in which a single nicotine dose was tested on cognitive tasks, minimal doses of nicotine tended to affect preferred cognitive strategies for problem-solving erasing initial task-related gender advantages. For example, greater speed and accuracy on vigilance tasks (e.g. CPT, RVIP) have been observed in males (e.g. Trimmel and Witteberger, 2004; File et al., 2002) and in one study transdermal nicotine treatment of abstaining smokers and non-smokers with a patch of only 5mg of nicotine / 16 hours after only 30 minutes of absorption normalized the above difference bringing females to the level of performance of males irrespective of their smoking status (Trimmel and Wittberger, 2004). At the same time these gender differences on a vigilance task (i.e. RVIP) remained in the nicotine condition but only for smokers after smoking a cigarette of their habitual yield (File et al., 2002). These findings suggest that female smokers may benefit from nicotine treatment on tasks that do not favor their preferred cognitive strategy only when treated with minimal nicotine doses, which may be lower than the habitual doses obtained from smoking a cigarette. At the same time male performance on preferred cognitive tests appears to be less dose-dependent.

Available imaging data, however, are somewhat more equivocal. For instance, in a PET study Fallon et. al. (2005) examined regional metabolic differences in the brains of male and female smokers and non-smokers in response to nicotine. The researchers found that both female smokers and non-smokers performing the CPT in the placebo condition showed higher brain metabolism than males especially in the prefrontal regions, mid and anterior temporal lobe, language cortices and related subcortical areas. The overall effect of transdermal nicotine was to decrease these gender differences in brain metabolism with only 3.5 mg of nicotine (but not 21mg) effective for non-smokers and both 3.5mg of nicotine and 21mg of nicotine effective in erasing metabolic gender differences for female smokers. Cognitive performance on the measures of the CPT, however, was not reported. It is thus not clear whether nicotine dose effects on regional metabolism in the brains of men and women correspond to similar differences in performance on behavioral measures of the CPT.

The gender-dose relationship observed in some studies may be reversed on tasks favoring cognitive strategies of women. On verbal and recognition tasks, for example, Burton et al., 2004 reported that female smokers outperformed male smokers after smoking a cigarette of their usual yield (e.g. Algan et al., 1997; File et al., 2002). Furthermore, on verbal tasks men have been found to show significantly greater recall of affective rather than neutral prose material while no such differences have been observed in women (Burton et al., 2004). To the author's knowledge these gender differences have not been tested in response to nicotine, but a large dose of transdermal nicotine (35mg) has been found to attenuate an emotional Stroop effect in abstaining smokers on the first day of a smoking cessation program when they completed a modified Stroop task on which affective words were related to smoking (e.g. tobacco, cigarette, smoke etc) (Waters et al., 2003). Although female subjects were also used in the study by Waters et al. (2003) no gender comparisons were reported.

Thus, indications that there might be dose-dependent gender differences in cognitive effects of nicotine in smokers as well as evidence suggesting that acute dose responses to nicotine replacement in the affective domain may also vary as a function of gender, it could be of interest to compare correspondence of dose and gender effects in both areas as improvement in one at a particular dose level may not necessarily correspond to similar improvements in the other. These findings may, therefore, have potential clinical implications for NRT use in women especially in view of the fact that transdermal nicotine patch doses higher than 22 mg are now considered to be somewhat more beneficial for smoking cessation than standard doses (e.g. 21 mg; Silagy et al., 2004). At the same time strong caution against using such high doses of transdermal nicotine as 42mg / 24 hours in smoking cessation trials with women has already been voiced, as women smokers (15 + cig/day) were reported to experience a significantly greater number of side effects which were also of significantly greater intensity than those observed in men (Evans et al., 2006). Additionally, McClure and Swan (2006) in their review of factors that may further enhance treatment outcomes and smoking safety have recently suggested a more discriminate approach to NRT use by individual tailoring of NRT type and dose to match smokers' needs and preferences.

Conclusion

Recapitulating the reviewed studies it appears that female smokers may not be as successful as men in their quit attempt when undergoing nicotine replacement therapy. Such differences can be related to the form of NRT used, nicotine dose and its combination with other forms of therapy (behavioral counseling and pharmacotherapy). Additionally, currently existing smoking cessation programs may not take into consideration an interplay of affective and cognitive factors that may be uniquely important for women trying to abstain from smoking. Specifically, female smokers may be more susceptible to experiencing prolonged negative affect associated with exposure to stressors in their environment than male smokers, and consequently, to relapsing in order to alleviate withdrawal symptomatology. They may also be more physiologically sensitive to different nicotine doses currently used in NRTs while at the same time being less accurate than men in the assessment of their own physiological states. Furthermore, observed NRT dose interactions with mood, cigarette cravings and withdrawal in women may be more disparate from the same dose effects on their cognitive functions than are seen in men, which may bear relevance for women pursuing cognitively challenging careers especially in the fields that favor cognitive strategies of men. This complexity can be further exacerbated by variability in mood and smoking rates of women in relation to stages of the menstrual cycle with the late luteal phase being the least auspicious for smoking abstinence due to increased negative affect and cigarette cravings. The use of oral contraceptives adds yet another facet to the multifarious issue of female tobacco addiction with abstaining OC-users in the late luteal phase of the menstrual cycle being most likely candidates for a relapse. The likelihood of a relapse appears to be further augmented by the presence of a particular genotype CC for the dopamine receptor D_2 in female smokers, as such women have a genetically-enhanced capacity for dopamine binding and may thus, be capable of experiencing greater nicotine reward resulting in greater cigarette consumption.

It thus appears that the most promising future research directions in the area of gender differences and tobacco addiction should incorporate measures of physiological response to nicotine challenge in addition to self-report measures of affect and cigarette withdrawal. Investigators ought to utilize different nicotine doses while juxtaposing performance on tests involving exposure to stress- and smoking-related cues with that observed on cognitive measures. Cognitive batteries should comprise instruments that favor cognitive strategies of both genders. Moreover, researchers should also control for or directly compare performance and self-reports of women in different stages of the menstrual cycle while also taking into consideration their use of oral contraceptives. Such methodologically rigorous studies will further assist in elucidation of the mechanism of gender differences in tobacco addiction and may help better explain the contribution of non-physiological factors to its maintenance which could result in development of better smoking cessation programs attuned to the unique needs of women.

References

Allen, S. S., Hatsukami, D., Christianson, D., Brown., S. (2000). Effects of transdermal nicotine on craving, withdrawal and premenstrual symptomatology in short-term smoking abstinence during different phases of the menstrual cycle. *Nicotine and Tobacco Research, 2,* 231-241.

Algan, O., Furedy, J. J., Demirgoren, S., Vincent, A., and Pogun, S. (1997). Effects of tobacco smoking and gender on interhemispheric cognitive function: performance and confidence measures. *Behavioral Pharmacology, 8 (5),* 416-428.

Balfour, D. J. (2004). The neurobiology of tobacco dependence: a preclinical perspective on the role of the dopamine projections to the nucleus. *Nicotine and Tobacco Research, 6,* 899-912.

Berthier, M. L. (2005). Poststroke aphasia: epidemiology, pathophysiology and treatment. *Drugs Aging, 22,* 163-182.

Biondi, M. and Picardi, A. (1999). Psychological stress and neuroendocrine function in humans: The Last two decades of research. *Psychotherapy and Psychosomatics, 68 (3),* 114 – 150.

Brody, A. L., Mandelkern, M. A., Jarvik, M. E., Lee, G.S., Smith, E. C., Huang, J.C., Bota, R. G., Bartzokis, G., London, E. D. (2004). Differences between smokers and non-smokers in regional gray matter volumes and densities. *Biological Psychiatry, 55,* 77-84.

Burton, L. A., Rabin, L., Bernstein-Vardy, S., Frohlich, J., Wyatt, Dimitri, D., Constante, S., and Guterman, E. (2004). Gender differences in implicit and explicit memory for affective passages. *Brain and Cognition, 54,* 218-224.

Cepeda-Benito, A., Reynoso, J. T., and Erath, S. (2004). Meta-analysis of the efficacy of nicotine replacement therapy for smoking cessation: Differences between men and women. *Journal of Consulting and Clinical Psychology, 72,* 712-722.

Cervo, L., Carnovali, F., Stark, J. A., Mennini, T. (2003). Cocaine-seeking behavior in response to drug-associated stimuli in rats: involvement of D3 and D2 dopamine receptors. *Neuropsychopharmacology, 28,* 1150-1159.

Cheeta, S., Kenny, P. J., and File, S. E. (2000). The role of 5-HT$_{1A}$ receptors in mediating the anxiogenic effects of nicotine following lateral septal administration. *European Journal of Neuroscience, 12,* 3797-3802.

Colamussi, L., Bovbjerg, D. H., Erblich, J. (2007). Stress-and cue-induced cigarette craving: Effects of a family history of smoking. *Drug and Alcohol Dependence* [In Press].

Collins, A. C., Romm, E., and Wehner, J. M. (1990). Dissociation of the apparent relationship between nicotine tolerance and up-regulation of nicotinic receptors. *Brain Research Bulletin, 25, 373-379.*

Crombag, H. S., Grimm, J. W., Shaham, Y. (2002). Effect of dopamine receptor antagonists on renewal of cocaine seeking by reexposure to drug-associated contextual cues. *Neuropsychopharmacology, 27,* 1006-1015.

Davis, L. J., Hurt, R. D., Offord, K. P., Lauger, G. G., Morse, R.M., Bruce, B. K. (1994). Self-administered Nicotine-Dependence Scale (SANDS): item selection, reliability estimation, and initial validation. *Journal of Clinical Psychology, 50,* 918-930.

Domino, E.F., Minoshima, S., Guthrie, S.K., Ohl, L., Ni, L., Koeppe, R. A., Cross, D. J., Zubieta, J. (2000a). Effects of nicotine on regional cerebral glucose metabolism in awake resting tobacco smokers. *Neuroscience, 101,* 277-282.

Domino, E.F., Minoshima, S., Guthrie, S.K., Ohl, L., Ni, L., Koeppe, R. A., Zubieta, J. (2000b). Nicotine effects on regional cerebral blood flow in awake, resting tobacco smokers. *Synapse, 38,* 313-321.

Evans, S. E., Blank, M., Sams, C., Weaver, M. F., and Eissenberg, T. (2006). Transdermal Nicotine-Induced Tobacco Abstinence Symptom Suppression: Nicotine Dose and Smokers' Gender. *Experimental and Clinical Psychopharmacology, 14,* 121-135.

Fallon, J. H., Keator, D. B., Mbogori, J., Taylor D., Potkin, S. G. (2005). Gender: a mojor determinant of brain response to nicotine. *International Journal of Neuropsychopharmacology, 8 (1),* 17 – 26.

File, S. E., Dinnis, A. K., Heard, J. E., Irvine, E. E. (2002). Mood differences between male and female light smokers and non-smokers. *Pharmacology, Biochemistry and Behavior, 72,* 681 – 689.

File, S. E., Cheeta, S., Kenny, P. J., Ouagazzal, A. M. and Gonzalez, L. E. (1999). Roles of the dorsal raphe nucleus, lateral septum and dorsal hippocampus in nicotine's effects on anxiety. *Society for Neuroscience Abstracts, 25,* 1981.

Franklin, T. R., Napier, K., Ehrman, R., Gariti, P., O'Brien, C. P., Childress, A. R. (2004). Retrospective study: Influence of menstrual cycle on cue-induced cigarette craving. *Nicotine and Tobacco Research, 6,* 171-175.

Fujii, S., Ji, Z., Morita, N., Sumikawa, K. (1999). Acute and chronic nicotine exposure differentially facilitate the induction of LTP. *Brain Research, 846,* 137 – 143.

Furedy, J. J., Algan, O., Vincent, A., Demirgoren, S., and Pogun, S. (1999). Sexually Dimorphic effect of an acute smoking manipulation on skin resistance but not on heart rate during a cognitive verbal task. *Integrative Physiological and Behavioral Science, 34* (4) 219 – 226.

Gal, K., and Gyertyan, I. (2006). Dopamine D3 as well as D2 receptor ligands attenuate the cue-induced cocaine-seeking in a relapse model of rats. *Drug and Alcohol Dependence, 81,* 63-70.

Gourlay, S. G., Forbes, A., Marriner, T., Pethica, D., and McNeil, J. J. (1994). Prospective study of factors predicting outcome of transdermal nicotine treatment in smoking cessation. *British Medical Journal, 309,* 1437-1438.

Hogle, J. M., and Curtin, J. J. (2006). Sex differences in negative affective response during nicotine withdrawal. *Psychophysiology, 43,* 344-356.

Hughes, J. R., Lesmes, G. R., Hatsukami, D. K., Richmond, R. L., Lichtenstein, E., Jorenby, D. E., Broughton, J. O., Fortmann, S. P., Leischow, S. J., McKenna, J. P., Rennard, S. I., Wadland, W. C., and Heatley, S. A. (1999). Are higher doses of nicotine replacement more effective for smoking cessation? *Nicotine and Tobacco Research, 1,* 169-174.

Juraska, J.M. (1998). Neural plasticity and the development of sex differences. *Annual Review of Sex Research, 9,* 20-38.

Jensvold, M. F., Hamilton, J. A., and Halbreich, U. (1996). Future research directions: Methodological considerations for advancing gender-sensitive statistics. In M. F. Jensvold, U. Halbreich, and J. A. Hamilton (Eds.), *Psychopharmacology and women: Sex, gender, and hormones*. Washington, DC: American Psychiatric Press.

Johnstone, E.C., Yudkin, P. L., Hey, K., Roberts, S. J., Welch, S. J., Murphy, M.F. et al (2004). Genetic variation in dopaminergic pathways and short-term effectiveness of the nicotine patch. *Pharmacogenetics, 14,* 83-90.

Killen, J. D., Fortmann, S. P., Varady, A., and Kraemer, H.C. (2002). Do men outperform women in smoking cessation trials? Maybe but not by much. *Experimental and Clinical Psychopharmacology, 10,* 295-301.

Killen, J. D., Fortmann, S. P., Davis, L., and Varady, A. (1997). Nicotine patch and self-help video for cigarette smoking cessation. *Journal of Consulting and Clinical Psycology, 65,* 663-672.

Koob, G.F., and Le Moal, M. (1997). Drug abuse: hedonic homeostatic dysregulation. *Science, 278:* 52-58.

Koylu, E., Demirgören, S., London, E. D., Pögun, S. Sex difference in up-regulation of nicotinic acetylcholine receptors in rat brain. (1997). *Life Sciences, 61 (12),* 185-190.

Krebs, S. J., Petros, T.V., Beckwith, B.E. (1994). Effects of smoking on memory for prose passages. *Physiology and Behavior ,4,* 723 – 7.

Kroyan, T. V., Barrett-Larimore, R. L., Rowlett, J. K., Spealman, R. D. (2000). Dopamine D1- and D2-like receptor mechanisms in relapse to cocaine-seeking behavior: effects of selective antagonists and agonists. *Journal of Pharmacology and Experimental Therapeutics, 294,* 680-687.

Kumari, V., Gray, J. A., Ffytche, D. H., Mitterschiffthaler, M. T., Das, M., Zachariah, E., Vythelingum, G.N., Williams, S.C.R., Simmons, A., Scharma, T. (2003). Cognitive effects of nicotine in humans: an fMRI study. *Neuroimage, 19,* 1002-1013.

Kunz-Ebrecht, S. R., Kirschbaum, C., Marmot, M., Steptoe, A. (2004). Differences in cortisol awakening response on work days and weekends in women and men from the Whitehall II cohort. *Psychoendocrinology, 29,* 516 – 528.

Lerman, C., Jepson, C., Wileyto, E. P., Epstein, L. H., Rukstalis, M., Patterson, F., Kaufmann, V., Restine, S., Hawk, L., Niaura, R., and Berrettini, W. (2006). Role of functional genetic variation in the dopamine D2 receptor (DRD2) in response to bupropion and nicotine replacement therapy for tobacco dependence: Results of two randomized clinical trials. *Neuropsychopharmacology, 31,* 231-242.

Levin, E. D. (2002). Nicotinic receptor subtypes and cognitive function. *Journal of Neurobiology, 53,* 633-640.

Levin, E. D., Conners, C. K., Silvia, D., Hinton, S. C., Meck, W. H., March, J., and Rose, J. E (1998). Transdermal nicotine effects on attention. *Psychopharmacology, 140,* 135-141.

Masson, C., and Gilbert (1999). Cardiovascular and mood responses to quantified doses of cigarette smoke in oral contraceptives users and non-users. *Journal of Behavioral Medicine, 22 (6),* 589 – 604.

McDowell, S., Whyte, J., D'Esposito, M. (1998). Differential effect of a dopaminergic agonist on prefrontal function in traumatic brain injury patients. *Brain, 121,* 1155-1164.

McClure, J. B., and Swan, G. E. (2006). Tailoring nicotine replacement therapy: rationale and potential approaches. *CNS Drugs, 20,* 281-291.

Mirowsky, J., and Ross, C. E. (1995). Sex differences in distress: Real or artifact? *American Sociological Review, 60,* 449-468.

Morissette, M., and Di Paolo, T. (1993). Sex and estrous cycle variations of rat striatal dopamine uptake sites. *Neuroendocrinology, 58,* 16 – 22.

Munafo, M., Bradburn, M., Bowes, L., and David, S. (2004). Are there sex differences in transdermal nicotine replacement therapy patch efficacy? A meta-analysis. *Nicotine and Tobacco Research, 6,* 769 – 776.

Netter, P., Henning, J., Huwe, S., and Olbrich, R. (1998). Personality related effects of nicotine, mode of application, and expectancies on performance, emotional states, and desire for smoking. *Psychopharmacology, 135,* 52-62.

Neuhaus, A., Bajbouj, M., Kienast, T., Kalus, P., von Haebler, D., Winterer, G., Gallinat, J. (2006). Persistant dysfunctional frontal lobe activation in former smokers. *Psychopharmacology* [In Press].

Newhouse, P. A., Potter, A., and Singh, A. (2004). Effects of nicotinic stimulation on cognitive performance. *Current Opinion in Pharmacology, 4,* 36 – 46.

Newhouse, P. A., Sunderland, T., Narang, P. K., Mellow, A. M., Fertig, J. B., Lawlor, B. A., and Murphy, D. L. (1990). Neuroendocrine, physiologic, and behavioral responses following intravenous nicotine in non-smoking healthy volunteers and in patients with Alzheimer's disease. *Psychoendocrinology, 15,* 471-484.

Niaura, R., Shadel, W. G., Abrams, D. B., Monti, P. M., Rohsenow, D. J., and Sirota, A. (1998). Individual differences in cue reactivity among smokers trying to quit:effects of gender and cue type. *Addictive Behaviors, 23,* 209-224.

Nisell, M., Nomikos, G. G., Svensson, T. H. (1994). Infusion of nicotine in the ventral tegmental area or the nucleus accumbens of the rat differentially affects accumbal dopamine release. *Pharmacology and Toxicology, 75,* 348 – 352.

Paoletti, P., Fornai, E., Maggiorelli, F., Puntoni, R., Viegi, G., Carrozzi, L., Corlando, A., Gustavsson, G., Sawe, U., and Giuntini, C. (1996). Importance of baseline cotinine plasma values in smoking cessation: results from a double-blind study with nicotine patch. *The European Respiratory Journal, 9,* 643-651.

Parrott, A. C. and Garnham, N. J. (1998). Comparative mood states and cognitive skills of cigarette smokers, deprived smokers and non-smokers. *Human Psychopharmacology, 13,* 367 – 376.

Perkins, K. A. (2001). Smoking cessation in women: Special considerations. *CNS Drugs, 15,* 391-411.

Perkins, K. (1996). Sex differences in nicotine versus non-nicotine reinforcement as determinants of tobacco smoking. *Experimental and Clinical Psychopharmacology, 4 (2),* 166- 177.

Perkins, K. A., Doyle, T., Ciccocioppo, M., Conklin, C., Sayette, M., and Caggiula, A. (2006). Sex differences in the influence of nicotine dose instructions on the reinforcing and self-reported rewarding effects of smoking. *Psychopharmacology, 184,* 600 -607.

Perkins, K. A., Grobe, J. E., Stiller, R. L., Fonte, C., and Goettler, J. E. (1992). Nasal spray nicotine replacement suppresses cigarette smoking desire and behaviour. *Clinical Pharmacology and Therapeutics, 52,* 627 – 634.

Poltavski, D. V., and Petros, T. (2005). Effects of transdermal nicotine on prose memory and attention in smokers and nonsmokers. *Physiology and behavior, 83,* 833–843.

Pontieri, F., Tanda, G., Orzi, F., and Di Chiara, G. (1996). Effects of nicotine on the nucleus accumbens and similarity to those of addictive drugs. *Nature, 382,* 255 – 257.

Razani, J., Boone, K., Lesser, I., Weiss, D. (2004). Effects of cigarette smoking history on cognitive functioning in healthy older adults. *American Journal of Geriatric Psychiatry, 12,* 404-411.

Rezvani, A. H., and Levin, E. D. (2001). Cognitive effects of nicotine. *Biological Psychiatry, 49 (3),* 258-267.

Robinson, J. D., Cinciripini, P. M., Tiffany, S. T., Carter, B. L., Lam, C. Y., and Wetter, D. W. (2007). Gender differences in affective response to acute nicotine administration and deprivation. *Addictive Behaviors, 32,* 543-561.

Sallette, J., Pons, S., Devillers-Thiery, A., Soudant, M., Prado de Carvalho, L., Changeux, J.P., Corringer, P.J. (2005). Nicotine upregulates its own receptors through enhanced intracellular maturation. *Neuron, 46 (4),* 595-607.

Sayette, M. A., and Hufford, M. R. (1995). Urge and affect: A facial coding analysis of smokers. *Experimental and Clinical Psychopharmacology, 3,* 417-423.

Shiffman, S., Sweeney, C. T., Dresler, C. M. (2005). Nicotine patch and lozenge are effective for women. *Nicotine and Tobacco Research, 1,* 119-127.

Shiffman, S., Waters, A. J., Hickcox, M. (2004). The Nicotine Dependence Syndrome Scale: A multidimensional measure of nicotine dependence. *Nicotine and Tobacco Research, 6 (2),* 327-348.

Silagy, C., Lancaster, T., Mant, D., Fowler, G. (2004). Nicotine replacement therapy for smoking cessation (Review). *Cochrane Database of Systematic Reviews, 3,* 1-25.

Stein, E. A., Pankiewicz, J., Harsch, H.H., Cho, J. K., Fuller, S. A., Hoffman, R. G., Hawkins, M., Rao, S. M., Bandettini, P.A., Bloom, A. S. (1998). Nicotine-induced limbic cortical activation in the human brain: a functional MRI study. *American Journal of Psychiatry, 155,* 1009-1015.

Steptoe, A., Ussher, M. (2006). Smoking, cortisol and nicotine. *International Journal of Psychophysiology, 59,* 228 – 235.

Swan, G. E., Jack, L. M., Ward, M. M. (1997). Subgroups of smokers with different success rates after use of transdermal nicotine. *Addiction, 92,* 207-218.

Takahashi, H., Kato, M., Hayashi, M., Okubo, Y., Takano, A., Ito, H., Suhara, T. (2007). Memory and frontal lobe functions: possible relations with dopamine D2 receptors in the hippocampus. *Neuroimage, 34,* 1643-1649.

Trimmel, M. and Wittberger, S. (2004). Effects of transdermally administered nicotine on aspects of attention, task load, and mood in women and men. Pharmacology, *Biochemistry and Behavior, 78,* 639-645.

VanderKaay, M. M., and Patterson, S. M. (2006). Nicotine and acute stress: Effects of nicotine versus nicotine withdrawal on stress-induced hemoconcentration and cardiovascular reactivity. *Biological Psychology, 71,* 191-201.

West, R., Hajek, P., Nilsson, F., Foulds, J., May, S., and Meadows, A. (2001). Individual differences in preferences for and responses to four nicotine replacement products. *Psychopharmacology, 153,* 225-230.

Wetter, D. W., Kenford, S. L., Smith, S. S., Fiore, M. C., Jorenby, D. E., Baker, T. B. (1999). Gender differences in smoking cessation. *Journal of Consulting and Clinical Psychology, 67,* 555 – 562.

Yilmaz, O., Kanit, L., Erdem, B., and Pogun, S. (1997). Effects of nicotine on active avoidance learning in rats: sex differences. *Behavioral Pharmacology, 8,* 253 – 260.

Yudkin, P., Munafo, M., Hey, K., Roberts, S., Welch, S., Johnstone, E., Murphy, M., Griffiths, S., and Walton, R. (2004). Effectiveness of nicotine patches in relation to genotype in women versus men: randomized controlled trial. *British Medical Journal, 328,* 989-990.

In: Smoking and Women's Health
Editors: M.K. Wesley and I.A. Sternbach, pp.165-181 ISBN 978-1-60456-148-7
© 2008 Nova Science Publishers, Inc.

Chapter 6

Effect of Gender and Smoking on Incidence of Cardiovascular Disease and Peptic Ulcer in A Japanese Population: The Radiation Effects Research Foundation Adult Health Study

Michiko Yamada[41] *and F. Lennie Wong*[2]
Departments of [1] Clinical Studies and [2] Statistics,
Radiation Effects Research Foundation, Japan
([2] current affiliation: Division of Population Sciences, City of Hope National Medical Center, Duarte, CA) USA

Abstract

Background: Studies on the effects of gender and smoking on cardiovascular and peptic ulcer disease have been reported in Western countries, but data from Asian countries are limited and inconsistent.

Methods: We examined the effects of gender and smoking on cardiovascular and peptic ulcer disease using the longitudinal data of the Adult Health Study collected during biennial health examinations from 1 July 1958 to 30 June 1998. The examinations included medical history, chest x-ray, ultrasonography, and fluoroscopy or endoscopy. Smoking histories were obtained from 5 questionnaires self-administered during different time periods. We estimated the relative risks for being female and for "ever" versus "never" smoking after adjusting for significant effects of age, city, birth cohort, calendar time, alcohol intake, and radiation dose. We also examined the interaction between gender and smoking.

---

4 Corresponding author: Departments of Clinical Studies, Radiation Effects Research Foundation, 5-2 Hijiyama Park, Minami-ku,Hiroshima 732–0815, Japan, Telephone: +81-82-261-3131, Fax: +81-82-263-7279, e-mail: yamada@rerf.or.jp.

Results: Eight hundred and fifty four strokes, 215 aortic aneurysms, 1093 gastric ulcers, and 437 duodenal ulcers were detected between 1958 to 1998: and, from 1978 to 1998, 125 myocardial infarction were detected. The incidence of myocardial infarction, stroke, and gastric and duodenal ulcer was significantly higher in men than in women, but we found no gender difference for aortic aneurysm incidence after adjustment for smoking status. We detected positive associations of smoking with myocardial infarction (RR for ever smoked to never smoked, 1.96), stroke (RR, 1.26), aortic aneurysm (RR, 1.80), gastric ulcer (RR, 2.06), and duodenal ulcer (RR, 1.32). The interaction between gender and smoking status was not significant for any of the diseases.

Conclusions: Male gender and smoking were significant risk factors for cardiovascular and peptic ulcer disease in a Japanese population.

KeyWords: *Gender differences, smoking, myocardial infarction, stroke, aortic aneurysm, gastric ulcer, duodenal ulcer*

Introduction

Many epidemiological studies in Western populations have reported gender differences for, and smoking effects on, cardiovascular disease and peptic ulcers.[1-5] Studies regarding stroke and coronary heart disease from Asian populations are limited, however, and the results are inconsistent.[6-10] Incidence and risk factor studies on peptic ulcers and aortic aneurysm in Asia are also limited.

Previous investigations on the relationship between cardiovascular disease and smoking in Japan varied by design (cross-sectional, case-control, and prospective studies), study population (gender, age, general population, and outpatient), or endpoint (mortality and incidence). The 23-year follow-up of the Hisayama study (a long-term prospective study of rural Japanese subjects followed since 1961) showed that cigarette smoking was an independent and significant risk factor for coronary heart disease, but not for non-embolic cerebral infarction.[6] Other pre-1980 Japanese epidemiological studies found no association between smoking and stroke.[7, 11, 12] The 32-year follow-up of the Hisayama study reported that smoking was a risk factor for lacunar stroke, the most common type of cerebral infarction in their study.[8] Studies published after the 1980s showed that smoking raised the risk of stroke [9, 13] and myocardial infarction (MI).[14] Only the Hisayama study reported gender differences in the incidence of all types of cardiovascular disease[6] and the prevalence of coronary atherosclerosis in the Japanese population.[15]

The Honolulu heart program, a long-term prospective study that has been following Japanese-American men in Hawaii since 1965, provided evidence that smoking was a risk factor for stroke, coronary heart disease, aortic aneurysm, and peptic ulcer.[16-19]

Although many studies report gender-specific estimates of incidence and mortality rates and gender-specific smoking effects on cardiovascular disease and peptic ulcer, gender differences have not been examined formally. In this study, we examined the effects of gender and smoking on the incidence of MI, stroke, aortic aneurysm, gastric ulcer, and duodenal ulcer in the Radiation Effects Research Foundation (RERF) Adult Health Study

(AHS) cohort. The AHS has health data spanning from 1958 to1998 for one of the largest existing cohorts of middle-aged and elderly men and women,[20, 21] and it is still ongoing.

Subjects and Methods

Subjects

The AHS was begun in 1958 by the Atomic Bomb Casualty Commission and was succeeded in 1975 by the Radiation Effects Research Foundation (RERF). By providing biennial clinical examinations to atomic-bomb survivors and their controls in Hiroshima and Nagasaki, the AHS has tracked the long-term clinical effects of exposure to atomic-bomb radiation.[20, 21]

The subjects of the present analysis are the 11,982 who attended at least two AHS examinations between 1 July 1958 and 30 June 1998 (about half of the original AHS subjects had died by then). About 62% of the participants were women and 69% were Hiroshima residents (Table 1). A high participation rate (75% to 90%) has been maintained, and more than half of the study participants underwent 11 or more routine clinical examinations.

Table 1. Characteristics of study subjects

		Hiroshima		Nagasaki	
		Men	Women	Men	Women
Total		2984	5265	1561	2172
Age in 1945	Mean	31.0	30.0	25.5	23.6
S.D.		15.9	14.6	14.7	13.0
Age at examination	Range	13 – 92	13 – 98	14 – 98	14 – 97
Smoking	Never smoked	300 (10%)	3709 (70%)	205 (13%)	1658 (76%)
	Ever smoked	2366 (79%)	996 (19%)	1258 (80%)	364 (17%)
	Missing data	318 (11%)	560 (11%)	98 (6%)	150 (7%)
Drinking	Never drank	472 (16%)	3180 (60%)	272 (17%)	1530 (70%)
	Ever drank	2076 (70%)	1440 (27%)	1132 (73%)	464 (21%)
	Missing data	436 (15%)	645 (12%)	157 (10%)	178 (8%)
Number of cases	Total				
Myocardial infarction[a]	125	50	40	17	18
Stroke	854	291	312	142	109
Aortic aneurysm	215	60	88	31	36
Gastric ulcer	1093	394	394	182	123
Duodenal ulcer	438	169	115	94	59
Radiation dose	Dose=0	1003 (34%)	1746 (33%)	514 (33%)	691(32%)
	Mean (Sv)	0.38	0.33	0.41	0.40
	Missing	286 (10%)	388 (7%)	450 (29%)	519 (24%)

[a] for incidence during 1978-1998.
Parenthetical values represent %.

Clinical Procedures and Selection of Diseases for Study

All participants provided informed consent, and the study complied with institutional guidelines regarding research ethics and the welfare of human subjects. A detailed description of the clinical procedures is available elsewhere.[20, 21] Briefly, the biennial AHS examination includes a clinical history taking, a physical examination, blood pressure measurements, urinalysis, blood cell count, biochemical tests, a chest X-ray, an electrocardiogram, and ultrasonography. Diagnoses were encoded according to the International Classification of Diseases (ICD)[22] and entered into the AHS database. The first 3 digits of the ICD codes (up to 6 diagnoses per person) were stored until June 1986, and 4-digit codes (up to 12 per person) were stored thereafter (appendix). MI was determined by history of hospitalization or angiography with a diagnosis of MI, episode of chest pain, and development of ischemic change on electrocardiogram. Stroke was determined by history of hospitalization or CT/MRI examination with a diagnosis of stroke and episode of neurological deficit. MI was not ascertained prior to July 1978 because ICD codes for acute MI and old MI did not exist then. Aortic aneurysm (thoracic and abdominal aortic aneurysm and aortic dissection) was diagnosed by medical history, chest x-ray examination, and ultrasonography. Ultrasonography was used optionally from 1981 to 1990 in Hiroshima and from 1984 to 1990 in Nagasaki. Since 1991, it has been performed routinely. It should be noted that this study includes only survivors of MI, stroke, ruptured aortic aneurysm, and aortic dissection who underwent subsequent examinations, as death certificate data were not considered. About 5% of participants, however, underwent clinical examinations at home or in a nearby hospital or an institution where they were residing because of severe illness or advanced age. Peptic ulcer was diagnosed by medical history and fluoroscopy or endoscopy, which were conducted optionally for subjects whose stool occult blood test was positive in a routine examination.

Cigarette Smoking and Alcohol Consumption Data

We obtained cigarette smoking history from 5 questionnaires self-administered to men in 1965, to women in 1969-1970, and to both men and women in 1965-1966, 1979-1980, and 1991. The response rate was over 95% for all surveys. Due to differences in the questionnaires and the make-up of the survey participants, the subjects were classified simply as "never smoked" (i.e., indicated in all the surveys that they had never smoked), "ever smoked" (indicated in any survey that they had smoked some quantity of cigarettes), or "missing smoking data" (did not participate in any of the smoking surveys).

Alcohol intake information was obtained from 3 questionnaires self-administered to both sexes in 1965-1966, 1979-1980, and 1991. The same classifications were applied: never drank, ever drank, and missing data. Non-drinkers were subjects who did not drink any beer, whiskey, shochu (Japanese distilled liquor), wine (including sake), or other liquor.

Statistical Methods

We applied Poisson regression methods for the longitudinal analysis of incidence data using AMFIT from the EPICURE program package.[23] We based person-year calculations on the subject's follow-up period, which began at the initial AHS visit and ended on the last disease-free visit or the date of disease onset, whichever came earlier. We estimated the disease onset date as the midpoint between the date of the initial AHS exam with a positive diagnosis and the date of the previous disease-free examination. For each disease, we excluded prevalent cases at the initial visit. We cross-tabulated person-years and case counts by stratifying the following covariates: city (Hiroshima, Nagasaki), sex (male, female), age at examination in years (0–39, 40–49, 50–59, 60–69, 70+), age at the time of the atomic bombings in years (0–9, 10–19, 20–29, 30–39, 40+), calendar time (1 July 1958 to 30 June 1978, 1 July 1978 to 30 June 1998), cigarette smoking (never smoked, ever smoked, missing data), alcohol consumption status (never drank, ever drank, missing data), and atomic-bomb radiation dose using the DS86 weighted stomach dose in Sv (missing, 0, 0.001–0.49, 0.5–1.49, 1.50+). Significant dose effects were not demonstrated in the previous AHS report for the diseases considered here.[20, 21] A detailed description of the dose estimation is available elsewhere.[21]

We modeled the disease incidence rates (γ) parametrically using the exponential function, $\gamma(x_1, ..., x_c) = \exp\{\sum_i \beta_i x_i\}$, where x_i is a covariable. We treated covariates as categorical except for age at the time of the bombings and age at examination, for which we used the cell-specific means. We included up to the third power of mean age at examination and at the time of the bombings in order to adjust for potential non-linear age effects. We allowed only the significant covariates in the model and considered first order interactions. We computed the relative risks (RRs) of a covariate using models that did not include its interactions with age at time of the bombings or age at examination. We calculated the RR based on indicator variables for the covariates in the models. We used the likelihood ratio method to test the significance of the coefficients of the covariates using Type I error rate of .05, in a forward step-wise algorithm, and to compute the 95% confidence intervals.

Results

Table 1 shows the characteristics of study subjects by gender and city. Overall among men, 11% never smoked, 80% ever smoked, and smoking data were missing for 9%; 16% never drank, 70% ever drank, and drinking data were missing for 13%. Overall among women, 72% never smoked, 18% ever smoked, and smoking data were missing for 10%; 63% never drank, 26% ever drank, and drinking data were missing for 11%. The distribution of smokers by atomic bomb radiation exposure did not vary significantly for men ($P = 0.14$), but there were significantly more smokers among the exposed women than among the non-exposed women (23% vs. 17%; $P < 0.0001$). The distribution of drinkers did not vary significantly by radiation exposure for either sex (data not shown).

Table 2 shows the number of incident cases and crude incidence rates for MI, stroke, aortic aneurysm, gastric ulcer, and duodenal ulcer by each variable and the multivariate adjusted RRs. Crude incidence rates were higher for men for all diseases, and RRs were significantly lower for women for all diseases, except aortic aneurysm. Risk for aortic aneurysm was same in males and females. Although the incidence of aortic aneurysm was significantly lower for women when smoking was not included in the model ($P = 0.008$), the gender difference was not significant when smoking status was included ($P = 0.42$).

Table 2. Multivariate adjusted relative risks for myocardial infarction, stroke, aortic aneurysm, gastric ulcer, and duodenal ulcer

Disease	Myocardial infarction[a]	Stroke	Aortic aneurysm	Gastric ulcer	Duodenal ulcer
Number of cases	125	854	215	1093	437
Males	67	433	91	576	263
Females	58	421	124	517	174
Person-years	111930	289629	293634	279650	287700
Males	36382	100183	102330	94738	98279
Female	75548	189446	191304	184912	189421
Crude incidence rate (10,000 PY) Males	11.2	29.5	7.3	39.1	15.2
	18.4	43.2	8 9	60.8	26.8
Females	7.7	22.2	6.5	28.0	9.2
Relative risk					
Sex (Female to Male, age 50)	0.59	0.54	0.99	0.71	0.43
(95% confidence interval)	(0.37 – 0.94)	(0.46 – 0.64)	(0.70 – 1.39)	(0.61 – 0.83)	(0.33 – 0.56)
P-value	0.025	<0.001	0.97	<0.001	<0.001
Smoking (Ever to Never)	1.96	1.26	1.80	2.06	1.32
(95% confidence interval)	(1.20 – 3.16)	(1.05 - 1.51)	(1.37 – 2.37)	(1.75 - 2.42)	(1.01 - 1.72)
P-value	0.018	0.013	<0..001	<0.001	0.043
City (Nagasaki to Hiroshima)	0.75	1.04	1.14	0.76	0.95
P-value	0.14	0.62	0.38	<0.0001	0.62
Period (late to early[b])	-	1.11	0.92	0.92	0.95
P-value	-	0.15	0.57	0.60	0.84
Drinking (Ever to Never)	0.83	0.93	0.90	1.01	1.06
P-value	0.39	0.36	0.50	0.38	0.50
Age in 1945					
15	1.00	1.00	1.00	1.00	1.00
25	0.74	0.95	1.06	0.90	0.86
35	0.54	0.90	1.13	0.81	0.74
45	0.40	0.86	1.20	0.73	0.63
P-value	0.17	0.16	0.42	0.003	0.010
Age at examination					
45	1.00	1.00	1.00	1.00	1.00
55	1.76	3.71	2.91	1.19	0.91
65	3.10	10.57	8.51	1.25	0.66
75	5.46	18.21	16.88	1.17	0.39
P-value	<0.0001	<0.0001	<0.0001	<0.0001	<0.0001

[a] Incidence, 1978-1998; [b] Early period, 7/58 – 6/78; late period, 7/78 – 6/98.

We detected a significantly increased RR for ever smokers compared with never smokers for all diseases, while the interaction between gender and smoking status was not significant for any of diseases (p-values=0.29, 0.81, 0.41, 0.16, and 0.44, respectively for MI, stroke, aortic aneurysm, gastric ulcer, and duodenal ulcer). Hiroshima residents showed a higher incidence of gastric ulcer. The younger birth cohort showed a higher incidence of gastric ulcer and duodenal ulcer. A higher incidence among older subjects was found for all diseases except duodenal ulcer, which displayed a convex risk curve (Figure 1).

Figure 1 shows the fitted age-specific incidence curves for MI, stroke, and gastric and duodenal ulcer by gender and smoking status. Because gender difference was significant for aortic aneurysm before, but not after adjustment for smoking status, age-specific incidence for aortic aneurysm by gender is shown unadjusted for smoking. The incidence curves by smoking status are also shown. The effects were significant, independent of gender. Adjusted for the significant covariates for each disease, we plotted the incidence of MI and duodenal ulcer in both cities, and of gastric ulcer for Hiroshima, for men and women aged 15 in 1945. Incidence of MI, stroke, aortic aneurysm, and gastric ulcer increased significantly with age. Incidence of duodenal ulcer peaked in the 4th and 5th decades of life and then declined. Incidence of duodenal ulcer peaked later in older cohorts.

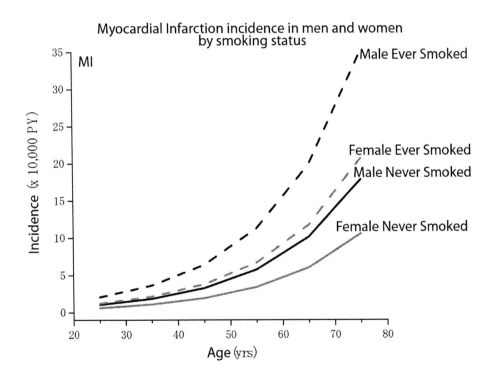

Figure 1. Continued on next page.

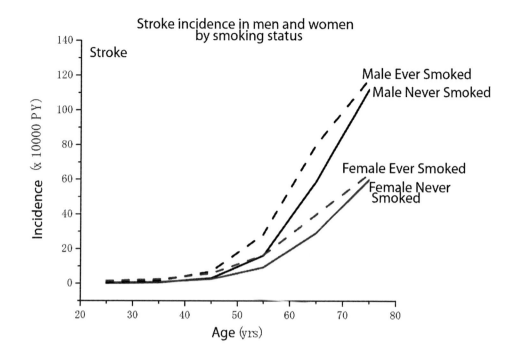

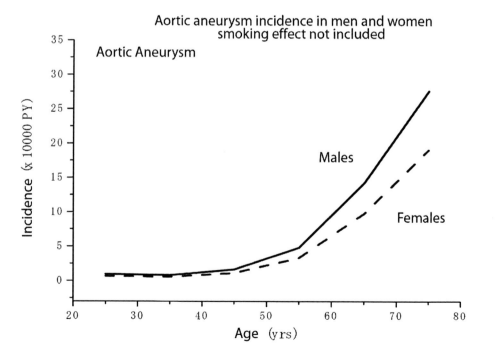

Figure 1. Continued on next page.

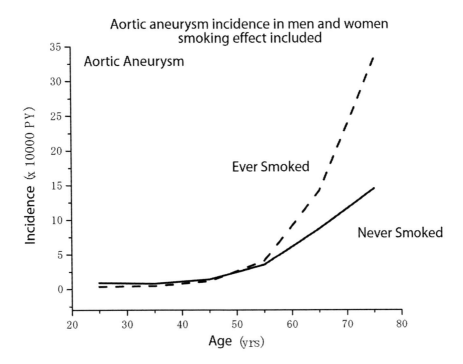

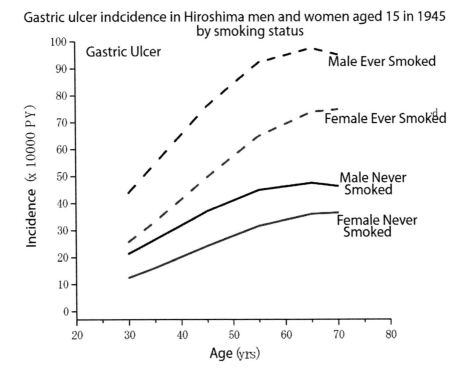

Figure 1. Continued on next page.

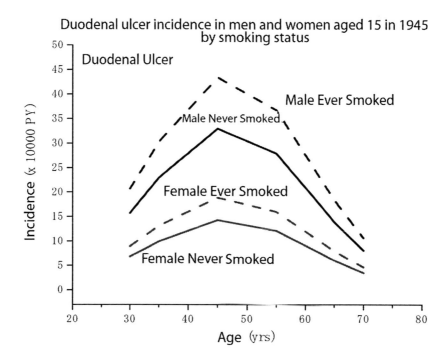

Figure 1. Gender-age specific incidence for myocardial infarction, stroke, aortic aneurysm, gastric ulcer, and duodenal ulcer.

Discussion

In this prospective study of a large Japanese cohort, the crude incidence rates for MI, stroke, and aortic aneurysm were higher for men than for women, but the RR was higher only for MI and stroke after adjustment for smoking status. Similar RRs for stroke were reported previously in Japan [6, 24] and Europe, [25, 26] and a smaller RR was reported in the US.[27] Although the gender difference in MI morbidity tended to diminish after menopausal age in the Framingham study, [28] we found no such tendency. A limitation in our study, however, was that some cases of silent MI, and all cases of fatal MI and stroke, were not included because some medical charts were not validated and death certificate data were not considered. The MI incidence in the AHS in 1958 and 1984 was calculated using a stringent set of criteria, including a review of medical history, electrocardiogram results, death certificate data, and autopsy information, was 1.6 times higher in men than in women.[29] In another AHS study that used similar criteria, the incidence of stroke and coronary heart disease, including asymptomatic and fatal cases, was twice as high in men as in women.[30] The risk of abdominal aortic aneurysm was about two times higher for men than for women in the Chicago Heart Association cohort.[31] The mortality rate of aortic aneurysm in Japan and its incidence rate (based on ultrasound scanning) in Malaysia were also more than twice as high in men.[32, 33] To clarify the disparity in the gender effect on aortic aneurysm that depended on smoking adjustment in this study, we examined the gender-specific crude incidence rates in the never smoked and the ever smoked groups. Whereas the crude incidence rate was higher for male never smokers than for female never smokers (7.97 vs. 5.32 per 10,000 py), it was lower for male ever smokers than for female ever smokers (8.96 vs. 11.36). A plausible explanation for our not detecting a gender difference in aortic aneurysm incidence after adjustment for smoking is that the proportion of fatal cases might have been higher among male smokers than among female smokers. The explanation is supported by the observation that male smokers have an increased risk of aneurysm rupture and poorer long-term survival.[34, 35] A future analysis that includes fatal cases should serve to clarify gender differences in cardiovascular disease within this cohort.

We found the incidence of peptic ulcer to be higher among men than among women, which is consistent with previous studies of Japanese and Koreans in Japan.[36, 37] Although more pronounced risks were seen in men in Western societies before the 1970s, [38] recent studies in Europe and in the US show a more equal distribution of peptic ulcer incidence between the sexes.[39, 40]

The smoking information we used in this study was obtained from multiple questionnaires administered over some time and could reflect changing habits. The lack of detailed temporal information necessitated our lumping current and past smokers into an "ever smoked" category. However, it is possible that the never smoked group may have contained a few subjects who started smoking after the last questionnaire was administered and that the ever smoked group included subjects who quit smoking over 5 years previously. Moreover, since the number of cigarettes smoked was not available in this study, we could not perform dose-response analyses.

The disease incidences for the ever smoked in this study were significantly higher than that for the never smoked, although the RR estimates (Table 2) were lower than those for current smoker versus nonsmoker reported in other studies.[3, 13, 14, 18, 19, 36, 41] Since smoking cessation and fewer smoking years are important for reducing the risk of cardiovascular disease and peptic ulcer,[4, 42-46] the lower RRs seen in this study may be due to the ever smoked category containing some current smokers.

Case ascertainment in this study was limited to participants whose illness was not fatal or too severe to preclude study participation. This may have led to an underestimation of smoker risk since illnesses in smokers tend to be of greater severity.[15, 47, 48] Although we did not consider in this analysis hypertension and diabetes, both well-known risk factors for cardiovascular disease, higher blood pressure among smokers has been observed in our cohort,[49] and smoking is associated with an increased risk of type 2 diabetes among middle-aged and elderly Japanese men and women.[50] Thus the smoking effects estimated in this study included both direct effects and indirect effects of confounding risk factors. Despite those limitations, we believe that our data clearly show that smoking negatively impacts the health of the cohort through the onset of these diseases.

Lederle's systematic review [51] of studies that examined smoking effects on aortic aneurysm and other smoking-related diseases showed that association of aortic aneurysm with smoking was greater than for MI or stroke. The RR estimate for aortic aneurysm in the present study was much lower than in previous studies based on both mortality and incidence. Further, there was no pronounced effect of smoking on aortic aneurysm.

The RR for individuals in the ever smoked category, relative to the never smoked category was higher for gastric ulcer than for duodenal ulcer, which is consistent with findings from other studies of Japanese [36, 37] and Japanese-Americans in Hawaii.[19] On the other hand, the RR was slightly greater for duodenal ulcer than for gastric ulcer among European countries.[52, 53] Our finding that the crude incidence rate was higher for gastric ulcer than for duodenal ulcer was consistent with reports from other Japanese populations [36, 37] and Japanese-Americans,[19] but not those from European countries.[53, 54] The US National Health Interview Survey [40] reported that duodenal ulcer was more common in whites than non-whites, while gastric ulcer was more common in non-whites. *Helicobacter pylori* infection, a major risk for peptic ulcer, [53] may be an important factor for interpreting apparent racial differences, since the prevalence of *H. pylori* infection is much higher in Japan and Asia than in Europe.[55] In Japan, the prevalence of *H. pylori* infection was high for those born before 1950 and decreased in later birth cohorts as Japan became more Westernized.[56, 57] Our study participants were all born in, or before 1945,. In this cohort, the prevalence of a positive IgG antibody response to *H. pylori* was about 60% in 2000 and 2002.[58] Since early acquisition of *H. pylori* increases the risk for developing gastric but not duodenal ulcer,[59] the higher prevalence of early *H. pylori* infection in Japan might have led to an increase in gastric ulcer incidence. Further analysis is required to fully elucidate the difference in incidence patterns and smoking effects on gastric and duodenal ulcer.

Although we found a greater incidence rate for MI, stroke, and peptic ulcer in men, the effects of smoking were comparable in both sexes. The incidence of MI, and its associated mortality, increased similarly among male and female smokers of European countries, as well as Japan.[5, 60] Other studies, by contract, showed a higher RR of MI for female smokers[26] and male smokers.[61] Many prospective studies in Europe and the US provided similar, strong evidence of an excess risk of stroke among male and female smokers,[3, 62-64] but data from Japanese populations are limited and results are not consistent.[6, 8, 9, 13] Many epidemiological and clinical studies of men[2, 19] and some of women [65] in Europe and the US demonstrate a similar increased risk of peptic ulcer in men and women who smoke.[66] However, there have been few Japanese and Asian prospective studies that have examined gender differences on the effects of smoking on peptic ulcer incidence. Our study was unusual in that we examined gender differences on the effects of smoking on several cardiovascular diseases, as well as peptic ulcer disease.

Participants in the present study--atomic bomb survivors and their controls--may not be representative of the general Japanese population, but we believe that the results might be extrapolated to the general population, due to the fact that one third of the participants were minimally exposed (estimated radiation dose, zero), and that the radiation exposure effects were fully accounted for by including radiation dose as a covariate in the analysis. The agreement of our findings on the effects of demographic variables such as age and gender with the findings of others [6, 37] further supports for the validity of our results.

The proportion of men who are current smokers is higher in Japan than in Western countries [9, 44] while the reverse is true for women, although a rise in smoking frequency among young to middle-aged Japanese women since 1990 has been reported.[67] The present results provide further support for smoking cessation as a way to prevent cardiovascular disease and peptic ulcer in Japan.

Appendix

International Classification of Diseases Codes			
	ICD edition		
Disease	7th	8th	9th
Myocardial infarction	-	410	410,412
Stroke	330-332,334	430,431,433,434,436	430,431,433,434,436
Aortic aneurysm	451	441	441
Gastric ulcer	540	531	531
Duodenal ulcer	541	532	532

Acknowledgments

This publication is based on research performed at the Radiation Effects Research Foundation (RERF), Hiroshima and Nagasaki, Japan. RERF is a private non-profit foundation funded equally by the Japanese Ministry of Health, Labour and Welfare and the US Department of Energy (DOE), the latter through the National Academy of Sciences. This publication was supported by RERF Research Protocol RP 2-75 and in part by a grant from the Japan Arteriosclerosis Prevention Fund.

References

[1]   Andersen IB, Jorgensen T, Bonnevie O et al.: Smoking and alcohol intake as risk factors for bleeding and perforated peptic ulcers: a population-based cohort study. *Epidemiology* 2000;11:434-439.

[2]   Doll R, Peto R, Wheatley K et al.: Mortality in relation to smoking: 40 years' observations on male British doctors. *Bmj* 1994;309:901-911.

[3]   Wolf PA, D'Agostino RB, Kannel WB et al.: Cigarette smoking as a risk factor for stroke. The Framingham Study. *Jama* 1988;259:1025-1029.

[4]   Hozawa A, Houston T, Steffes MW et al.: The association of cigarette smoking with self-reported disease before middle age: the Coronary Artery Risk Development in Young Adults (CARDIA) study. *Prev. Med.* 2006;42:193-199.

[5]   Nilsson S, Carstensen JM, Pershagen G: Mortality among male and female smokers in Sweden: a 33 year follow up. *J. Epidemiol. Community Health* 2001;55:825-830.

[6]   Kiyohara Y, Ueda K, Fujishima M: Smoking and cardiovascular disease in the general population in Japan. *J. Hypertens. Suppl.* 1990;8:S9-15.

[7]   Tanaka H, Ueda Y, Hayashi M et al.: Risk factors for cerebral hemorrhage and cerebral infarction in a Japanese rural community.. *Stroke* 1982;13:62-73.

[8]   Tanizaki Y, Kiyohara Y, Kato I et al.: Incidence and risk factors for subtypes of cerebral infarction in a general population: the Hisayama study. *Stroke* 2000;31:2616-2622.

[9]   9..Ueshima H, Choudhury SR, Okayama A et al.: Cigarette smoking as a risk factor for stroke death in Japan: NIPPON DATA80. *Stroke* 2004;35:1836-1841.

[10]   Liu XF, van Melle G, Bogousslavsky J: Analysis of risk factors in 3901 patients with stroke. *Chin. Med. Sci. J.* 2005;20:35-39.

[11]   Okada H, Horibe H, Yoshiyuki O et al.: A prospective study of cerebrovascular disease in Japanese rural communities, Akabane and Asahi. Part 1: evaluation of risk factors in the occurrence of cerebral hemorrhage and thrombosis. *Stroke* 1976;7:599-607.

[12]   Takeya Y, Popper JS, Shimizu Y et al.: Epidemiologic studies of coronary heart disease and stroke in Japanese men living in Japan, Hawaii and California: incidence of stroke in Japan and Hawaii. *Stroke* 1984;15:15-23.

[13]   Mannami T, Iso H, Baba S et al.: Cigarette smoking and risk of stroke and its subtypes among middle-aged Japanese men and women: the JPHC Study Cohort I. *Stroke* 2004;35:1248-1253.

[14]   Tokuda Y: Risk factors for acute myocardial infarction among Okinawans. *J. Nutr. Health Aging* 2005;9:272-276.

[15]   Okumiya N, Tanaka K, Ueda K et al.: Coronary atherosclerosis and antecedent risk factors: pathologic and epidemiologic study in Hisayama, Japan. *Am. J. Cardiol.* 1985;56:62-66.

[16]   Benfante R, Yano K, Hwang LJ et al.: Elevated serum cholesterol is a risk factor for both coronary heart disease and thromboembolic stroke in Hawaiian Japanese men. Implications of shared risk. *Stroke* 1994;25:814-820.

[17]   Yano K, MacLean CJ, Reed DM et al.: A comparison of the 12-year mortality and predictive factors of coronary heart disease among Japanese men in Japan and Hawaii. *Am. J. Epidemiol.* 1988;127:476-487.

[18]   Goldberg RJ, Burchfiel CM, Benfante R et al.: Lifestyle and biologic factors associated with atherosclerotic disease in middle-aged men. 20-year findings from the Honolulu Heart Program. *Arch. Intern. Med.* 1995;155:686-694.

[19]   Kato I, Nomura AM, Stemmermann GN et al.: A prospective study of gastric and duodenal ulcer and its relation to smoking, alcohol, and diet. *Am. J. Epidemiol.* 1992;135:521-530.

[20]   Wong FL, Yamada M, Sasaki H et al.: Noncancer disease incidence in the atomic bomb survivors: 1958-1986. *Radiat. Res.* 1993;135:418-430.

[21]   Yamada M, Wong FL, Fujiwara S et al.: Noncancer disease incidence in atomic bomb survivors, 1958-1998. *Radiat. Res.* 2004;161:622-632.

[22]   International Classification of Diseases, 9th Revision (ICD 9). Geneva: WHO; 1977.

[23]   Preston D, Lubin J, Pierce D. Epicure User's Guide. Seattle: Hirosoft *International Corp.*; 1993.

[24]   Suzuki K, Kutsuzawa T, Takita K et al.: Clinico-epidemiologic study of stroke in Akita, Japan. *Stroke* 1987;18:402-406.

[25]   Rozenthul-Sorokin N, Ronen R, Tamir A et al.: Stroke in the young in Israel. Incidence and outcomes. *Stroke* 1996;27:838-841.

[26] Prescott E, Hippe M, Schnohr P et al.: Smoking and risk of myocardial infarction in women and men: longitudinal population study. *Bmj* 1998;316:1043-1047.

[27] Sacco RL, Benjamin EJ, Broderick JP et al.: American Heart Association Prevention Conference. IV. Prevention and Rehabilitation of Stroke. Risk factors. *Stroke* 1997;28:1507-1517.

[28] Lerner DJ, Kannel WB: Patterns of coronary heart disease morbidity and mortality in the sexes: a 26-year follow-up of the Framingham population. *Am. Heart J.* 1986;111:383-390.

[29] Kodama K, Sasaki H, Shimizu Y: Trend of coronary heart disease and its relationship to risk factors in a Japanese population: a 26-year follow-up, Hiroshima/Nagasaki study. *Jpn. Circ. J.* 1990;54:414-421.

[30] Robertson T, Shimizu H, Kato K et al. Incidence of stroke and coronary heart disease in atomic bomb survivors living in Hiroshima and Nagasaki. 1958-74. Hiroshima: Radiation *Effects Research Foundation*; 1979.

[31] Rodin MB, Daviglus ML, Wong GC et al.: Middle age cardiovascular risk factors and abdominal aortic aneurysm in older age. *Hypertension* 2003;42:61-68.

[32] Yii MK: Epidemiology of abdominal aortic aneurysm in an Asian population. *ANZ J. Surg.* 2003;73:393-395.

[33] Hu YH, Shimizu H, Kawakami N et al.: Increasing trends in mortality rate of aortic aneurysms in Japan, 1955-90. *Tohoku J. Exp. Med.*1993;171:221-228.

[34] Smoking, lung function and the prognosis of abdominal aortic aneurysm. The UK Small Aneurysm Trial Participants. *Eur. J. Vasc. Endovasc. Surg .*2000;19:636-642.

[35] Ballaro A, Cortina-Borja M, Collin J: A seasonal variation in the incidence of ruptured abdominal aortic aneurysms. *Eur. J .Vasc. Endovasc. Surg.* 1998;15:429-431.

[36] Kato I, Tominaga S, Ito Y et al.: Comparative case-control analysis of gastric and duodenal ulcers. *Jpn. J. Public Health* 1990;37:919-925.

[37] Watanabe Y, Kurata JH, Kawamoto K et al.: Epidemiological study of peptic ulcer disease among Japanese and Koreans in Japan. *J. Clin. Gastroenterol.* 1992;15:68-74.

[38] Friedman GD, Siegelaub AB, Seltzer CC: Cigarettes, alcohol, coffee and peptic ulcer. *N. Engl. J. Med.* 1974;290:469-473.

[39] Sonnenberg A: Smoking and mortality from peptic ulcer in the United Kingdom. *Gut* 1986;27:1369-1372.

[40] Sonnenberg A, Everhart JE: The prevalence of self-reported peptic ulcer in the United States. *Am. J. Public Health* 1996;86:200-205.

[41] Sauvaget C, Nagano J, Allen N et al.: Intake of animal products and stroke mortality in the Hiroshima/Nagasaki Life Span Study. *Int. J. Epidemiol.* 2003;32:536-543.

[42] Kawachi I, Colditz GA, Stampfer MJ et al.: Smoking cessation in relation to total mortality rates in women. A prospective cohort study. *Ann. Intern. Med.* 1993;119:992-1000.

[43] Tornwall ME, Virtamo J, Haukka JK et al.: Life-style factors and risk for abdominal aortic aneurysm in a cohort of Finnish male smokers. *Epidemiology* 2001;12:94-100.

[44] Kawachi I, Colditz GA, Stampfer MJ et al.: Smoking cessation and decreased risk of stroke in women. *Jama* 1993;269:232-236.

[45] Iso H, Date C, Yamamoto A et al.: Smoking cessation and mortality from cardiovascular disease among Japanese men and women: the JACC Study. *Am. J. Epidemiol.* 2005;161:170-179.

[46] Kawachi I, Colditz GA, Stampfer MJ et al.: Smoking cessation and time course of decreased risks of coronary heart disease in middle-aged women. *Arch. Intern. Med.* 1994;154:169-175.

[47] Clavier I, Hommel M, Besson G et al.: Long-term prognosis of symptomatic lacunar infarcts. A hospital-based study. *Stroke* 1994;25:2005-2009.

[48] Ovbiagele B, Weir CJ, Saver JL et al.: Effect of smoking status on outcome after acute ischemic stroke. *Cerebrovasc. Dis.* 2006;21:260-265.

[49] Sasaki H, Wong FL, Yamada M et al.: The effects of aging and radiation exposure on blood pressure levels of atomic bomb survivors. *J. Clin. Epidemiol.* 2002;55:974-981.

[50] Sairenchi T, Iso H, Nishimura A et al.: Cigarette smoking and risk of type 2 diabetes mellitus among middle-aged and elderly Japanese men and women. *Am. J. Epidemiol.* 2004;160:158-162.

[51] Lederle FA, Nelson DB, Joseph AM: Smokers' relative risk for aortic aneurysm compared with other smoking-related diseases: a systematic review. *J. Vasc. Surg.* 2003;38:329-334.

[52] Johnsen R, Forde OH, Straume B et al.: Aetiology of peptic ulcer: a prospective population study in Norway. *J. Epidemiol. Community Health* 1994;48:156-160..

[53] Rosenstock S, Jorgensen T, Bonnevie O et al.: Risk factors for peptic ulcer disease: a population based prospective cohort study comprising 2416 Danish adults. *Gut* 2003;52:186-193.

[54] Susser M: Causes of peptic ulcer. A selective epidemiologic review. *J. Chronic Dis.* 1967;20:435-456.

[55] Graham DY: Helicobacter pylori: its epidemiology and its role in duodenal ulcer disease. *J. Gastroenterol. Hepatol.* 1991;6:105-113.

[56] Asaka M, Kimura T, Kudo M et al.: Relationship of Helicobacter pylori to serum pepsinogens in an asymptomatic Japanese population.. *Gastroenterology* 1992;102:760-766.

[57] Asaka M: [Epidemiology of Helicobacter pylori infection in Japan]. *Nippon Rinsho* 2003;61:19-24.

[58] Hakoda M, Kasagi F, Kusunoki Y et al.: Levels of antibodies to microorganisms implicated in atherosclerosis and of C-reactive protein among atomic bomb survivors. *Radiat. Res.* 2006;166:360-366.

[59] Blaser MJ, Chyou PH, Nomura A: Age at establishment of Helicobacter pylori infection and gastric carcinoma, gastric ulcer, and duodenal ulcer risk. *Cancer Res.* 1995;55:562-565..

[60] LaCroix AZ, Lang J, Scherr P et al.: Smoking and mortality among older men and women in three communities. *N. Engl. J. Med.* 1991;324:1619-1625.

[61] Seltzer CC: Framingham study data and "established wisdom" about cigarette smoking and coronary heart disease. *J. Clin. Epidemiol.* 1989;42:743-750.

[62] Hart CL, Hole DJ, Smith GD: Comparison of risk factors for stroke incidence and stroke mortality in 20 years of follow-up in men and women in the Renfrew/Paisley Study in Scotland. *Stroke* 2000;31:1893-1896.

[63] Hankey GJ: Smoking and risk of stroke. J Cardiovasc Risk 1999;6:207-211.

[64] Shinton R, Beevers G: Meta-analysis of relation between cigarette smoking and stroke. *Bmj* 1989;298:789-794.

[65] Anda RF, Williamson DF, Escobedo LG et al.: Smoking and the risk of peptic ulcer disease among women in the United States. *Arch. Intern. Med.* 1990;150:1437-1441.

[66] Ashley MJ: Smoking and diseases of the gastrointestinal system: an epidemiological review with special reference to sex differences. *Can. J. Gastroenterol* .1997;11:345-352.

[67] Ministry of Health, Labor and Welfare.. Tobacco or Health. Cited 2007 July 6 available from hrrp://www.health-net.or.jp/tobacco/product/pd090000.html.

In: Smoking and Women's Health   ISBN 978-1-60456-148-7
Editors: M.K. Wesley and I.A. Sternbach, pp.183-198   © 2008 Nova Science Publishers, Inc.

Chapter 7

Longitudinal Patterns of Cigarette Use Among Girls in Cape Town, South Africa

*Lori-Ann Palen[1], Edward A. Smith[1], Linda L. Caldwell[1]
and Alan J. Flisher[2]*

1. The Pennsylvania State University, USA
2. University of Cape Town, South Africa and University of Bergen, Norway

Abstract

The current study used latent class analysis to describe longitudinal patterns of regular cigarette use among a sample of 1,214 high school girls from a low-income township in Cape Town, South Africa. It also sought to test whether participation in a comprehensive leisure, life skills and sexuality education program was related to these patterns. There was support for the presence of three patterns of regular cigarette use: non-smokers, initiators, and consistent smokers. Intervention participants were more likely to be non-smokers than were control group students. In addition, girls with the highest risk in a number of domains (academics, peer norms, use of other substances) were more likely to be consistent smokers and less likely to be non-smokers, as compared to girls with less risk. These results suggest that smoking prevention efforts need to begin prior to or early in high school and that there may be concrete markers that allow for the targeting of intervention to those most at risk of early smoking initiation.

Introduction

Smoking is more common in South Africa than in most other countries in Southern Africa (Flisher et al., 2001; Global Youth Tobacco Survey Collaborative Group, 2002, 2003; Steyn, Bradshaw, Norman, Laubscher, and Saloojee, 2002; Townsend, Flisher, Gilreath, and King, 2006). National mortality data have linked cigarette use with heightened risk for a number of diseases of the respiratory, circulatory, and digestive systems, including lung cancer, tuberculosis, and ischaemic heart disease (Sitas et al., 2004). In 2003, these diseases were the documented causes of approximately 40% of South African deaths (Statistics South Africa, 2005).

Among U.S. adults, smoking has been shown to be highly addictive and cessation difficult (e.g., Smith and Fiore, 1999). While nicotine dependence is somewhat less prevalent among youth, it is still a condition that affects approximately half of adolescent smokers in the United States, South Africa, and elsewhere (Colby, Tiffany, Shiffman, and Niaura, 2000; DiFranza et al., 2002; Panday, Reddy, Ruiter, Bergström, and de Vries, 2007). Particularly troubling is that symptoms of dependence often emerge in youth who smoke at low frequencies (DiFranza et al., 2002; Panday et al., 2007). Because the addictive nature of nicotine makes cessation challenging, a more feasible goal is to prevent tobacco use before its onset. However, the timing of prevention efforts requires knowledge of when smoking is typically initiated. In addition, not all youth smoke, so it may be more cost-effective to deliver intervention targeted at only those youth who are at the highest risk for smoking initiation. If one wants to use this type of strategy, it requires knowledge of the characteristics and needs of youth who are at risk for smoking.

Smoking in Adolescence and Young Adulthood

Most research on adolescent smoking in the South African context has been cross-sectional. In South Africa, about 40% of teenagers have smoked cigarettes in their lifetime, with more than half of this group made up of current smokers (Global Youth Tobacco Survey Collaborative Group, 2003; Reddy et al., 2003). These figures differ somewhat by gender, which we will address below. A review of South African youth tobacco use (Townsend et al., 2006) found evidence of racial, age, and residence differences in smoking prevalence; Colored youth (derived from Asian, European, and African ancestry), older youth, and urban youth were the most likely to smoke.

Smoking can have a direct impact on health and well-being, but previous research with this population also suggests that cigarette use may be related to adolescent outcomes through its association with the initiation of marijuana and inhalant use (Patrick et al., in press). In addition, cigarette smoking has been associated with numerous risky non-substance-related outcomes for South African youth including school absence, grade retention, sexual activity, carrying weapons to school, and suicide attempts (Flisher, Parry, Evans, Muller, and Lombard, 2003; Flisher, Ziervogel, Chalton, Leger, and Robertson, 1996; Taylor, Dlamini, Kagoro, Jinabhai, and de Vries, 2003).

While cross-sectional data may provide information on prevalence of smoking and characteristics of smokers at one particular point in time, it is less helpful for elucidating timing of initiation and how this relates to risk factors and outcomes. The bulk of longitudinal research on smoking in adolescence and young adulthood has been conducted with samples from the United States. These studies have typically yielded between three and six distinct patterns of use over time (Abroms, Simons-Morton, Haynie, and Chen, 2005; Chassin, Presson, Pitts, and Sherman, 2000; Colder et al., 2001; Fergus, Zimmerman, and Caldwell, 2005; Juon, Ensminger, and Sydnor, 2002; Maggi, Hertzman, and Vaillancourt, 2007; Orlando, Tucker, Ellickson, and Klein, 2004; Soldz and Cui, 2002; White, Pandina, and

Chen, 2002). These trajectories are fairly similar across studies, despite the fact that the variables with which they are constructed often differ. The simplest smoking variable used in defining trajectories is a dichotomous indicator of lifetime use (e.g., Maggi et al., 2007). Other studies examine frequency of use (Maggi et al., 2007), amount of use during a designated time period (Colder et al., 2001; Fergus et al., 2005; Soldz and Cui, 2002), or some combination of the two (Chassin et al., 2000; Orlando et al., 2004; White et al., 2002).

The most common longitudinal smoking pattern appears to be abstinence, with as many as 75% of participants reporting being non-smokers or light smokers across time. Previous research has also consistently identified a group who initiates or accelerates their smoking in mid-adolescence and tends to smoke over subsequent assessments; these youth have represented up to half of participants across various studies. Most studies have identified a group who initiate smoking early (either prior to the beginning of a study or shortly thereafter) and remain smokers, representing up to a quarter of youth. Finally, most studies have evidence of a small group of youth who either smoke erratically over the course of the study or begin as smokers and later quit.

There is some evidence that patterns of smoking differ by demographic characteristics. One study found that consistent smokers and quitters tended to be older that non-smokers or those who accelerated in their smoking behavior (Fergus et al., 2005). There is mixed evidence for the association between cigarette use and socioeconomic status, with some studies finding no association (Fergus et al., 2005; Juon et al., 2002; White et al., 2002) but one study finding that youth whose parents had more education were more likely to be non-smokers or have a late-onset smoking trajectory than to have patterns of early use (Orlando et al., 2004). There is also some evidence for gender differences in trajectories, which will be described below.

Several theories underscore the importance of social context for the initiation and continuation of cigarette use. Social learning theory (e.g., Akers, 1977) asserts that substance-specific cognitions are learned from role models, and these cognitions in turn drive substance use. In a related vein, social control theories (e.g., Elliott, Huizinga, and Menard, 1989; Hawkins and Weis, 1985; Hirschi, 1969) suggest that adolescents become attached to influential deviant peers when they have weak connections to conventional social institutions (e.g., school, family, work, religion). These theories have received some support in longitudinal smoking research that examines parent, school, free-time activity, and peer domains, as is discussed below.

Several studies have examined smoking and available family support. Youth with stable trajectories of smoking are most likely to come from single-parent households. Non-smokers and those with late-onset smoking trajectories are most likely to live with both parents, and those with early onset or quitting trajectories fall somewhere in the middle (Orlando et al., 2004). Youth who do not smoke also report significantly more parental support and monitoring than those with early-onset patterns of smoking (Abroms et al., 2005; Chassin et al., 2000).

In terms of attachment to school, several studies have shown that non-smokers have higher grades, especially when compared to those with early-onset or stable trajectories of smoking (Orlando et al., 2004; White et al., 2002). Abroms and colleagues (2005) also found that non-smokers were higher than all other trajectories on school engagement, school adjustment, and perceptions of a supportive school climate.

It is possible for adolescents to develop pro-social attachments through their free-time activities; however, it is also possible that activities are a venue for youth to be exposed to substance-using role models. Fergus and colleagues (2005) found that involvement in several types of free time activities at baseline (9th grade) was unrelated to subsequent smoking trajectory. However, youth who were more involved in sports at the end of the study (12th grade) were more likely to have been non- or light smokers and less likely to have been quitters. Those who were more involved in non-school extracurriculars in the 12th grade were most likely to have been non-smokers and least likely to have been consistent smokers across high school. Soldz and Cui (2002) found that there was no longitudinal association between amount of time spent watching television and pattern of smoking behavior. One study found that church attendance was related to smoking trajectory (Juon et al., 2002), with non-smokers being the most likely to attend services weekly; other studies have failed to find an association (Fergus et al., 2005; Soldz and Cui, 2002).

Several studies have examined the roles of peers in smoking. Consistent with social learning and control theories, they have found that youth with early-onset patterns of smoking tend to have the most friends who smoke while non-smokers have the fewest smoking friends (Chassin et al., 2000; Orlando et al., 2004).

In Jessor's Problem Behavior Theory (Jessor and Jessor, 1977), risk behaviors are hypothesized to co-occur because of their shared intra- and inter-personal etiologies. Consistent with this theory, a number of studies have found that trajectories of adolescent smoking behavior have differential associations with a number of other risk behaviors. Frequency of alcohol, marijuana, and other drug use appears to be lowest among non-smokers and especially high among those with early-onset or stable patterns of use (Fergus et al., 2005; Orlando et al., 2004; Soldz and Cui, 2002). In addition, early adopters of cigarettes are most likely to have a diagnosis of drug abuse or dependence (Juon et al., 2002). There is also some suggestion that smoking patterns are related to frequency of delinquent acts (Fergus et al., 2005).

While longitudinal patterns of cigarette use have been well-studied with U.S. samples, little is known about smoking over time in South African populations. Nichter (2003) suggests that there are many ways in which culture can influence longitudinal patterns of cigarette use. More proximal aspects of culture that can influence smoking include differences in parenting style and influence and differences in peer norms and rules for acceptable behavior. At the societal level, culture can influence smoking via the role of tobacco in the economy, the political influence of tobacco companies, and cultural views of what is attractive or stylish. Therefore, if one hopes to implement effective tobacco-prevention programs in South Africa, it is crucial to base them on epidemiological data from that nation specifically.

Smoking and Gender

Researchers have advocated incorporating gender into analyses of adolescent substance use onset. Flisher and colleagues (2001) suggest that it is possible that the timing of initiation may differ for boys and girls, and this may or may not be reflective of differing etiologies of substance use. In particular, there is evidence that the psychopharmacology of cigarette use may differ by gender, with girls reporting faster onset and more severe tobacco dependence (DiFranza et al., 2002; Panday et al., 2007). Therefore, in the current study, we are choosing to focus on adolescent girls.

National adult prevalence data show that South African women are less likely to smoke than men (Steyn et al., 2002). However, evidence among adolescent cohorts is mixed. In the data from the 2002 South African National Youth Risk Behavior Survey, boys were more likely to have initiated cigarette use, to have initiated it prior to age 10, and to be current smokers (Reddy et al., 2003). Similarly, in South African data from the 2002 Global Youth Tobacco Survey, as compared to girls, boys were twice as likely to be current smokers (Global Youth Tobacco Survey Collaborative Group, 2003). Alternatively, data from the Cape Town area show that boys and girls had similar incidence of smoking (Flisher et al., 2001). The authors of the latter study suggest possible area-specific explanations, including minimal disparity in disposable income by gender and a decrease in the influence of gender roles on substance use (Flisher et al., 2001).

A number of US studies have examined whether there are gender differences in longitudinal patterns of cigarette use. At least two studies have found that the girls began smoking earlier and smoked at higher rates as compared to boys (Abroms et al., 2005; White et al., 2002). However, other studies have found that trajectory membership is similar for boys and girls (Fergus et al., 2005; Juon et al., 2002; Orlando et al., 2004).

Healthwise South Africa

There is currently a lack of research on programs designed to prevent substance use among South African youth. In an attempt to address this problem, a US program was recently adapted for use with South African adolescents.

TimeWise: Taking Charge of Leisure Time (Caldwell, Baldwin, Walls, and Smith, 2004) is a school-based intervention that aims to increase participants' involvement in positive free-time activities by increasing awareness of various leisure opportunities and their benefits/drawbacks, enhancing self-awareness, and developing leisure-related decision-making skills. Early findings revealed that program participants did become more involved in leisure and develop their leisure-related skills and awareness (Caldwell, Baldwin et al., 2004). These proximal effects were related to longer-term reductions in risk behaviors, including a reduction in the use of some substances (Caldwell, Smith, Ridenour, and Maldonado-Molina, 2005).

The original TimeWise curriculum, plus added components on substance use, sexuality, and general life skills, was adapted to be culturally appropriate (Wegner, Flisher, Caldwell, Vergnani, and Smith, in press) and delivered as *HealthWise: Life Skills for Young Adults*

(Caldwell, Smith et al., 2004). HealthWise consists of 12 lessons presented to 8th graders and 6 lessons presented to 9th graders. Each lesson takes approximately three class periods to deliver. This curriculum, combined with an effort to connect youth with community resources, aims to increase healthy free time use, reduce substance use, delay onset of sexual activity, and increase condom use among sexually active youth. While the curriculum does not directly address smoking behavior, we anticipated that the positive health messages conveyed in the curriculum would seek to reduce and prevent cigarette use.

The Current Study

The current study aims to describe longitudinal patterns of regular cigarette use among South African adolescent girls. Specifically, we will examine how many and which patterns of smoking are evident in the data. We will then test whether participation in the HealthWise program impacts the probability of exhibiting given smoking patterns. We will also explore various predictors of these patterns, including demographic characteristics, academics, peers, activities, and use of other substances.

Method

Sample

Participants were from Mitchell's Plain, a low-income township in Cape Town that was established during the apartheid era. Data were drawn from the randomized control trial of HealthWise South Africa. Four high schools implemented the HealthWise program, and five other high schools served as controls. At baseline, fifty-one percent of the 2,204 participants were female. Most participants were Colored (86%), with the remaining students being Black (9%), White (4%), Indian or other (1%).

Procedure

Beginning in 8th grade, participants completed biannual assessments of their substance use and other behaviors. Questionnaires were administered via personal digital assistants (PDAs) during school hours. Over the course of three academic years, 1,214 high school girls completed up to six assessments. However, school absence and drop-out is fairly high among the target population, so the mean number of completed assessments for each participant was four.

Measures

Regular cigarette use. At each assessment, participants were asked how many cigarettes they had smoked in their lifetime. Participants who indicated that they had used more than one cigarette were presented with a follow-up question asking whether they had smoked cigarettes in the four weeks preceding the current assessment. Participants who responded in the affirmative answered an item about the number of cigarettes that they had smoked in the preceding four weeks, with response options consisting of 1 or less, 2-9, or 10 or more cigarettes. For the purposes of the present study, participants who had used 10 or more cigarettes in the past month were coded as regular cigarette users at that assessment. Participants who had never used cigarettes or had used less than 10 cigarettes in the past month were coded as not being regular cigarette users at the assessment.

Demographic covariates at baseline. Year of birth was used to compute age at the time of the baseline assessment. We had *a priori* hypotheses that Muslim students would exhibit different patterns of substance use than students from other religious traditions (in this study, Catholic, other Christian, and other). Therefore, if a student reported practicing Islam, they were coded as being Muslim; all other students were coded as being non-Muslim. Participants responded to two separate items about whether their mother and whether their father lived with them. Participants also answered three items that served as indicators of their socioeconomic status: whether their home had electricity, whether it had tap water, and whether the family owned a car. A count of these amenities is typically used to represent SES. However, given the small number of youth in the present study (about 5%) who did not have electricity or tap water, we used only the family car item as an indicator of SES.

Academic covariates at baseline. Participants reported on whether they had ever failed a grade in school. They answered a free-response item asking how many days they were absent from school during the last school term. They also responded "yes" or "no" to the question, "Do you think you will complete your schooling up to Grade 12?," which we have termed "intention to complete school."

Peer covariates at baseline. Participants responded as to whether they had spent time hanging out with friends after school or on weekends during the four weeks preceding the assessment. Those who responded in the affirmative (or who left this item blank) where presented with a follow-up item about the frequency of this behavior. Response options were: 1 = less than 1 hour per week, 2= 1-5 hours per week, 3 = 6-10 hours per week, and 4 = more than 10 hours per week. Participants who responded negatively to the lead item were coded as a fifth category (0).

Participants responded "yes" or "no" to the item "Do most of your friends think it's okay for someone your age to smoke cigarettes?" Smoking norms were measured with the following item: "Out of 100 learners your age at your school, how many do you think smoke cigarettes at least once a month?" Response options were: 0 = none of them, 1 = only a few of them, 2 = about half of them, and 3 = most of them.

Activity covariates at baseline. Participants responded as to whether or not they had done each of the following activities after school or over the weekends in the past four weeks: sports or physical activities, performing arts (musical instrument, singing, school drama or dance group), hobbies (e.g., artwork, drawing, woodwork, needlework, beadwork, collecting things), and volunteer work.

Risk behavior covariates at baseline. Participants responded to items about 4 different risk behaviors: sexual intercourse, alcohol use, marijuana use, and inhalant use. Participants indicated whether or not they had ever had vaginal sexual intercourse. They also responded about their frequency of lifetime alcohol, marijuana, and inhalant use. Participants who reported "none, or only sips in church services" for alcohol or "never" for marijuana or inhalants were coded as having no history of use of that particular substance. All other participants were coded as having used that substance in their lifetime. A summary of all baseline covariates appears in Table 1.

Table 1. Descriptive statistics at baseline

Variable	N	Frequency (%)
HealthWise participation	1,106	42
Demographics		
Age at baseline	1,104	mean = 13.9 (SD = .77)
Muslim	1,103	28
Family owns car	1,106	52
Live with mother	1,108	87
Live with father	1,106	67
Academics		
Failed grade	1,109	14
School absences	1,071	mean = 2.9 (SD = 3.51)
		range = 0-34
Intention to complete school	1,107	92
Peers		
Time spent with friends	1,108	mean = 1.2 (SD = 1.39)
Friends think smoking is okay	1,109	41
Learners smoking monthly	1,108	mean = 2.2 (SD = 1.02)
Activities in past month		
Sports/physical	1,108	47
Performing arts	1,108	50
Hobbies	1,109	54
Volunteering	1,108	42
Risk behavior in lifetime		
Sexually active	1,105	4
Alcohol use	1,099	38
Marijuana use	1,107	10
Inhalant use	1,107	5

Analytic Strategy

Latent class analysis (SAS PROC LCA) was used to determine the minimum number of profiles needed to accurately represent longitudinal patterns of smoking in the sample. Input data were each participant's dichotomous indicators of regular cigarette use across the six time points. PROC LCA uses the Expectation Maximization (EM) algorithm to arrive at maximum likelihood (ML) parameter estimates, however, there is evidence that ML and EM can yield multiple solutions (e.g., Boomsma, 1985; Rubin and Thayer, 1982). Therefore, each model was estimated using 100 different sets of random starting values.

Overall model fit was assessed using the G^2 statistic, with lower values representing a better fit than higher values and a G^2 close to a model's degrees of freedom indicating acceptable model fit. Comparisons between models with differing numbers of classes were made using the Akaike information criterion (AIC) and Bayesian information criteria (BIC), two statistics that reflect fit with a penalty for the number of estimated parameters (Lanza, Flaherty, and Collins, 2002). Following model-fitting, each baseline covariate was entered independently in the final model to assess its relation with the various patterns of cigarette use.

Given that PROC LCA uses the EM algorithm, missing data on the smoking indicators can be accounted for in the models (Lanza, Lemmon, Schafer, and Collins, 2007). However, cases with missing covariates are excluded from analysis. About 9% of participants ($n = 105$) were missing at the baseline assessment but participated in one or more subsequent assessments. Therefore, while these cases were included in preliminary model-building, they were not included in analyses involving baseline covariates.

Results

We estimated models with two, three, and four classes. Both the two- and three-class models replicated across the 100 sets of starting values, but the three-class solution offered a significantly better model fit (see Table 2). Probabilities of class membership and item responses for this model appear in Table 3. The largest class in this model (65% of cases) was made up with girls who had extremely low probabilities of regular smoking at all time points (hereafter referred to as non-smokers). There was a class in which girls had a high probability of regular smoking at all time points (consistent smokers; 17%). Finally, there was a class in which girls had a low probability of regular smoking for the first three assessments and a high probability for the final three assessments (initiators; 18%).

Beginning with the four-class model, the 100 replications yielded multiple solutions. Specifically, the 4-class model had 5 different solutions. Only one of the solutions (25% of starts; $G^2 = 35$, AIC = 89, BIC = 226) yielded a lower AIC than the 3-class solution, and no solution yielded a lower BIC. Given that AIC can lead to the selection of a model with too many classes (Lin and Dayton, 1997) and in light of the instability in the 4-class solution, we selected the 3-class model as our final solution and followed it up with covariate analyses (Table 4).

Comparisons between Non-Smoker, Initiator, and Consistent Smoker Classes

As compared to students in the control group, participants in the HealthWise program had higher odds of being in the non-smoker class and lower odds of being in the initiator and consistent smoker classes. In other words, among youth who were not regular smokers at baseline, HealthWise participants were more likely to remain non-smokers than were control students.

As compared to younger girls, older girls were more likely to be classified as consistent smokers and less likely to be classified as non-smokers or initiators. Those who lived with their mother and lived with their father at baseline were also more likely to be non-smokers than were youth with absent parents. Religion and socioeconomic status (car ownership) did not distinguish among the three classes.

Table 2. Measures of model fit

Model	Loglikelihood	G^2	df	AIC	BIC
2 class	-1932.50	235.67	50	261.67	327.99
3 class	-1843.12	56.90	43	96.90	198.93
4 class	-1832.01	34.69	36	88.69	226.43

Note. The best-fitting 4-class solution (25% of random starts) is tabled here.

Table 3. Class membership probabilities and item endorsement probabilities

	Class Label		
	Non-smoker	Initiator	Consistent
3-class solution			
Class membership probabilities	.65	.18	.17
Item endorsement probabilities			
Beginning of 8th grade	.00	.07	**.63**
End of 8th grade	.02	.07	**.90**
Beginning of 9th grade	.02	.21	**.93**
End of 9th grade	.03	**.60**	**.98**
Beginning of 10th grade	.02	**.86**	**.86**
End of 10th grade	.06	**.82**	**.86**

Note. Item endorsement probabilities greater than .5 are in bold.

Those who had failed a grade in school at baseline had heightened odds of being initiators or consistent smokers. In addition, those with the most school absences were more likely to be consistent smokers and less likely to be non-smokers or initiators. While those who believed that they would complete high school were more likely to be non-smokers, this finding was not statistically significant.

Girls who spent more time with friends had higher odds of being classified in one of the two classes of smokers. Those whose friends thought that smoking was okay had higher odds of being smokers, consistent smokers especially. In addition, those who perceived that a greater proportion of their classmates were smokers were more likely to be consistent smokers.

There were no statistically significant differences in baseline activity involvement, with participants in sports, performing arts, hobbies, or volunteerism all having about the same odds of belonging to each of the three classes as non-participants.

Girls who were sexually active at baseline were more likely to be consistent smokers and less likely to be initiators, as compared to virgins. Those who had used alcohol or marijuana at baseline were significantly more likely to be in the initiator or consistent smoker classes, with the difference in odds being especially large between the non-smokers and the consistent smokers. There was no significant difference in class membership by baseline inhalant use.

Table 4. Unconditional odds ratios for model covariates by latent class, 3-class model

| Baseline covariates | Latent class | | p-value |
	Initiator	Consistent	
HealthWise participation	0.6	0.8	.051
Demographics			
Age	0.9	1.5	< .001
Muslim	1.3	1.0	.558
Family owns car	0.8	0.9	.695
Live with mother	0.8	0.6	.052
Live with father	1.1	0.6	.007
Academics			
Failed grade	1.2	2.2	.004
School absences	1.0	1.1	.006
Intention to complete school	0.6	0.8	.368
Peers			
Time spent with friends	1.3	1.4	< .001
Friends think smoking is okay	1.3	2.2	< .001
Smoking norms	1.0	1.3	.010
Activities in past month			
Sports/physical	1.3	1.0	.365
Performing arts	1.2	1.4	.147
Hobbies	1.0	0.8	.472
Volunteering	1.1	0.8	.308
Risk behavior in lifetime			
Sexually active	0.2	1.6	.067
Alcohol use	2.5	8.1	< .001
Marijuana use	4.1	16.1	< .001
Inhalant use	1.1	2.0	.201

Note. The non-smoker class is the reference group.

Conclusion

This study provided evidence for three longitudinal patterns of regular cigarette smoking among South African high school girls. The majority of girls in this sample did not engage in regular smoking during their early high school years. There was a smaller group of girls who smoked consistently across the whole time period under study. Finally, there was a group of girls who initiated regular smoking in the 9th grade. These general patterns have all been evidenced in previous U.S. studies, and they appear in roughly the same proportions as have been found previously.

Participation in the HealthWise intervention was related to heightened odds of being a non-smoker, and odds of initiating smoking were especially low for this group. This suggests that HealthWise is a promising strategy for preventing the onset of regular cigarette use and underscores the need to deliver prevention programs before smoking begins. Also, as mentioned previously, there is evidence that smoking tends to precede the use of other substances in a portion of this sample (Patrick et al., in press). Therefore, it is possible that by preventing cigarette use, HealthWise may also be effective in either preventing or delaying the use of alcohol, marijuana, and inhalants. However, this will require further investigation.

In terms of the covariates examined here, the non-smoker group was characterized by a profile of low risk in almost all domains. They were more likely to live with both parents and less likely to be absent from school or experience school failure. They perceived norms of less smoking, and they were less likely to have tried alcohol and marijuana.

Consistent with previous research, the girls who smoked across the full course of the study had numerous markers of risk. They were the group most likely to be living apart from one or both parents. They had experienced the most school absence and failure. They spent the most time with friends, and they were more likely to believe that these friends were permissive of smoking. This group was also most likely to be sexually active and to have tried alcohol and marijuana.

The findings for the consistent smoking group have several implications for intervention. First, prevention efforts targeted at these girls need to begin early, before the beginning of high school. One solution would be to deliver universal intervention to younger students. However, it is unclear whether very early smoking interventions would still be relevant (and therefore effective) for the bulk of adolescents who initiate smoking in 9th grade or later. Therefore, it may be possible and preferable to deliver targeted intervention to only students most at risk for early smoking onset. These girls do have several concrete risk markers (e.g., single-parent home, school absence and failure) that should be relatively noticeable to teachers, parents, coaches, or other adults in a child's life. Assuming that these risk markers also existed before the onset of smoking, they could represent ways for adults to determine who was in greatest need of early smoking intervention.

The initiation group evidenced in this study was characterized by levels of risk factors that typically fell between those of the non-smokers and the consistent smokers. As compared to the non-smokers, initiators had somewhat higher rates of school failure, and they had friends with more permissive smoking attitudes. They were also more likely to have tried alcohol and marijuana. However, initiators perceived the lowest level of smoking among their peers, and they were also least likely to have been sexually active at baseline.

The legal age for tobacco purchase and use in South Africa is 16 years. Increased accessibility, either on one's own or through slightly older friends, may help to explain why the timing of regular smoking onset was in the middle of 9th grade (mean age of between 15 and 16 years). Beyond issues of accessibility, social norms and values may play a role in the timing of initiation. Tobacco policy may have stemmed from, or be resulting in, smoking being more socially acceptable behavior around age 16 years as compared to younger ages. This may help to explain why the initiators have a profile of less risk than consistent smokers; they are engaging in a behavior that is "normal" rather than "deviant." However, the degree of awareness and enforcement of tobacco regulations in South Africa is unclear. Also, the patterns of smoking initiation evidenced in this study are fairly similar to those in studies from the US, where the legal age for tobacco purchase is 18. This suggests that underlying patterns of adolescent physical, psychological, and social development also have a role in the timing of regular smoking initiation.

The results from initiators also suggest that programmatic intervention at the beginning of high school may be early enough to prevent cigarette use for a subset of would-be smokers. Programming may be particularly effective if it addresses normative reasons for smoking, although this hypothesis must be examined empirically.

Limitations and Future Directions

The data used in the present study cover a three year span, from approximately ages 14 to 16. This represents only a portion of individual smoking histories. Among South African adolescents, a small minority begin smoking before age 10 (Reddy et al., 2003), and national data on adult smokers show that the average reported age of smoking initiation is about 20 (Steyn et al., 2002). Therefore, to capture the complete range of smoking trajectories, it will be important to collect longitudinal data on samples that begin in late childhood and continue through early adulthood and beyond. In addition, it will useful to examine differences in the long-term health outcomes of various smoking trajectories.

It should also be noted that cigarette smoking is not the only tobacco-use behavior that puts the health of South African women at risk; about 10% of this population reports having used smokeless tobacco products (Global Youth Tobacco Survey Collaborative Group, 2003; Steyn et al., 2002). Therefore, analyses to inform tobacco-related public health efforts are not complete without considering the onset and continuation of smokeless tobacco use.

These limitations aside, the current study is the first to describe longitudinal smoking trajectories among South African girls, as well as to explore predictors of these trajectories. It suggests that preventative intervention should be implemented prior to the 9th grade and even earlier for a high-risk subset of youth. We have demonstrated that HealthWise is a promising universal approach for preventing the onset of regular cigarette smoking, however, further research is needed on targeted intervention and smoking cessation programs.

Acknowledgements

This research was funded by NIH Grants R01 DA01749 and T32 DA017629-01A. Lisa Wegner, John Graham, Tania Vergnani, Catherine Mathews, Inshaaf Evans, and Xavier September played roles in the collection and/or analysis of the HealthWise data. The authors also wish to thank Bethany Bray and Eric Loken for their assistance with the specific analyses presented here.

References

Abroms, L., Simons-Morton, B., Haynie, D. L., and Chen, R. (2005). Psychosocial predictors of smoking trajectories during middle and high school. *Addiction, 100*, 852-861.

Akers, R. L. (1977). *Deviant behavior: A social learning approach* (2nd ed.). Belmont, CA: Wadsworth.

Boomsma, A. (1985). Nonconvergence, improper solutions, and starting values in LISREL maximum likelihood estimation. *Psychometrika, 50*(2), 229-242.

Caldwell, L. L., Baldwin, C. K., Walls, T., and Smith, E. (2004). Preliminary effects of a leisure education program to promote healthy use of free time among middle school adolescents. *Journal of Leisure Research, 36*(3), 310-335.

Caldwell, L. L., Smith, E., Wegner, L., Vergnani, T., Mpofu, E., Flisher, A. J., et al. (2004). HealthWise South Africa: Development of a life skills curriculum for young adults. *World Leisure, 3*, 4-17.

Caldwell, L. L., Smith, E. A., Ridenour, T. A., and Maldonado-Molina, M. (2005). A three-year randomized control study on the effects of a leisure-based intervention on substance use. *Manuscript submitted for publication.*

Chassin, L., Presson, C. C., Pitts, S. C., and Sherman, S. J. (2000). The natural hustory of cigarette smoking from adolescence to adulthood in a Midwestern community sample: Multiple trajectories and their psychosocial correlates. *Health Psychology, 19*(3), 223-231.

Colby, S. M., Tiffany, S. T., Shiffman, S., and Niaura, R. S. (2000). Are adolescent smokers dependent on nicotine? A review of the evidence. *Drug and Alcohol Dependence, 59*(Suppl. 1), S83-S95.

Colder, C. R., Mehta, P., Balanda, K., Campbell, R. T., Mayhew, K. P., Stanton, W. R., et al. (2001). Identifying trajectories of adolescent smoking: An application of latent growth mixture modeling. *Health Psychology, 20*(2), 127-135.

DiFranza, J. R., Savageau, J. A., Rigotti, N. A., Fletcher, K., Ockene, J. K., McNeill, A. D., et al. (2002). Development of symptoms of tobacco dependence in youths: 30 month follow up data from the DANDY study. *Tobacco Control, 11*, 228-235.

Elliott, D. S., Huizinga, D., and Menard, S. (1989). *Multiple problem youth: Delinquency, substance use, and mental health problems*. New York: Springer-Verlag.

Fergus, S., Zimmerman, M. A., and Caldwell, C. (2005). Psychosocial correlates of smoking trajectories among urban African American adolescents. *Journal of Adolescent Research, 20*(4), 423.

Flisher, A. J., Butau, T., Mbwambo, J. K., Kaaya, S. F., Kilonzo, G. P., Aarø, L. E., et al. (2001). Substance us by students in South Africa, Tanzania and Zimbabwe. *African Journal of Drug and Alcohol Studies, 1*(2), 81-97.

Flisher, A. J., Parry, C. D. H., Evans, J., Muller, M., and Lombard, C. (2003). Substance use by adolescents in Cape Town: Prevalence and correlates. *Journal of Adolescent Health, 32*(1), 58-65.

Flisher, A. J., Ziervogel, C. F., Chalton, D. O., Leger, P. H., and Robertson, B. A. (1996). Risk-taking behaviour of Cape Peninsula high-school students: Part IX. Evidence for a syndrome of adolescent risk behaviour. *South African Medical Journal, 86*, 1090-1093.

Global Youth Tobacco Survey Collaborative Group. (2002). Tobacco use among youth: A cross country comparison. *Tobacco Control, 11*, 252-270.

Global Youth Tobacco Survey Collaborative Group. (2003). Differences in worldwide tobacco use by gender: Findings from the Global Youth Tobacco Survey. *The Journal of School Health, 73*(6), 207-215.

Hawkins, J. D., and Weis, J. G. (1985). The Social Development Model: An integrated approach to delinquency prevention. *Journal of Primary Prevention, 6*, 73-97.

Hirschi, T. (1969). A control theory of delinquency. In *Causes of delinquency* (pp. 16-34). Berkeley, CA: University of California Press.

Jessor, R., and Jessor, S. L. (1977). The social-psychological framework. In *Problem behavior and psychosocial development: A longitudinal study of youth* (pp. 17-42). New York: Academic Press.

Juon, H., Ensminger, M., E., and Sydnor, K. D. (2002). A longitudinal study of developmental trajectories to young adult smoking. *Drug and Alcohol Dependence, 66*, 303-314.

Lanza, S. T., Flaherty, B. P., and Collins, L. M. (2002). Latent class and latent transition analysis. In J. Schinka and W. Velicer (Eds.), *Handbook of psychology* (Vol. 2, pp. 663-685). New York: Wiley.

Lanza, S. T., Lemmon, D. R., Schafer, J. L., and Collins, L. M. (2007). *PROC LCA and PROC LTA User's Guide*. University Park, PA: The Methodology Center.

Lin, T. H., and Dayton, C. M. (1997). Model selection information criteria for non-nested latent class models. *Journal of Educational and Behavioral Statistics, 22*(3), 249-264.

Maggi, S., Hertzman, C., and Vaillancourt, T. (2007). Changes in smoking behaviors from late childhood to adolescence: Insights from the Canadian Longitudinal Survey of Children and Youth. *Health Psychology, 26*(2), 232-240.

Nichter, M. (2003). Smoking: What does culture have to do with it? *Addiction, 98*(Suppl 1), 139-145.

Orlando, M., Tucker, J. S., Ellickson, P. L., and Klein, D. J. (2004). Developmental trajectories of cigarette smoking and their correlates from early adolescence to young adulthood. *Journal of Consulting and Clinical Psychology, 72*(3), 400-410.

Panday, S., Reddy, S. P., Ruiter, R. A. C., Bergström, E., and de Vries, H. (2007). Nicotine dependence and withdrawal symptoms among occasional smokers. *Journal of Adolescent Health, 40*, 144-150.

Patrick, M. E., Collins, L. M., Smith, E. A., Caldwell, L. L., Flisher, A. J., and Wegner, L. (in press). A prospective longitudinal model of substance use onset among South African adolescents. *Substance Use and Misuse.*

Reddy, S. P., Panday, S., Swart, D., Jinabhai, C. C., Amosun, S. L., James, S., et al. (2003). *Umthenthe Uhlaba Usamila: The South African Youth Risk Behaviour Survey 2002.* Cape Town: South African Medical Research Council.

Rubin, D. B., and Thayer, D. T. (1982). EM algorithms for ML factor analysis. *Psychometrika, 47*(1), 69-76.

Sitas, F., Urban, M., Bradshaw, D., Kielkowski, D., Bah, S., and Peto, R. (2004). Tobacco attributable deaths in South Africa. *Tobacco Control, 13*, 396-399.

Smith, S. S., and Fiore, M. C. (1999). The epidemiology of tobacco use, dependence, and cessation in the United States. *Primary Care, 26*(3), 433-461.

Soldz, S., and Cui, X. (2002). Pathways through adolescent smoking: A 7-year longitudinal analysis. *Health Psychology, 21*(5), 495-504.

Statistics South Africa. (2005). *Mortality and causes of death in South Africa, 1997-2003.* Pretoria.

Stcyn, K., Bradshaw, D., Norman, R., Laubscher, R., and Saloojee, Y. (2002). Tobacco use in South Africans during 1998: The first demographic and health survey. *Journal of Cardiovascular Risk, 9*, 161-170.

Taylor, M., Dlamini, S. B., Kagoro, H., Jinabhai, C. C., and de Vries, H. (2003). Understanding high school students' risk behaviors to help reduce the HIV/AIDS epidemic in KwaZulu-Natal, South Africa. *Journal of School Health, 73*(3), 97-100.

Townsend, L., Flisher, A. J., Gilreath, T. D., and King, G. (2006). A systematic review of tobacco use among sub-Saharan African youth. *Journal of Substance Use, 11*(4), 245-269.

Wegner, L., Flisher, A. J., Caldwell, L. L., Vergnani, T., and Smith, E. A. (in press). HealthWise South Africa: Cultural adaptation of a school-based risk prevention programme. *Health Education Research.*

White, H. R., Pandina, R. J., and Chen, P. (2002). Developmental trajectories of cigarette use from early adolescence into young adulthood. *Drug and Alcohol Dependence, 65*, 167-178.

In: Smoking and Women's Health
Editors: M.K. Wesley and I.A. Sternbach, pp.199-215

ISBN 978-1-60456-148-7
© 2008 Nova Science Publishers, Inc.

Chapter 8

Smoking and Suicide: Another Concern in Women's Mental Health

Iulian Iancu[5] and Ehud Bodner
Rehovot Mental Health Clinic, Rehovot and the Sackler Faculty of Medicine,
Tel Aviv University, Israel
Interdisciplinary Department of Social Sciences, Bar Ilan University,
Ramat Gan, Israel

Abstract

Cigarette smoking among women is unfortunately still very frequent despite its negative consequences. In addition to its economic and medical implications, smoking might affect women's mental health, inducing cases of dependence, depression and anxiety disorders, and even suicidal behavior.

In this paper we will describe the epidemiology of smoking among women, present several psychiatric complications frequently reported in smokers, and will elaborate on the link between smoking and suicide. Smoking has been related to increased risk of suicidal behavior in the general population, in a cohort of nurses, among male soldiers and in psychiatric patients. We also report the results of our study on the link between smoking and suicide risk, in patients with schizophrenia.

It is unclear, however, whether the abovementioned connection results from a causal effect of smoking or whether it derives from the confounding effect of low mental well-being, impulsivity or of mental disorders, clustering with other substance abuse. The link may result from the effect of smoking on brain serotonin levels or from lower monoamine oxidase activity found in smokers. The link between suicide, psychopathology and smoking is important due to its potential ramifications and due to the frequent use of nicotine in today's culture. Further studies in males and in females are crucial to clarify the role of smoking in mental health.

---

5 Correspondence address: Iulian Iancu, M.D. Director Rehovot Mental Health Clinic Remez 80, Rehovot, Israel, Fax: 972-8-9258389, e-mail: iulian1@bezeqint.net.

Keywords: *smoking, nicotine, depression, anxiety, schizophrenia, suicide.*

Introduction

The prevalence of smoking has decreased in the last 40 years from 51.9% and 33.9% among males and females respectively (1965), to 37.5% and 29.9% (1979), and to a nadir of 26.4% and 22% in 1998 (Surgeon General's Report, 2001). Smoking is nearly three times higher among women who have only 9 to 11 years of education (32.9%) than among women with 16 or more years of education (11.2%). Despite a decrease in the rate of smoking among adults, smoking prevalence in the 1990s increased among both boys and girls. In 2000, 29.7% of high school senior girls and 32.8% of high school senior boys reported having smoked within the past 30 days (Surgeon General's Report, 2001).

Girls who initiate smoking have parents or friends who smoke, have weaker attachments to parents and family, and stronger attachments to peers. They are inclined to risk-taking and rebelliousness, believe that smoking can control weight and negative mood, and have a positive image of smokers (Surgeon General's Report, 2001). Tobacco marketing and the tobacco companies, which produce brands specifically for women, had been extensively targeted to some of these beliefs. Tobacco marketing is dominated by themes of social desirability and independence, which are conveyed through ads featuring slim, attractive, athletic models. This marketing is an obvious factor influencing the susceptibility of women to initiate and continue smoking, resulting in approximately 3 million U.S. women who have died since 1980 prematurely from smoking-related medical disorders, and 2.1 million years of life were lost due to these deaths (Surgeon General's Report, 2001). Unfortunately, while women who stop smoking greatly reduce their risk of dying prematurely, many refrain or fail in quitting their habit.

In the following chapter we will examine gender effects as regards smoking and evaluate the complex relationship between smoking and suicide through clinical and epidemiological studies, and the linkage between smoking and various psychiatric conditions that might also result in cases of suicide.

Gender Differences in Smoking

Several gender differences exist regarding smoking, such as the smaller smoking rate among women (Jha et al., 2002), as well as the somewhat different psychological and biological roots of the initiation and persistence of smoking behavior across genders (Acierno et al., 1996; Perkins et al., 1999). Interestingly, as social roles of men and women changed, so have gender differences in smoking become less apparent even in young age.

A survey on full-time employees in a bank (N=2139) and in a university (N=1611) (Emslie, Hunt, and Macintyre, 2002) showed that in both organizations there were no significant gender differences in smoking. Also, high masculinity scores among both men and women were associated with smoking. The authors concluded that men and women occupying similar social roles are equally likely to smoke, and that there is an association between high masculinity scores and health-damaging behaviors in both men and women. In a mail survey with 2934 daily smokers (1533 women and 1401 men) in Switzerland (Etter, Prokhorov, and Perneger, 2002) men reported of significantly higher quota of cigarettes per day (22 vs 18). These studies suggest that smoking behavior might be regulated by similar psychological mechanisms in men and women, and that smoking habits in both men and women reflect the importance of gender role orientation, rather than the role of biological gender.

Having said that, there are also evidences that point at a differential effect that smoking has on females. Males show greater sensitivity to the rewarding and reinforcing effect of nicotine as compared to females (Perkins et al. 1999), who under high stress smoke for the sedative and calming effects (Acierno et al., 1996). Teenage girls that smoke frequently cite as a reason for their smoking a calming or anxiety-reducing effect (Crisp et al. 1999), and are more likely than males to smoke to relieve negative withdrawal symptoms (Stanton, Lowe and Silva, 1995).

According to File et al. (1999) the anxiolytic effects of smoking are mediated by presynaptic 5-HT1a receptors, and females are more sensitive than males to the anxiolytic effects mediated by these receptors. Additionally, cigarettes decreased ratings of anxiety and sadness only in female smokers with low neuroticism scores, but even increased these ratings in those with high scores (Netter et al., 1998).

File and associates (2001) examined the effects of nicotine (2 mg administered by inhalator) in healthy young adults (N=32) who were exposed to moderate stress.

Stress resulted in significantly increased ratings of anxiety, discontent and aggression, while nicotine blocked these mood changes in females, but enhanced them in males (File et al, 2001). This study supports the notion that women start regular smoking as a form of stress self-medication.

The prevalence of smoking among psychiatric patients (Hughes et al, 1986; Istvan and Matarazzo, 1984; Glassman et al.,1990, Covey and Tam, 1990), and especially in patients who suffer from Major depressive disorder (MDD) (Breslau, Kilbey, and Andreski, 1991; Glassman et al.,1990; Glassman, 1993; Kendler et al., 1993; Breslau, Kilbey, and Andreski, 1993; Breslau, 1995; Anda et al, 1990) appears to be substantially higher than among the general population. Some studies (Anda et al., 1990; Glassman et al., 1990; Perez-Stable et al., 1990) suggested that the relationship between smoking and depression in adult women, and between smoking and the development of depressive symptoms in adolescent girls (Choi et al., 1997) may be stronger than for males. Patton and colleagues (1998) found that depression and anxiety symptoms among adolescents were associated with a higher risk for smoking initiation through increased susceptibility to the effect of peer smoking, especially among girls. However, the relationship between MDD and cigarette smoking in women had not been universally proven (Breslau, 1995; Breslau et al., 1998).

The association of smoking and MDD seems particularly important in women because they are more likely to be diagnosed with MDD than men (Johnson et al., 1992). According to Kendler and associates (1993), the association between smoking and MDD among women may result from inherited, neurobiological factors that predispose to both conditions. In addition, some association was found between anxiety disorders in women and smoking cessation, so that women with anxiety disorders were more likely than men with anxiety disorders to stop or reduce smoking (Covey et al., 1994). Also, Pohl and associates (1992) found a significantly higher prevalence of smoking only among women with panic disorder, but not among men. A link between smoking and gender was also found with regarding to Schizophrenia with De Leon and colleagues (1995) showing that smoking was less prevalent among women with schizophrenia than among men with schizophrenia.

Smoking and Suicidality

During the last 15 years, epidemiological studies inquired the link between smoking and different manifestations of suicidality. These studies were conducted in Finland (Tanskanen et al., 1998, Tanskanen et al., 2000; Riala et al, 2007), Sweden (Hemmingsson and Kriebel, 2003), Greece (Beratis et al., 1997), Japan (Moriya and Hashimoto, 2005) and the US (Miller et al., 2000; Hemenway et al.,1993).

These studies have found high positive correlations between smoking and different manifestations of suicidal behavior. Tanskanen et al. (1998) studied the relationship between smoking and suicidality among 1,217 Finnish psychiatric patients, and found that the odds of at least one previous suicide attempt were 100% higher in current smokers than in nonsmokers. Smokers had a 43% higher risk of experiencing mild to severe suicidal ideation than nonsmokers. These findings remained even after controlling for several confounding factors (i.e., sex, age, marital status, education, income level, employment status, psychiatric diagnosis, alcohol drinking and level of depression). Similar findings were reported by the same group (Tanskanen et al., 2000), on the link between smoking and completed suicide (sample of 36,689 healthy adults, aged 25-64 years, men and women who participated in population surveys between 1972 and 1992, of which 169 committed suicides). Riala et al (2007) investigated the relationship between adolescents' regular smoking and later suicides in a prospective longitudinal birth cohort in Finland from 1966 to 2001 (N=10934). After adjusting for socio-demographic factors in adolescence and psychiatric morbidity, regular smokers were at a 4.05–fold hazard for committing suicide at a younger age. Corresponding associations were not found among females. Further- more, the proportion of suicide attempts was significantly higher among regular daily smokers, both boys and girls.

Hemmingsson and Kriebel (2003) found a significant trend of increasing suicide risk with increasing intensity of smoking in 49323 Swedish male conscripts of which 810 committed suicide in the 25 years after their military service. In Greece, Beratis et al. (1997) compared the number of smoked cigarettes per day among 100 suicide attempters, 100 matched controls and 60 psychiatric controls, aged 30-46, with the same psychiatric disorders as diagnosed in the corresponding attempters. They found that consumption of 40-50 cigarettes per day was significantly more frequent in suicide attempters than in the controls.

Moriya and Hashimoto (2005) performed forensic autopsies and found significant higher levels of nicotine and cotinine in the blood and urine of eight smokers who committed suicide compared with the levels found in eight smokers who did not commit suicide.

Hemenway et al. (1993) examined over 121,700 American female registered nurses (30 to 55 years of age) over a period of 12 years (1976-1988). The authors found a positive association between completed suicide (N=136) and cigarette smoking, so that in comparison with never smokers, women who smoked 1-24 cigarettes per day had twice the chance to commit suicide, and women who smoked 25 and more cigarettes per day, had four times the likelihood for such an act. Miller et al. (2000) examined the relation between cigarette smoking and suicide by conducting a cohort study of 300,000 male US Army personnel, of which 113 have committed suicides during a period of 10 years since the first survey. They also reported that the risk of suicide increased significantly with the number of cigarettes smoked daily.

As the link between smoking and suicidality is complex, there is also a lack of knowledge regarding the role of gender in the association smoking-suicidality (suicide ideation, attempted and completed suicide). For example, a recent study with 3357 men and 4004 women aged 17 to 39, found smoking to be significantly associated with attempted suicide in men, but not in women (Zhang et al., 2005).

Beratis et al (1997) found unique connections in women between smoking and suicide attempts. They reported that the mean number of cigarettes smoked was particularly greater for women attempters versus controls. In addition, female attempters without a psychiatric disorder smoked more frequently than the corresponding controls, and female attempters with psychiatric disorders smoked more frequently than the psychiatric controls. The authors explained these significant differences as indicating that the greater prevalence of smoking among female suicide attempters did not result from the higher prevalence of psychiatric disorders (i.e., MDD, schizophrenia) in this group. Moreover, an earlier initiation of cigarette smoking was observed in female suicide attempters, whereas male suicide attempters initiated smoking at an almost identical mean age as smokers in the control group. Beratis et al (1997) concluded that there is a proclivity to suicidal attempts in women, which results from shared predispositions, genetic or environmental, in the personality of the suicide attempter. They also claimed that the stronger association between smoking and suicide attempts in females compared with males could at least in part, result from the lower smoking rate among females Nevertheless, they admitted that the etiology which underlies beneath the association between smoking and suicide attempts, especially among females, remains as yet obscure.

The prospective study by Hemenway et al. (1993) examined only women and the authors explained the association found between smoking and completed suicide, by the hypothesis of self-medication of depression with nicotine, by the poor personal health habits of the smokers that may lead to depression, and because of the low social status of smokers that may also increase depression. Since this study lacks a comparison group of men, it cannot be concluded that these explanations are relevant among women.

Explanations for the Smoking-Suicide Association

It is not yet known whether the association between smoking and suicide is causal or whether it is affected by other risk factors for suicide. Some of the risk factors that have frequently been shown to be more common among smokers are depression (Korhonen et al., 2007), alcohol consumption (Yamasaki et al., 2005), social isolation

(Berkman et al., 2004), impulsivity (Malone et al., 2003), and poor marital status (Miller et al., 2000). All of the above are frequent in suicide attempters and completers.

Korhonen et al. (2007) used the Finnish Twin Cohort to follow up 24,053 respondents from 1975 until 1990, and found that even when family and genetic background were controlled, smoking remained a predictor of depression. Yamasaki et al. (2005) tested the influence of policies designed to reduce the tobacco and alcohol consumption in Switzerland in 1965-1994 on suicide rates, and found that the tax on tobacco correlated significantly negatively with male standardized suicide rate.

Finally, Miller et al. (2000) reported that there are more unmarried individuals among smokers who commit suicide than among smokers who do not commit suicide, but also claimed that the smoking-suicide connection is not entirely due to the greater tendency among smokers to be unmarried.

In multivariable-adjusted analyses, smokers of more than 20 cigarettes a day, compared with never smokers, were more than twice as likely to commit suicide. For male active-duty army personnel, the dose-related association between smoking and suicide was not entirely explained by the greater tendency of smokers to be white, drink heavily, have less education, and exercise less often. In order to explain the smoking-suicide association, Hemmingsson and Kriebel (2003), in their study on conscripts in Sweden, adjusted for psychiatric diagnosis, parental divorce, low emotional control, medication for nervous problems, contact with police and childcare, heavy alcohol consumption, drug use and education, and found there was no longer an increased relative risk for heavy smokers. They concluded that the tobacco consumption itself is not a causal factor for suicide.

The principal pathway suggested for the plausible relationship between smoking and suicide is the effect of smoking on serotonin levels in the brain or on lower MAO activity in smokers. Lower serotonin levels are associated with lower serotonin function and impulsive/aggressive traits, which are associated with suicidal acts and completed suicide (Malone et al, 2003). In a study with 162 patients with depression, an inverse relationship was observed between the amount of cigarette smoking and both indices of serotonin function. Malone et al (2003) concluded that the association between cigarette smoking and the presence and severity of suicidal behavior across major psychiatric disorders may be related to lower brain serotonin function. The finding of increased suicidal behavior associated with smoking parallels the observation reported by Whitfield et al (2000) of a lower MAO activity in current smokers, but not in ex-smokers.

Smoking and Schizophrenia

The prevalence of smoking is very high among patients with schizophrenia, but the mechanisms underlying this association are not yet understood. Smoking may reduce cognitive deficits and negative symptoms in schizophrenia, alleviate medication side effects, and also decrease boredom. Unsurprisingly, smoking has also been recently related to the higher suicide risk in patients with schizophrenia (Potkin et al, 2003).

Weiser et al (2004) demonstrated higher rates of cigarette smoking in male adolescents before the onset of schizophrenia and postulated that an impaired nicotinic neurotransmission is involved in the pathophysiology of schizophrenia. Indeed, a decrease in the $\alpha_4\beta_2$ nicotinic receptors was found in the caudate nucleus and cortex of schizophrenia patients, two brain regions that are essentially enervated by the dopaminergic and cholinergic systems (Breese et al, 2000). It is possible that the nicotinic derangement occurs before the overt development of delusions and hallucinations, thus causing a tendency to smoke *to increase dopamine levels*

(Davidson, personal communication, 2007). Alternatively, Weiser et al (2004) speculated that nicotine causes chronic activation of the mesolimbic dopaminergic neurotransmission, which in predisposed individuals might increase the risk for the development of schizophrenia. Such putative chronic activation of mesolimbic dopaminergic system (Pontieri et al, 1996) may explain the increased severity of psychotic symptoms observed in smoking patients compared to non-smokers (Corvin et al, 2001). Indeed, a recent PET in vivo study has demonstrated dopamine release in response to smoking and craving alleviation (Brody et al, 2004).

In a study by our group (Iancu et al, 2006) with 61 patients with schizophrenia, smokers exhibited significantly higher Suicide Risk Scale (SRS) scores and a trend for higher impulsivity. Women that smoked had significantly higher SRS scores compared with female non-smokers and also higher than in males (both smokers and nonsmokers) (See Figure 1). Smoking and a history of suicide attempt predicted a higher SRS score.

Despite the fact that in our sample, males comprised of more smokers (75% vs 40% among the females), this male over-representation was not the reason for our overall finding that schizophrenia patients that smoke have increased SRS scores. As mentioned above, in our female group, the SRS score among the female smokers was even higher as compared to the female non-smokers, a discrepancy much higher than among the males.

_Women with schizophrenia might attempt to self-medicate with nicotine, since nicotine possesses mood-elevating and hedonic properties, but possibly fail in the emotional regulation and retain higher despair and suicidal score. The reason for this trend among women is not clear. We did have difficulty to recruit non-smoker patients as the majority of schizophrenia patients do smoke, thus leading to a potential bias. It is also possible that a divergent distribution occurred among the male patients, who were mainly heavy smokers. This might have caused a limited range effect, resulting in a lack of correlation between smoking and suicide. Nonetheless, it is possible that women with schizophrenia who smoke constitute a specific phenotype, characterized by more substance abuse, more impulsivity and suicidality (i.e. higher rates of psychopathology according to the self-medication model) (Dinn et al, 2004). The results of our regression analysis among the females regarding the contribution of the number of pack-years smoked by the female patients and the SRS score is in partial support of this postulation (without ascertaining the direction of the linkage). But still, the higher SRS scores among the female smokers are not supported by clinical experience or reports in the literature of schizophrenia, and it might result from a bias in the female group in our study (i.e. more depression, which is more frequent among smokers, see Murphy et al, 2003) or from an inclination among female patients to over-report suicidal/frustration issues on self-report assessments, such as the SRS). Indeed, women afflicted with schizophrenia are known to suffer from more prominent mood symptoms, a possible reason for increased suicidal risk.

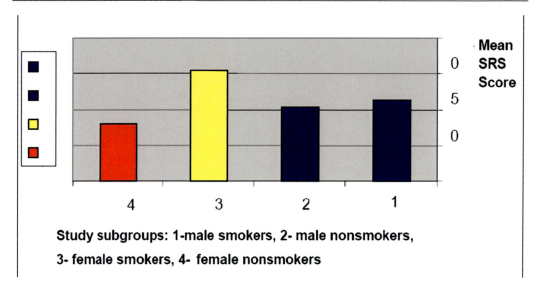

Figure 1. Mean Suicide Risk Scale Scores in 61 schizophrenia patients.

Smoking and Major Depressive Disorder (MDD)

The World Health Organization estimates that one-third of the global adult population smokes (Dani and Harris, 2005), and the National Institute of Mental Health assessed the prevalence of MDD in the United States in 2000, between 5 and 10.3 percent of the population (Nichols et al., 2007). Depression carries a high suicide risk and this could be another reason for the smoking-suicidality connection. Smoking could induce depression and this might lead to suicidal behavior. The association of smoking and depression is particularly important among women because they are more liable to be diagnosed with depression than are men. The high prevalence of smoking and MDD, the economic burden they inflict on health systems (Wang, Simon, and Kessler, 2003; Collins and Escobar, 2006), and the gradual accumulation of findings about the connections between depression and smoking during the nineties (Carmody, 1989; Covey, Glassman, and Stetner, 1998; Hall, Munoz, Reus, and Sees, 1993), instigated a comprehensive investigation of the reciprocal connections between the two phenomena. Findings showed that smokers suffer more of MDD than nonsmokers (Tanskanen et al., 1998; Haukkala, et al., 2000; Hamalainen et al., 2001; Williams and Ziedonis, 2004). For example, around a third of smokers seeking treatment at university-based cessation clinics have a history of MDD (Hall et al., 1993; Borrelli et al., 1996). In addition, more people who suffer from psychiatric disorders, and MDD among them, are smokers, compared with healthy controls (Kaylene and Pradhan, 2001; Glassman et al., 2001). For example, Hamalainen et al. (2001) interviewed a random sample of 5993 non-institutionalized Finnish people aged 15-75 years, in order to investigate the associations of cigarette smoking with MDD. Smoking 10 or more cigarettes daily was found as a risk factor for MDD, even after adjusting for other major risk factors (marital status, education, unemployment and chronic diseases). Based on findings about the prevalence and incidence of MDD over a 40-year period, Murphy et al. (2003) used logistic regression models and survival regressions to analyze data from interviews with adult population samples (1952, 1970, and 1992) and followed cohorts (1952-1970 and 1970-1992). In 1992 (and not in previous years) the odds that a smoker would be depressed were three times the odds that a nonsmoker would be depressed. In the cohort analysis, smoking at baseline did not predict depression, but subjects who became depressed were more likely to start or continue smoking and less likely to quit than those who never had a depression. Breslau, Novak and Kessler (2004) examined the role of DSM-III-R psychiatric disorders in predicting the subsequent onset of daily smoking, and found higher risk for daily smoking for persons with MDD.

In addition, reciprocal neuro-chemical mechanisms had been reported and some evidence exists regarding a shared genetic component for smoking and MDD (Kendler et al., 1993; Bergen and Caporaso, 1999; Williams and Ziedonis, 2004) although this is more evident in men, than in women (Korhonen et al., 2007). For example, Korhonen et al. (2007) characterized 4164 men and 4934 women, based on surveys in 1975 and 1981, as never smokers, persistent former smokers, quitters, recurrent smokers and persistent smokers. When family and genetic background were controlled, smoking remained a predictor of MDD, and genetic modeling among the men suggested a modest correlation between genetic components of smoking and MDD.

Moreover, clinical and epidemiological investigations have shown the link between MDD and inability to stop smoking (Glassman et al., 1990; Breslau, Kilbey, and Andreski, 1991; Kendler et al., 1993; Covey et al., 1994; Ginsberg et al., 1995; Hall et al., 1993), so that a history of MDD decreased the rate of successful cessation of smoking (Covey, Glassman, and Stetner, 1997; Hall et al., 1993).

Some explain the depressive patients' persistent smoking as a way to relieve depressive symptoms. This hypothesis is referred to as the "self-medication" hypothesis, although this is not an exhaustive explanation for the link. The hypothesis regards nicotine dependence as aiding in a context of self-regulation vulnerabilities, such as difficulties in regulating affects, self-esteem, relationships, and self-care (Khantzian, 1997). Nicotine has been described as having antidepressant effects and may reduce the dysphoric emotions which result from difficulties in self-regulation (Glassman et al., 1990; Hemenway et al., 1993, Hughes et al., 1988; Khantzian, 1997). Others explain the difficulty of the depressive patients to stop smoking as stemming from their indifference to risks, and from their view that life is not worthwhile (Murphy et al., 2003). Accordingly, in contrast to people who are not depressive and care about their health, the awareness of the MDD patients' for the risk associated with smoking may not reduce their incentive to smoke. Hughes (1988) proposed that there may be a common predisposition to both smoking and depression, either because of cognitive factors such as low self-esteem or because of a common genetic effect. Kendler and associates (1993) likewise minimized the causal element, arguing that the strong association between smoking and MDD in women derives from inherited, neurobiological factors that predispose to both conditions. Finally, the frequency and intensity of depressive mood was higher after smoking cessation among smokers with past depression, compared with smokers with no such history (Covey, Glassman, and Stetner, 1990). An examination of this link was carried out by Glassman et al. (2001) who examined during a period of two months, 76 smokers (42 successful abstainers and 34 continuous smokers) with a history of past major depression, who were free from MDD and had not been on antidepressant medications for at least six months. The reoccurrence of MDD was assessed by structured clinical interviews, three and six months after the end of treatment. A significantly higher risk of developing a new episode of MDD was found among the abstainers (seven times more than for those who continued to smoke), that remained high for at least six months. Therefore, the researchers recommended that doctors should inquire about smoking habits when a patient presents with MDD.

Anxiety and Smoking

Nicotine probably modulates the function of pathways involved in stress response and anxiety in the normal brain, which results in alterations in anxiety levels. Some studies found that smokers smoke more under stressful conditions and also reported an increased smoking prevalence among patients with anxiety disorders (Surgeon General's Report, 2001), while others found that smokers suffer from high anxiety (McCrae et al, 1978; Patton et al, 1996). However, the direction of the connection between smoking and anxiety in general, and specific anxiety disorders in particular, has not been as yet determined. Does nicotine use result in anxiety or does anxiety make us smoke? Is nicotine anxiogenic or rather anxiolytic, as some studies have shown that smoking may reduce anxiety (Pomerleau et al, 1984; Gilbert et al, 1989)? Is smoking suicidogenic? Unfortunately, there are no studies on this issue.

In the upstate New York study, 688 youths were prospectively followed up since 1985-6 (mean age of 16) to 1991-1993. Heavy cigarette smoking (≥ 20/d) during adolescence was associated with higher risk of agoraphobia (OR= 6.79), Generalized Anxiety Disorder (OR=5.53) and panic disorder (OR=15.58) during adulthood after controlling for age, sex, alcohol and drug abuse, anxiety and depressive disorders during adolescence, etc. Anxiety disorders during adolescence were however not associated with chronic cigarette smoking during early adulthood (Johnson et al, 2000). Thus, this study supports the notion that smoking may increase the risk of anxiety disorders.

Patton et al (1998) found in a prospective study that anxiety and depression symptoms were associated with higher risks for initiation of smoking, through an increased susceptibility to peers. Anxiety sensitivity (AS; the fear of anxiety sensations which arises from beliefs that these sensations have harmful somatic, social, or psychological consequences) was shown to have a role as heavy smokers high in AS had the highest levels of avoidance and greatest increase in anticipatory anxiety (McLeish, Zvolensky and Bucossi, 2007). AS also moderated the link between smoking and depressive symptoms, with gender, alcohol and past month stress controlled for (Zvolensky et al, 2006). High AS smokers smoked more often to manage negative mood and tolerated less withdrawal symptoms, during early stages of a quit attempt (Brown et al, 2001).

Data from the Oregon Adolescent Depression Project (N=1709) show that daily smoking at adolescence was associated with a significantly increased risk of panic attacks (OR=2.6) and panic disorder (PD) (OR=4.2) at young adulthood (Goodwin et al, 2005). The association decreased partially after controlling for parental anxiety disorder and parental smoking, but remained significant for PD (OR=3.7). These findings replicate previous results showing that smoking in adolescence is associated with a higher risk of panic attacks and PD in early adulthood.

A greater proportion of PD patients (40%) reported smoking compared to the Social Phobia (SP) (20%) and Obsessive Compulsive Disorder (22.4%) groups. Those in the PD group were more likely to be heavy smokers (McCabe et al, 2004). Subjects who smoked had significantly higher scores than non-smokers on measures of depression, general anxiety and distress.

Data from the Early Developmental Stages of Psychopathology Study (N=3021 adolescents and young adults) showed that at baseline 35.7% were regular smokers and 18.7% were dependent on nicotine, whereas 7.2% met criteria for DSM-IV SP most of whom reported first onset of social fears prior to smoking initiation (different form other anxiety disorders). Social fears and SP were both associated with higher rates of nicotine dependence (Sonntag et al, 2000). The authors suggested that social fears could lead to heavy tobacco use as smoking is a socially acceptable behavior that relieves anxiety in social situations.

Patients with traumatic experiences and with Posttraumatic Stress Disorder also display higher rates of smoking, and a recent study (Feldner et al, 2007) reported that levels of posttraumatic stress symptoms were associated with smoking to reduce negative affect; this relation was observed after controlling for variance accounted for by number of cigarettes smoked per day and gender. Posttraumatic stress symptoms appeared particularly related to smoking to reduce negative affect and smoking for stimulation. The authors concluded that further understanding of this relation may be critical in developing specialized smoking cessation interventions for persons with trauma-related symptomatology, which may need to include a specific focus on *substituting alternative affect regulation strategies for smoking.*

Conclusion

An early theory postulated that initial experimentation with smoking is motivated by psychosocial factors and curiosity, but quickly the "pharmacological rewards" of nicotine in the form of "indulgent", "sedative", or "stimulation" smoking provide the motivation for use, prior to dependence (see Difranza et al, 2007).

Smoking became prevalent among women after it did among men, and smoking has always been lower among women, although the gender gap has recently narrowed. Smoking is still a prevalent behavior among women. It can lead to various medical problems and plays a major role in the mortality of women. In recent decades it has become clearer that smoking is associated with depression, anxiety and schizophrenia, and even with suicidal behavior. Smokers are more likely to be depressed, a finding that may reflect the effect of smoking on the risk for depression, the use of smoking for self-medication, or the influence of common genetic or biopsychosocial factors on both depression and smoking. Although the causality in this connection is not always clear, the phenomena of smoking, mood disorders and suicidal behavior are important and frequent, and deserve additional scrutiny in research.

While it is possible that women smoke more in order to "self-medicate" or to get social desirability and control weight, the later psychiatric complications seem to be similar among males and females. It is possible that smoking could cause impulsivity and suicidal tendencies, either through a direct effect or indirect one through various confounding variables. Having said that, it seems that in other individuals smoking might induce serenity and reduce mental anguish.

Recent studies (DiFranza et al, 2007) show that some susceptible youths lose autonomy over tobacco within a day or two of first inhaling from a cigarette, leading to a long-term use and even dependence on nicotine. The appearance of tobacco withdrawal symptoms and failed attempts at cessation can precede daily smoking (Difranza et al, 2007). Thus, attempts to prevent smoking during childhood and adolescence are necessary. It is unclear why smoking prevalence increased among teenagers in the 1990s despite the upsurge of data on negative medical consequences. Youths must be warned that it may take only 1 cigarette to initiate life-long dependence on tobacco. The medical and psychiatric complications of smoking should be explained to all females, adolescents and adults, from high as well as from low socioeconomic strata, and especially in women populations that traditionally refrained from smoking but nowadays are displaying increased smoking.

Jurisdictions can make additional progress in reducing tobacco use, particularly by further increasing taxes on tobacco products, expanding smoke-free public places, and pervasive anti-tobacco advertising and well-funded media campaigns. Campaigns that promote smoking are targeted to women with prevailing themes of social desirability and independence, as well as slimness, attractiveness, sportive life. These themes are in deep contrast to the consequences of smoking. Clinicians and public health officials should aid in women's anti-tobacco advocacy efforts and publicize that most women are non-smokers. Examples of famous women who refrain from smoking should be stressed, for the young susceptible generation.

While some researchers see the strong association found between anxiety and depressive symptoms and youth smoking, they also suggest reducing these symptoms, as a major preventive step against the onset of addictive smoking and against self-medication attempts (Dudas, Hans and Barabas, 2005). Additional research on gender differences in susceptibility to psychiatric disorders and suicidal behavior are needed. Research on smoking prevention and smoking cessation (pharmacological and behavioral) are mandatory in order to better understand and reduce this problematic human behavior. Additionally, studies on gender susceptibility to nicotine addiction and the magnitude of the effects of smoking on disorders outcome might elucidate the role of nicotine in health and in illness.

It is important to remember, however, that smoking is used by some persons who would otherwise manifest psychiatric symptoms to manage these symptoms. For such persons the cessation of smoking may lead to the emergence of depression or other psychopathology, and a psychiatric evaluation should be required before the attempt to abstain from this bad habit.

References

Acierno, R.A., Kilpatrick, D.G., Resnick, H.S., Saunders, B.E., Best, C.L. (1996). Violent assault, posttraumatic stress disorder, and depression. Risk factors for cigarette use among adult women. *Behavior Modification* 20(4):363-84.

Anda, R.F., Williamson, D.F., Escobedo, L.G., Mast, E.E., Giovino, G.A., Beratis, S., Lekka, N. P., and Gabriel, J. (1997). Smoking among suicide attempters.*Comprehensive Psychiatry*, 38, 74-79.

Bergen, W. and Caporaso, N. (1999). Cigarette smoking. *Journal of the National Cancer Institute*, 91, 1365-1375.

Berkman, L.F., Melchior, M., Chastang, J.F., Niedhammer, I., Leclerc, A., Goldberg, M. (2004). Social integration and mortality: a prospective study of French employees of Electricity of France-Gas of France: the GAZEL Cohort. *American Journal of Epidemiology*, 159(2):167-174.

Borrelli, B., Niaura, R., Keuthen N. J. et al. (1996). Development of major depressive disorder during smoking-cessation treatment. *The Journal of Clinical Psychiatry*, 57, 534-538.

Breese, C.R., Lee, M.J., Adams, C.E. et al. (2000). Abnormal regulation of high affinity nicotinic receptors in subjects with schizophrenia. *Neuropsychopharmacology*, 23(4), 351-364.

Breslau, N. (1995). Psychiatric comorbidity of smoking and nicotine dependence. *Behavioral Genetics* 25:95–101

Breslau, N., Kilbey, M., and Andreski, P. (1991). Nicotine dependence, major depre- ssion, and anxiety in young adults. *Archives of General Psychiatry*, 48, 1069-1074.

Breslau, N., Kilbey, M., Andreski, P. (1993). Nicotine dependence and major depression. New evidence from a prospective investigation. *Archives of General Psychiatry* 50, 31–35.

Breslau, N., Peterson, E.L., Schultz, L.R., Chilcoat, H.D., Andreski, P. (1998). Major depression and stages of smoking. *A longitudinal investigation*, 55(2), 161-166.

Breslau, N., Novak, S. P., and Kessler R. C. (2004). Daily smoking and the subsequent onset of psychiatric disorders. *Psychological Medicine*, 34, 323-333.

Brody, A.L., Olmstead, R.E., London, E.D., et al. Smoking-induced ventral striatum dopamine release. *American Journal of Psychiatry*, 161(7), 1211-1218.

Brown, R.A., Kahler, C.W., Zvolensky, M.J., Lejuez, C.W., Ramsey, S.E. (2001).Anxiety sensitivity: relationship to negative affect smoking and smoking cessation in smokers with past major depressive disorder. *Addictive Behaviors* 26(6):887-99.

Carmody, T. P. (1989). Affect regulation, nicotine addiction, and smoking cessation. *Journal of Psychoactive Drugs,* 21, 331-342.

Choi, W.S., Patten, C.A., Gillin, J.C., Kaplan, R.M. and Pierce, J.P. (1997). Cigarette smoking predicts development of depressive symptoms among U.S. adolescents. *Ann. Behav. Med.* 19(1):42-50

Collins, R. L., and Escobar, J. I. (2005). Dialogues on depression management: the primary care and specialist perspectives. *Managed Care,* 15, 3-9.

Corvin, A., O'Mahony, E., O'Regan, M. et al. (2001). Cigarette smoking and psycho-tic symptoms in bipolar affective disorder. *British Journal of Psychiatry*. 179, 35-38.

Covey, L. S., Glassman, A. H., and Stetner, F. (1990). Depression and depressive symptoms in smoking cessation. *Comprehensive Psychiatry,* 31, 350-354.

Covey, L. S., Glassman, A. H. and Stetner, F. (1997). Major depression following smoking cessation. *American Journal of Psychiatry*, 154(2), 263-265.

Covey, L. S., Glassman, A. H., and Stetner, F. (1998). Cigarette smoking and major depression. *Journal of Addictive Diseases*, 17, 35-46.

Covey, L.S., Hughes, D.C., Glassman, A.H. et al. (1994). Ever-smoking, quitting and psychiatric disorders: Evidence from the Durham North Carolina, Epidemiological Catchment Area. *Tobacco Control*, 3, 222–227.

Covey, L.S., Tam, D. (1990). Depressive mood, the single-parent home, and adolescent cigarette smoking. American Journal of Public Health 80:1330–1333.

Crisp, A., Sedgwick, P., Halek, C., Joughin, N., Humphrey, H. (1999): Why may teenage girls persist in smoking? *Journal of Adolescence* 22:657-672.

Dani, J. A., and Harris,R. A. (2005). Nicotine addiction and comorbidity with alcohol abuse and mental illness. *Nature Neuroscience*, 8, 1465-1470.

De Leon, J., Dadvand, M., Canuso, C., White, A.O., Stanilla, J.K., Simpson, G.M. (1995) Schizophrenia and smoking: an epidemiological survey in a state hospital. American *Journal of Psychiatry* 152(3):453-5

DiFranza, J.R., Savageau, J.A., Fletcher, K. et al (2007). Symptoms of tobacco dependence after brief intermittent use. The development and assessment of nicotine dependence in youth-2 study. *Archives of Pediatric and Adolescent Medicine* 161(7), 704-710, 2007.

Dinn, W.M., Aycicegi, A., Harris, C.L. (2004). Cigarette smoking in a student sample: neurocognitive and clinical correlates. *Addictive Behaviors,* 29(1), 107-126.

Dudas, R.B., Hans, K., Barabas, K. (2005) Anxiety, depression and smoking in school children- implications for smoking prevention. *Journal of the Royal Society of Health*, 125(2), 87-92.

Emslie, C., Hunt, K., Macintyre, S. (2002). How similar are the smoking and drinking habits of men and women in non-manual jobs? *European Journal of Public Health.* 12(1), 22-28.

Etter, J.F., Prokhorov, A.V., and Perneger, T.V. (2002). Gender differences in the psychological determinants of cigarette smoking. *Addiction,* 97, 733-743.

Feldner, M.T., Babson, K.A., Zvolensky, M.J., Vujanovic, A.A., Lewis, S.F., Gibson, L.E., Monson, C.M., Bernstein, A. (2007). Posttraumatic stress symptoms and smoking to reduce negative affect: an investigation of trauma-exposed daily smokers. *Addictive Behaviors* 32(2):214-27.

File, S.E., Cheeta, S., Kenny, P.J., Ouagazzal, A-M, Gonzalez, L.E. (1999). Roles of the dorsal raphe nucleus, lateral septum and dorsal hippocampus in nicotine's e□ects on anxiety. *Society for Neuroscience Abstracts* 25, 1981.

File, S.E., Fluck, E., Leahy, A. (2001). Nicotine has calming effects on stress induced mood changes in females but enhances aggression in males, 4(4), 371–376.

Gilbert, D.G., Robinson, J.H., Chamberlin, C.L., Spielberger, C.D. (1989) Effects of smoking/nicotine on anxiety, heart rate, and lateralization of EEG during a stressful movie. *Psychophysiology.* 26(3):311-20.

Ginsberg, D., Hall, S. M., Reus, V. I. et al. (1995). Mood and depression diagnosis in smoking cessation. Experimental and Clinical Psychopharmacology, 3, 389-395.

Glassman, A.H. (1993). Cigarette smoking: Implications for psychiatric illness. *American Journal of Psychiatry* 150:546–553

Glassman, A.H., Covey, L.S., Stetner, F. et al. (2001). Smoking cessation and the course of major depression: a follow-up study. *Lancet,* 357, 1929-1932.

Glassman, A. H., Helzer, J.E., Covey, L.S. et al. (1990). Smoking, smoking cessation,and major depression. *Journal of the American Medical Association*, 264, 1546-1569.

Goodwin, R.D., Lewinsohn, P.M., Seeley, J.R. (2005) Cigarette smoking and panic attacks among young adults in the community: the role of parental smoking and anxiety disorders. *Biological Psychiatry*. 58(9):686-93.

Hall, S. M., Munoz, R. F., Reus, V. I. et al. (1993). Nicotine, negative affect and depression. *Journal of Consulting Clinical Psychology,* 61, 61-767.

Hamalainen, J., Kaprio, J., Isometsa, E. et al. (2001). Cigarette smoking, alcohol intoxication and major depressive episode in a representative population sample. *Epidemiology and Community Health*, 55, 573-576.

Haukkala, A., Uutela, A., Vartiainen, E. et al. (2000). Depression and smoking cessation: the role of motivation and self-efficacy. *Addictive Behaviors*, 25, 311-316.

Hemenway, D, Solnick, S.J., Colditz, G.A. (1993). Smoking and suicide among nurses. *American Journal of Public Health*, 83(2), 249-251.

Hemmingsson, T., and Kriebel, D. (2003). Smoking at age 18-20 and suicide during 26 years of follow-up-how can the association be explained? International *Journal of Epidemiology*, 32(6), 1000-1004.

Hughes, J.R., Arana, G., Amori, G., Stewart, F., Workman, R. (1988). Effect of tobacco withdrawal on the dexamethasone suppression test. *Biological Psychiatry*. 1;23(1):96-8.

Hughes, J.R., Hatsukami, D.K., Mitchell, J.E., Dahlgren, L.A. (1986) Prevalence of smoking among psychiatric outpatients. *American Journal of Psychiatry* 143:993–997.

Iancu, I., Sapir, A.P., Shaked, G., Poreh, A., Dannon, P.N., Chelben, J., Kotler, M. (2006). Increased suicidal risk among smoking schizophrenia patients. *Clinical Neuropharmacology* 29(4):230-7.

Istvan, J., Matarazzo, J. (1984). Tobacco, alcohol, and caffeine use: A review of their interrelationship. *Psychological Bulletin* 95:301– 326

Jha, P., Ranson, M.K., Nguyen, S.N., and Yach, D. (2002). Estimates of global and regional smoking prevalence in 1995, by age and sex. *American Journal of Public Health* 92(6), 1002–1006.

Johnson, J., Weissman, M.M. and Klerman, G.L. (1992). Service utilization and social morbidity associated with depressive symptoms in the community. *Journal of the American Medical Association* 267(11):1478-83

Johnson, J.G., Cohen, P., Pine, D.S., Klein, D.F., Kasen, S., Brook, J.S. (2000) Association between cigarette smoking and anxiety disorders during adolescence and early adulthood. *Journal of the American Medical Association*. 284(18):2348-51.

Kaylene, M., and Pradhan, S. C. (2001). Smoking cessation and major depression. *Lancet,* 358, 1011-1011.

Kendler, K.S., Neale, M.C., MacLean, C.J., Health, A.C., Eaves, L.J., Kessler, R.C. (1993) Smoking and major depression. A causal analysis. *Archives of General Psychiatry* 50:36–43

Khantzian, E. J. (1997). The self-medication hypothesis of substance use disorders: a reconsideration and recent applications. Harvard Review of Psychiatry, 4, 231-244.

Korhonen, T., Broms, U., Varjonen, J. et al. (2007). Smoking behavior as a predictor of depression among Finnish men and women: a prospective cohort study of adult twins. *Psychological Medicine,* 37, 705-715.

Malone, K.M., Waternaux, C., Haas, G.L. et al. (2003) Cigarette smoking, suicidal behavior, and serotonin function in major psychiatric disorders. *American Journal of Psychiatry,* 160, 773-779.

McCabe, R.E., Chudzik, S.M., Antony, M.M., Young, L., Swinson, R.P., Zolvensky, M.J. (2004) Smoking behaviors across anxiety disorders. *Journal of Anxiety Disorders* 18(1):7-18.

McCrae, R.R., Costa, P.T. Jr, Boss, R. (1978). Anxiety, extraversion and smoking.British *Journal of Social Clinical Psychology* 17(3):269-73.

McLeish, A.C., Zvolensky, M.J., Bucossi, M.M. (2007). Interaction between smoking rate and anxiety sensitivity: Relation to anticipatory anxiety and panic-relevant avoidance among daily smokers. *Journal of Anxiety Disorders.* 21(6):849-59.

Miller, V.M., Clouse, W.D., Tonnessen, B.H., et al. (2000). Time and dose effect of transdermal nicotine on endothelial function. American Journal of Physiology. *Heart and circulatory physiology,* 279(4):H1913-1921.

Moriya, F., Hashimoto, Y. (2005). Do smokers who commit suicide have high blood levels of nicotine? *American Journal of Psychiatry,* 162, 816-817.

Murphy, J.M., Horton, N. J., Monson, R.R. et al. (2003). Cigarette smoking in relation to depression: historical trends from the Stirling County Study. *American Journal of Psychiatry,* 160, 1663-1669.

Netter, P., Hennig, J., Huwe, S., Olbrich, R. (1998). Personality related e□ects of nicotine, mode of application, and expectancies on performance, emotional states, and desire for smoking. *Psychopharmacology* 135, 52–62.

Nichols, L., Barton, P. L., Glazner, J. McCollum M. (2007). Diabetes, minor depression and health care utilization and expenditures: a retrospective database study. *Cost Effectiveness and Resource Allocation,* 5, 4.

Patton, G.C., Hibbert, M., Rosier, M.J., Carlin, J.B., Caust, J., Bowes, G. (1996). Is smoking associated with depression and anxiety in teenagers? *American Journal of Public Health.* 86(2):225-30.

Patton, G.C., Carlin, J.B., Coffey, C., Wolfe, R., Hibbert, M., Bowes, G. (1998). Depression, anxiety, and smoking initiation: a prospective study over 3 years. *American Journal of Public Health.* 88(10):1518-22.

Perez-Stable, E.J., Marin, G., Marin, B.V., Katz, M.H. (1990). Depressive symptoms and cigarette smoking among Latinos in San Francisco. *American Journal of Public Health* 80(12):1500-2.

Perkins, K.A., Donny, E., Caggiula, A.R. (1999). Sex differences in nicotine effects and self-administration: review of human and animal evidence. *Nicotine and tobacco research,* 1(4), 301-315.

Pohl, R., Yeragani, V.K., Balon, R., Lycaki, H., McBride, R.(1992). Smoking in patients with panic disorder. *Psychiatry Research.* 43(3):253-62.

Pomerleau, O.F., Turk, D.C., Fertig, J.B. (1984).The effects of cigarette smoking on pain and anxiety. *Addictive Behavior.* 9(3):265-71.

Pontieri, F.E., Tanda, G., Orzi, F., Di Chiara, G.(1996). Effects of nicotine on the nuc- leus accumbens and similarity to those of addictive drugs. *Nature* 382(6588), 255-7.

Potkin, S.G., Alphs, L., Hsu, C., Krishnan, K.R., Anand, R., Young, F.K., et al. (2003). Predicting suicidal risk in schizophrenic and schizoaffective patients in a prospective two-year trial.*Biological Psychiatry*. 54(4),444-452.

Riala, K., Alaraisanen, A., Taanila, A., Hakko, H., Timonen, M., Rasanen, P. (2007). Regular daily smoking among 14-year-old adolescents increases the subsequent risk for suicide: The Nothern Finland 1966 Birth Cohort Study. *Journal of Clinical Psychiatry* 68(5):775-780.

Sonntag, H., Wittchen, H.U., Hofler, M., Kessler, R.C., Stein, M.B. (2000). Are social fears and DSM-IV social anxiety disorder associated with smoking and nicotine dependence in adolescents and young adults? *European Psychiatry*. 15(1):67-74.

Stanton, W.R., Lowe, J.B. and Silva, P.A. (1995). Antecedents of vulnerability and resilience to smoking among adolescents. *Journal of Adolescence Health*. 16(1):71-7.

Surgeon General's Report (2001). Centers for Disease Control and Prevention. *Women and Smoking*.

Tanskanen, A., Tuomilehto, J., Viinamaki, H. et al. (2000). Joint heavy use of alcohol, cigarettes and coffee and the risk of suicide. *Addiction,* 95, 1699-1704

Tanskanen, A., Viinamaki, H., Hintikka, J. et al. (1998). Smoking and suicidality among psychiatric patients. *American Journal of Psychiatry*, 155, 129-130 .

Wang, P. S., Simon, G., Kessler, R. (2003). The economic burden of depression and the cost-effectiveness of treatment. *International Journal of Methods in Psychiatric Research*, 12, 22–33.

Weiser, M., Knobler, H., Lubin, G., et al. (2004). Body mass index and future schizophrenia in Israeli male adolescents. *Journal of Clinical Psychiatry*, 65(11), 1546-1549.

Whitfield, J.B., Pang, D., Bucholz, K.K., et al. (2000). Monoamine oxidase: associations with alcohol dependence, smoking and other measures of psychopathology. *Psychological Medicine,* 30(2), 443-454.

Williams, J. M. and Ziedonis, D. (2004). Addressing tobacco among individuals with a mental illness or an addiction, *Addictive Behaviors* 29, 1067-1083.

Yamasaki, A., Chinami, M., Suzuki, M. et al. (2005). Tobacco and alcohol tax relationships with suicide in Switzerland. *Psychological Reports*, 97, 213-216.

Zhang, J., McKeown, R. E., Hussey, J. R. et al. (2005). Gender differences in risk factors for attempted suicide among young adults: findings from the Third National Health and Nutrition Examination Survey. *Annals of Epidemiology,* 15, 167-174.

Zvolensky, M.J., Kotov, R., Bonn-Miller, M.O., Schmidt, N.B., Antipova, A.V. (2006). Anxiety sensitivity as a moderator of association between smoking status and panic-related processes in a representative sample of adults. *Journal of Psychiatric Research*. Nov 10.

In: Smoking and Women's Health   ISBN 978-1-60456-148-7
Editors: M.K. Wesley and I.A. Sternbach, pp.217-229   © 2008 Nova Science Publishers, Inc.

Chapter 9

Smoking and Women's Health Research

G. A. Scardina and P. Messina

Department of Oral Sciences ,University of Palermo, Sicily, Italy

Abstract

Many studies have tried to evaluate the effects of smoking on women's oral health and women's oral microcirculation. Oral side effects of tobacco are: sticky tar deposits or brown staining on the teeth; 'smoker's palate' - red inflammation on the roof of the mouth; delayed healing of the gums; increased severity of gum disease; bad breath or halitosis; black hairy tongue; oral lesions; gum recession - with chewing tobacco at the site of the tobacco "wad", the gums react by receding along the tooth root, exposing the root; oral cancer, aesthetics: tobacco stains and discolours teeth, dentures and restorations.

A significant relationship between women's smoking and the presence of capillary tortuosity emerged too.

A pathological situation was characterized by architectural confusion or by the presence of clear morphological anomalies.

Smoking causes an abnormal pattern formation of chorioallantois membrane blood vessels in chicks, which alters the composition of the extracellular matrix in the chorioallantois membrane mesoderm.

According to these studies, nicotine has no direct effect on vascular caliber, but it may interact with certain intravenous substances (norepinephrine, acetylcholine, adenosine phosphate), consequently determining vascular constriction.

The microcirculation variations observed in correspondence with oral microcirculation can compromise the phlogistic defense response. In particular, it can compromise one of the first phases of phlogosis: vasodilatation and the resulting vasopermeabilization, with consequent impossibility on the part of defense mechanisms to react. Such events would make smoker women more sensitive towards exogenous noxae, since they cannot respond effectively. This could explain why smoking represents a risk factor, especially for women's oral health.

The Surgeon General's Report stated that "Cigarette smoking is the major single cause of cancer mortality in the United States" [2,9]. Because cigarette smoking and tobacco use is an acquired behavior, one that the individual chooses to do, smoking is the most preventable cause of premature death in our society. Each year, a staggering 440,000 people die in the US from tobacco use. Nearly 1 of every 5 deaths is related to smoking. Cigarettes kill more Americans than alcohol, car accidents, suicide, AIDS, homicide, and illegal drugs combined [9]. Cigarette smoking accounts for at least 30% of all cancer deaths. It is a major cause of cancers of the lung, larynx, oral cavity, pharynx, and esophagus, and is a contributing cause in the development of cancers of the bladder, pancreas, liver, uterine cervix, kidney, stomach, colon and rectum, and some leukemias [11]. The risk of having lung cancer and other smoking-related cancers is related to total lifetime exposure to cigarette smoke, as measured by the number of cigarettes smoked each day, the age at which smoking began, and the number of years a person has smoked [2]. The Office of the US Surgeon General released a long-awaited, detailed report entitled "Women and Smoking" along with the following statement: "When calling attention to public health problems, we must not misure the word "epidemic" [9,17]. But there is no better word to describe the 600-percent increase since 1950 in women's death rates for lung cancer, a disease primarily caused by cigarette smoking [11,17]. Clearly, smoking-related disease among women is a full-blown epidemic" [3]. According to the Centers for Disease Control and Prevention (CDC), smoking-related diseases caused the deaths of about 178,000 women in each year from 1995-1999. On average, these women died 14.5 years earlier because they smoked. The most recent CDC survey showed that about 1 in 5 American women aged 18 years or older (19%) smoked cigarettes. The highest rates were seen among American-Indian and Alaska-Native women (29%), followed by white (20%), African-American (17%), Hispanic (11%), and Asian women (5%) [3]. The less education a woman has, the more likely she will smoke. For instance, women with less than a high school education are twice as likely to smoke as college graduates. A literature review on changes in cigarette smoking by gender in different populations of the developed world after 1980 reveals that smoking is almost uniformly declining in men, but trends are much more diverse in women. In most northern European and North American populations women are smoking less, but in most middle and southern European populations, including Switzerland, the prevalence of current smoking among women is still on the rise. Compared to older women, younger women began smoking cigarettes at a much earlier age and smoked more. Moreover, absence of a decline in the age at smoking cessation among women indicates little will to stop smoking at the population level. The observed smoking increase among women are in general accord with lung cancer surveillance data collected. Women who smoke typically begin as teenagers -- usually before high school graduation. And the younger a girl is when she starts, the more heavily she is likely to use tobacco as an adult [5]. Teenage girls are just as likely to smoke as are boys. Why do we smoke cigarettes? Smoking is fun, smoking is a reward, smoking is oral pleasure, "with a cigarette I am not alone", "I like to watch the smoke", smoking memories, cigarettes help us to relax, "I blow my troubles away". While people become dependent on cigarettes for a number of reasons, addiction to the nicotine contained in cigarettes is the primary factor in smoking dependency. Its most immediate effect is a physiological "rush", an increase in blood pressure, respiration, and heart rate caused by stimulation of the adrenal glands to release epinephrine (adrenaline). Nicotine can also have a sedative effect. It leads to addiction primarily because of its effect on the neurotransmitter dopamine (chemical that activates the areas of the brain, called reward centers that control pleasure). Nicotine increases the levels of dopamine in the reward centers of the brain, similar to the action of other addictive substances, such as cocaine and heroine. Nicotine in tobacco is a particularly powerful and effective drug delivery system, and "hooks" the smoker quickly. The nicotine within a single puff of cigarette smoke reaches the brain within 10 seconds of inhalation. While the effects of the substance are experienced quickly, they fade within minutes, which leads the user to dose frequently with cigarettes. It is estimated that a person who smokes about 1 1/2 packs a day receives 300 doses of nicotine daily. This high-frequency dosing reinforces the addictive quality of the drug. Researches indicate that dependence on cigarettes is not the result of nicotine alone. Women, teenagers, and Caucasians experience more symptoms of tobacco dependence than other groups, even while using the same number, or fewer, cigarettes. According to a 2001 review of available research on women and smoking, nicotine replacement therapy is less effective for women [4,5]. Together, these findings may indicate that women's dependence on smoking is based in part on something in addition to nicotine. Cigarette smoking was rare among women in the early 20th century and became prevalent among women after it did among men. In 2005, 20.3 million (18.1 percent) of women smoked in the United States. Although fewer women smoke than men, the percentage difference between the two has continued to decrease year to year. Today, with a much closer gap between men's and women's smoking rates, women share a much larger burden of smoking-related diseases. Tobacco has a damaging affect on women's reproductive health and is associated with increased risk of miscarriage, early delivery (prematurity), stillbirth, infant death, and is a cause of low birth weight in infants. Women who smoke, especially after going through menopause, have lower bone density and a higher risk for fracture, including hip fracture, than women who do not smoke [5]. They may also be at higher risk for developing rheumatoid arthritis and cataracts (clouding of the lenses of the eyes). Tobacco use can damage a woman's reproductive health. Women who smoke have an increased risk for delayed conception and fertility problems. Smokers are younger at menopause than nonsmokers and may have more unpleasant symptoms while going through menopause. Smoking can also cause complications during pregnancy that can hurt both mother and baby. Smokers have a higher risk of the placenta growing too close to the opening of the uterus. Smokers are also more likely to have premature membrane ruptures and placentas that separate from the uterus too early. Bleeding, premature delivery, and emergency Caesarean section (C-section) may result from these problems. Smokers are also more likely to have miscarriages and stillbirths. More than 10% of pregnant women smoke throughout their pregnancies. Smoking is linked to an increased risk of preterm delivery and infant death. Research also suggests that infants of mothers who smoke during and after pregnancy are 2 to 3 times more likely to die from sudden infant death syndrome (SIDS) than babies born to nonsmoking mothers. Even of the women who are able to stop smoking during pregnancy, only one third of those remain quit one year after the delivery. The risk is somewhat less for infants whose mothers stop smoking during pregnancy and resume smoking after delivery. But infants of nonsmoking mothers have the lowest risk of SIDS. As many as 10% of all infant deaths could be prevented if pregnant women did not smoke.

Smoking during pregnancy is responsible for 20% or more of cases of low birth weight infants. Smoking during pregnancy slows fetal growth, often causing babies to have health problems as a result of being born underweight. Quitting smoking during pregnancy reduces this risk. Some harmful chemicals in tobacco smoke can also be passed on to a baby through breast milk. Cigarette smoking can affect women's fertility, pregnant women's health and the health of unborn and young children: '

1) Fertility: women who smoke may have reduced fertility. Studies found that 38% of non-smokers conceived in their first cycle compared with 28% of smokers. And Smokers were 3.4 times more likely than non-smokers to have taken more than one year to conceive. It was estimated that the fertility of smoking women was 72% that of non- smokers. Cigarette smoking can also affect male-fertility; spermatozoa from smokers are found to be decreased in density and motility compared with that of non-smokers. A new study found that sperm cells carrying Y-chromosome are more vulnerable to the toxins in cigarette smoke.

2) Smoking and oral contraceptives: for younger women, smoking and the use of oral contraceptives increase the risk of a heart attack, stroke or other cardiovascular disease by tenfold. This effect is more marked in women over 45.

3) Foetal growth and birth weight: babies born to women who smoke are on average 200 grams (8 ozs) lighter than babies born to comparable non-smoking mothers. Low birth weight is associated with higher risks of death and diseases in infancy and early childhood. The more cigarettes a woman smokes during pregnancy, the greater the probable reduction in birth weight. Recent research suggests that cigarettes can reduce the flow of blood in the placenta which limits the amount of nutrients that reach the foetus.

4) Spontaneous abortion: the rate of spontaneous abortion (miscarrage) is substantially increased in women who smoke by tenfold. Moreover, smokers have more complications of pregnancy and labour which include bleeding during pregnancy, premature detachments of the placenta and premature rupture of the membranes, and inadequate milk production. Perinatal mortality (defined as still birth or death of an infant within the first week of life) is increased by about one-third in babies of smokers.

5) Infant health and long term growth: infants of parents who smoke are twice as likely to suffer from serious respiratory infection than the children of nonsmokers. Smoking during pregnancy can also increase the risk of asthma in young children (before 1-year-old) by 2.8 times. Other disorders associated with smoking in pregnancy include an increased risk of infantile colic and cleft palate. Smoking in pregnancy also have implications for the long term physical growth and intellectual development of the child, such as reduced height, lower attainments in reading and mathematics up to age 16 and even the highest qualification achieved by the age of 23.

6) Smoking, cervial cancer and menopause: the natural menopause occurs up to two years earlier in smokers. The likelihood is related to the number of cigarettes

smoked, with those smoking more than ten cigarettes a day having an increased risk of an early menopause.

7)   Oral side effects of tobacco:

- sticky tar deposits or brown staining on the teeth (Figure1)
- 'smoker's palate' - red inflammation on the roof of the mouth (Figure2)
- delayed healing of the gums
- increased severity of gum disease
- bad breath or halitosis
- black hairy tongue
- oral lesions
- gum recession - with chewing tobacco at the site of the tobacco "wad", the gums react by receding along the tooth root, exposing the root
- oral cancer (Figure 3)
- aesthetics: tobacco stains and discolours teeth, dentures and restorations. Pipe smokers and smokeless tobacco users are prone to excessive wear on their teeth, which often become flat. The eventual exposing of tooth dentin can lead to deep tobacco staining. Tobacco, whether smoked or chewed, can cause halitosis. Cleft lips and palates are twice as common amongst children born to mothers who smoked during pregnancy. Heavy smoking can cause an overgrowth of the papilla of the tongue surface. This brown, furry growth traps germs and eventually creates a burning sensation on the tongue and exacerbates bad breath. Tobacco-associated bad breath is related to the strength of tobacco smoked. Pipes and cigar tobacco contain a higher concentration of sulphur that produces stronger bad breath. The use of breath freshening mints to alleviate the bad breath can themselves cause dental erosion due to the large quantities of sugar and citric acid contained in them.Smokers have higher levels of calculus formation than non-smokers. Calculus deposits make it easier for plaque to stick to teeth and cause gum disease and cavities to form [1].
- Dental caries: although smoking is a commonly included factor in the analysis of rates of caries there is still insufficient evidence for any aetiological relationship [1].
- Dental implants: tobacco can be damaging to both the initial and long-term success of dental implants.1 Indeed, in one study smoking was the most significant factor predisposing implant failure - rates were 4.8% in non-smokers and 11.3% in smokers [1].
- Healing of wounds: tobacco is a peripheral vasoconstrictor which influences the rate at which wounds heal within the mouth. Carbon monoxide and other chemicals produced during the combustion of tobacco can reduce the capillary blood flow within the mouth - research has suggested that a single cigarette can reduce the peripheral blood velocity by 40% for one hour. Consequently healing is much slower and not as successful following oral surgery on smokers. The resulting absence of blood clotting that follows the removal of teeth (referred to as dry sockets or localised osteitis) occurs 4-times more frequently in smokers

than in non-smokers. Studies have also shown that smokers have a 50-100% inhibition of the function of polymorphonuclear leukocytes (white blood cells which help fight infection) compared to non-smokers [1].

- Heart disease: there is increasing debate as to whether poor oral health (in particular periodontitis) can be a cause of pulmonary heart disease. Studies have shown that there is an association between the two: though the precise mechanisms of how this occurs are not fully understood. It is believed that certain oral bacteria, such as Streptococcus sanguis, play a major role: when the bacteria enter the bloodstream through diseased gum tissue they cause blood platelets to clump together and start clotting, which can eventually lead to a heart attack. In addition, inflammatory white blood cells and fibrinogen are found in higher concentrations in sufferers of periodontitis and these have been known to increase the risk of heart attack. However, more recent study concluded that people with and without dental infections had the same risk of heart disease. The University of Washington report claims that the link between oral health and heart disease only existed in the first place because earlier studies had not adjusted their data to take into consideration the effects of smoking. These studies showed "an association between gum disease and stroke, coronary heart disease, low birth weight, chronic obstructive pulmonary disease and lung cancer. All of these diseases are smoking-related". Despite the contradictions in the research, it is clear that the best way to ensure good oral health and to reduce the risk of heart disease is to stop smoking [1,6].

- Oral cancer: it is well documented that tobacco has a direct carcinogenic effect on the epithelial cells of the oral mucous membranes. The British Dental Association (BDA) defines oral cancer based on a series of risk factors and includes all cancers of the lip, tongue, gingiva, mouth floor, oropharynx and hypopharynx, but not cancers of the major salivary glands and nasopharynx [7].

- Oral mucosal diseases: Smoker's palate (nicotinic stomatitis): A change in the hard palate caused by heavy smoking. The palate turns white and can be littered with red dots located within small raised lumps. This condition is not pre-malignant and disappears after smoking is stopped, though some severe forms can progress to oral cancer. Smoker's melanosis: White caucasian smokers are 3 times as likely to show a melanin pigmentation of their mucous membranes. Again, the condition is not pre-malignant and is reversible, though it can take up to 1 year after the cessation of smoking for benefits to accrue [8].

- Oral Candidosis: Several reports have shown that smoking is a factor in the appearance of oral candidosis, although the actual pathogenic role of tobacco in this is unknown [1] (Figure 4).

- Chronic sinus infections: People who are especially sensitive to tobacco smoke can develop swelling in their nasal membranes and sinus cavities. Sinusitis occurs more regularly amongst smokers than non-smokers [1].

- Smoker's lip: This is created by burns caused by smoking unfiltered cigarettes to the end, but is generally rare unless people are under the influence of alcohol [1].

- Lichen Planus: A chronic inflammation that affects skin and the mucous membrane characterised by multiple white oral lesions that cannot be wiped away [1] (Figures 5,6).
- Salivary changes: it is thought that smoking increases the flow rate of the parotid gland 5 but most evidence on the subject of saliva and smoking is inconclusive [1].
- Smell and taste: the smell and taste functions of smokers can be acutely affected by the gasses and chemicals within tobacco and the ancillary particulate matter associated with smoking. The greater the amount smoked, the greater the impact, and only once smoking is stopped do these functions begin to improve again. A reduced ability to taste and smell may lead to potentially problematic changes in diet such as an increased use of salt[1,6].
- Oral microcirculation: the morphological-functional study of microcirculation is of fundamental importance. Our study shows that capillaroscopy is a reliable method for studying oral microcirculation; capillaroscopy makes it possible to study *in vivo* the microcirculatory characteristics of the oral mucosa and to highlight the significant difference between smokers and non-smokers. The smoking habit is an important risk factor in periodontal diseases. In recent years, many studies have tried to evaluate the effects of smoking on microcirculation. A knowledge of microscopic anatomy is fundamental for the interpretation of the oral vascular examination. In fact, the thickness and typology of the epithelial covering, as well as the presence or absence of keratinization, are directly involved in determining microcirculation visibility and capillary length. In our studies, significant relationship between smoking habit and the presence of capillary tortuosity emerged. A pathological situation is characterised by an architectural confusion or by the presence of evident morphological anomalies, as shown in fingernail capillaroscopic studies. The smoking habit causes an abnormal pattern formation of chorioallantois membrane blood vessels in chicks, which alters the composition of the extra-cellular matrix in the chorioallantois membrane mesoderm. Capillary calibre is significantly reduced in smokers; this statement agrees with the data present in literature. According to these studies, nicotine has no direct effect on vascular calibre, but it may interact with certain intravenous substances (norepinephrine, acetylcholine, adenosine phosphate), consequently determining vascular constriction. A greater number of capillary loops in marginal gingival was observed, and this must be related to capillary course with respect to the surface. Our researcges show that the chronic smoking habit induces significant changes in oral capillary morphology, calibre and number, which means that such a habit plays has a determining role as a risk factor in the etiopathogenesis of oral diseases [12,13,14,15,16] (Figure 7).

The US Surgeon General outlined the benefits of smoking cessation [17]:

- Smoking cessation has major and immediate health benefits for men and women of all ages. Benefits apply to persons with and without smoking-related disease.
- Former smokers live longer than continuing smokers. For example, persons who quit smoking before age 50 have one-half the risk of dying in the next 15 years compared with continuing smokers.
- Smoking cessation decreases the risk of lung cancer, other cancers, heart attack, stroke, and chronic lung disease.
- Women who stop smoking before pregnancy or during the first 3 to 4 months of pregnancy reduce their risk of having a low birth weight baby to that of women who never smoked.
- The health benefits of smoking cessation far exceed any risks from the average 5-pound (2.3-kg) weight gain or any adverse psychological effects that may follow quitting [11,17].

A number of studies have shown that women find it more difficult than do men to quit smoking cigarettes [10]. This is especially evident in studies of nicotine replacement therapies that use nicotine patches or nicotine gum. Now two separate NIDA-funded studies examining gender differences related to smoking suggest that something in addition to nicotine is involved in women's dependence on smoking tobacco [10,18].

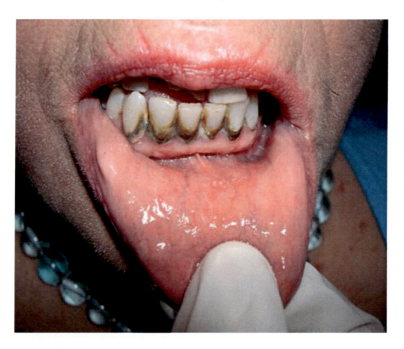

Figure 1. Periodontal disease.

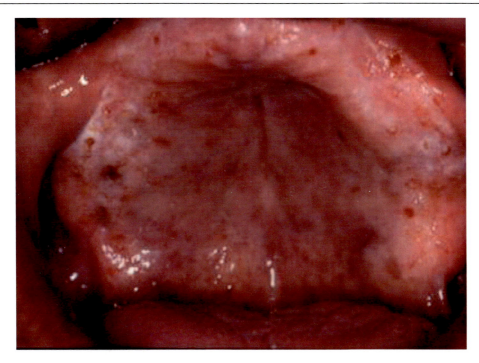

Figure 2. 'smoker's palate'.

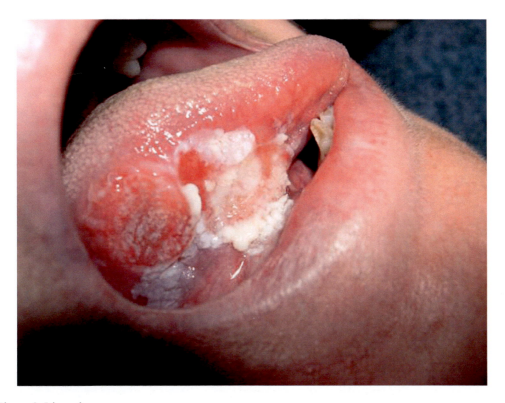

Figure 3. Lingual cancer .

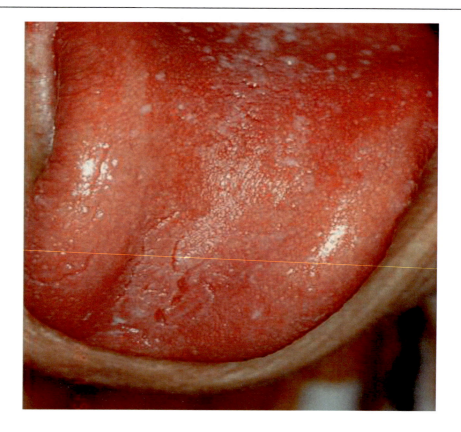

Figure 4. Oral candidiasis.

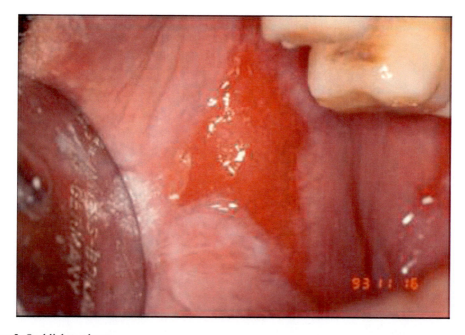

Figure 5. Oral lichen planus.

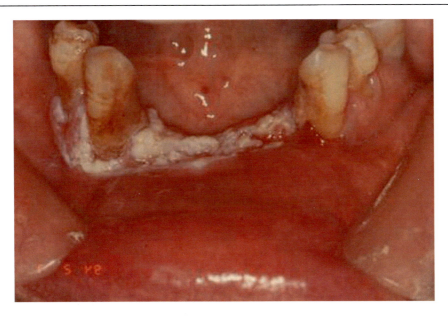

Figure 6. Oral iperkeratosis.

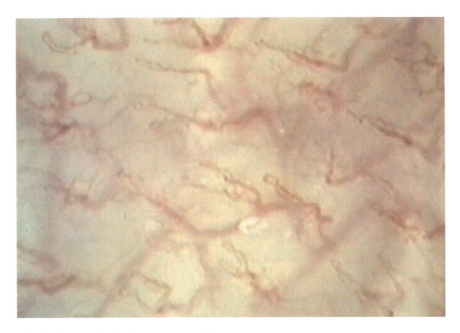

Figure 7. Oral microcirculation in women smoking.

These nonnicotine influences might include nondrug-induced sensory effects like seeing and smelling tobacco smoke, conditioned responses to these smoke stimuli, or social pleasures involved in smoking rituals. For example, one observer has noted that smokers may exhibit gender differences in the way they gather outside buildings to smoke. Male smokers tend to be loners; females tend to gather in social groups [18]. These behaviors may indicate critical gender-based differences relating to tobacco smoking that may have little to do with nicotine, observers theorize. It will be important to revise smoking cessation treatments for women trying to quit [10,18]. This would mean tailoring therapy for women to increase behavioral support and rely less on nicotine replacement. Women in the studies tend to be less successful in smoking cessation trials, especially those using nicotine replacement therapy. Lower cessation rates for women could be expected if women smoked more cigarettes or inhaled more nicotine than did men. Both are indicative of nicotine dependence, and smokers who are more strongly nicotine-dependent often have greater difficulty quitting. But women tend to smoke fewer cigarettes per day, to smoke brands with lower nicotine yields, and to be less likely to inhale deeply, compared to men, according to the researches review [10,18]. Thus, evidence indicates women smokers are less, not more, nicotine-dependent than are men. Thus, external stimuli appear to be more important to women than to men. It can be theorized, then, that women may be less responsive to internal stimuli such as nicotine and more responsive to external stimuli such as the sight and smell of tobacco and its smoke. For tobacco, more study is called for because studies of nonnicotine reinforcement may help develop more effective smoking cessation therapies for women [10,18].

References

[1] Allard R, Johnson N, Sardella A et al. Tobacco and Oral Diseases – Report of EU Working Group, 1999. *Journal of Irish Dental Association;* 1999; 4612-23.

[2] Center for Disease Control and Prevention. Morbidity and Mortality Weekly Report. *Tobacco Use Among Adults*---U.S., 2005. Vol. 42(42); 1145-1145.

[3] Centers for Disease Control and Prevention (CDC). Annual smoking-attributable mortality, years of potential life lost, and economic costs - United States, 1995-1999. MMWR Morb Mort Wkly Rep. 2002;51 300-303.

[4] Connett JE, Murray RP, Buist AS, Wise RA, Bailey WC, Lindgren PG, Owens GR. Changes in Smoking Status Affect Women More than Men: Results of the Lung Health Study, *American Journal of Epidemiology* 2003; 157: 973-979.

[5] Costanza MC, Salamun J, Lopez AD, Morabia A. Gender differentials in the evolution of cigarette smoking habits in a general European adult population from 1993–2003 BMC Public Health 2006, 6:130.

[6] Hujoel PP, Drangsholt M, Spiekerman C et al. Examining the link between coronary heart disease and the elimination of chronic dental infections. *J. Am. Dent. Assoc.;* 2001; 132: 883-9.

[7] Johnson N. Tobacco use and oral cancer: A global perspective. *Journal of Dental Education* 2001; 65: 328-339.

[8] Kawamurafk M, Wright AC, Sasahara L, Yamasaki Y, Suh O, Iwamoto Y. An Analytical Study on Gender Differences in Self-Reported Oral Health Care and Problems of Japanese Employees. *J. Occup. Health* 1999; 41: 104-111.

[9] Office of the US Surgeon General. The Health Benefits of Smoking Cessation: A Report of the Surgeon General. Centers for Disease Control and Prevention (CDC), *Office on Smoking and Health.* 1990.

[10]   Perkins KA. Sex differences in nicotine versus nonnicotine reinforcement as determinants of tobacco smoking. *Experimental and Clinical Psychopharmacology*; 1966; 4:166-177.

[11]   Peto R, Darby S, Deo H, Silcocoks P, Whitlety E, Doll R. Smoking, smoking cessation, and lung cancer in the UK since 1950: combination of national statistics with two case-control studies. *BMJ*. 2000; 321: 323-329 .

[12]   Scardina G.A., and Messina P. Study of the microcirculation of oral mucosa in healthy subjects. It. *J. Anat. Embryol.*2003; 108: 39-48.

[13]   Scardina GA, Fuca G, Messina P. Microvascular characteristics of the human interdental papilla. *Anat Histol Embryol.* 2007;36:266-8.

[14]   Scardina GA, Messina P. Morphologic changes in the microcirculation induced by chronic smoking habit: a videocapillaroscopic study on the human gingival mucosa. *Am. J. Dent.* 2005;18:301-4.

[15]   Scardina GA, Messina P. Smoking habit and labial microcirculation.*Ital. J. Anat. Embryol.* 2004;109:95-103.

[16]   Scardina GA. The effect of cigar smoking on the lingual microcirculation.*Odontology.* 2005;93:41-5.

[17]   U.S Department of Health and Human Services. Health Consequences of Smoking: *A Report of the Surgeon General,* 2004.

[18]   West R, McNeill A, Raw M. Smoking Cessation Guidelines for Health Professionals: An Update. *Thorax*; 2000; 55(12):987-99.

In: Smoking and Women's Health   ISBN 978-1-60456-148-7
Editors: M.K. Wesley and I.A. Sternbach, pp.231-243   © 2008 Nova Science Publishers, Inc.

Chapter 10

Increased Oxidation Injury in Children of Smoking Parents

Roswitha M. Wolfram[61, 2], *Alexandra C. Budinsky*[1, 2], *Heidemarie Pils*[2], *Anthony Oguogho*[2] *and Helmut Sinzinger*[2]

[1]Department of Angiology, Medical University of Vienna,
[2]Wilhelm Auerswald Atherosclerosis Research Group (ASF) Vienna,
Nadlergasse 1, A-1090 Vienna, Austria
*Dr. Anthony Oguogho was on sabbatical leave from the Faculty of Basic Medical Sciences, Edo State University, Ekpoma, Nigeria, supported by the Austrian Academic Exchange Division (ÖDAAD)

Abstract

Mortality rates from diseases related to environmental tobacco smoke exposure (ETS) are constantly increasing. The potential impact of ETS on the development of cardiovascular diseases has recently been under debate, but has so far remained uncertain among children. In order to address this issue we examined plasma and urinary levels of 8-epi-prostaglandin-$F_{2\alpha}$ (8-epi-$PGF_{2\alpha}$) as a measure of in-vivo oxidation injury in 158 children (71 boys, 87 girls, aged 3-15 years). Children were grouped according to smoking habits of their parents: one or both parents smoking, < 20, > 20, or > 40 cigarettes smoked a day, and compared to a non-smoking control group.

Plasma and urinary 8-epi-$PGF_{2\alpha}$ levels were elevated in children of smoking parents. An increased number of smoked cigarettes correlated with higher 8-epi-$PGF_{2\alpha}$ levels and smoking by mother had a trendwise more pronounced influence compared to smoking by father. These data clearly demonstrate a significant in-vivo oxidation injury in children of smoking parents and indicates that development and progression of later vascular disease may already be triggered in childhood by ETS. Considering that worldwide nearly half of

6 Corresponding Author: Prof. Dr. Roswitha Wolfram, Department of Angiology, Medical University of Vienna, Austria, Währinger Gürtel 18-20, 1090 Vienna, Austria, Tel: +43/1/40400/4670, Fax: +43/1/40400/4665, e-mail: rmwolfram@hotmail.com, roswitha.wolfram@meduniwien.ac.at.

the children are exposed to ETS these data clearly underline the importance of the implementation of preventive strategies.

Keywords: *environmental tobacco smoke - isoprostane - 8-epi-PGF   - oxidation, injury - cardiovascular risk.*

Introduction

Active cigarette smoking [1, 2] is known to be a major the risk factor for the development of cardiovascular disease. Recently not only active smoking but also ETS has gained increasing interest [3, 4] as passive smoking is known to cause death due to cardiovascular- [5], lung disease [5, 6], as well as cancer [7] in over 50.000 Americans every year.

The impact of ETS, due to parental smoking, on oxidation injury in children has not yet been addressed. ETS consists of sidestream smoke (SSS) (85%), mainstream smoke (MSS) (15%), exhaled and inhaled by the smoker and vaporphase components diffusing through the cigarette paper. SSS-, MSS and vaporphase components mainly differ in aspects of quantitative composition of gas- and particulate phase [8]. SSS for instance is composed of smaller particles and contains a 2.5 fold higher concentration of carbon monoxide.

Some constituents of SSS and MSS cause oxidative stress [9-12] with unfavorable effects an lipid levels and composition [13], on fibrinogen levels [14], and the prostaglandin system [15, 16] leading among others to increased platelet activation and endothelial dysfunction [17].

Development of atherosclerotic plaque, the pathomorphological substrate of Coronary Heart Disease (CHD), is triggered by increasing amounts of oxidized LDL (ox-LDL) [18]. Ox-LDL, in contrast to native LDL, is taken up by macrophages via the scavenger receptor in an uncontrolled manner [19]. The lack of feedback between intracellular cholesterol-content and cholesterol-uptake via the scavenger-pathway results in an intracellular LDL overload and thereby the transformation of macrophages into foam cells [20]. Free radicals, generated due to ETS, are favoring this process. Therefore the impact of passive smoking on vascular risk has recently been under discussion from an epidemiological [21, 22] as well as from a pathogenetic [23] point of view.

Methods to standardize ETS-exposure are difficult to establish, particularly in children. In adults, series of tests with exposure to ETS in standardized rooms revealed a significant influence on various parameters of platelet function and the prostaglandin system [24]. There is a considerable interest in the development of reliable non-invasive methods to assess the increase of oxidative stress by a quantifiable exposure to ETS. The formation of 8-epi-PGF$_{2\alpha}$ as an in-vivo indicator of oxidation injury resulting from free radical catalyzed per-oxidation of arachidonic acid during active smoking or passive exposure to smoke has already been described previously [25]. Its measurement in plasma and urine was reported to be a useful and reliable tool to assess oxidation injury [26]. Short-term exposure to ETS has been shown to exert no significant influence an LDL-oxidation via oxidative stress. The easy approach to assess 8-epi-PGF$_{2\alpha}$ in plasma and urine of children living together with cigarette smoking parents as a certain form of ETS exposure which is approximately quantifiable has not been evaluated yet. On the occasion of a cholesterol screening program performed at our institution, we therefore studied the effect of parental cigarette smoking (one or both parents) and of the total amount of cigarettes consumed and plasma and urinary 8-epi-PGF$_{2\alpha}$ of the children living in the shared household.

Material and Methods

Blood of a total of 158 children (71 boys, 87 girls, aged 3-15 years; for characteristics see table 1) was drawn from the cubital vein using a 1.2 mm diameter butterfly needle after an at least 30 minutes rest and avoiding venous occlusion for cholesterol screening. Blood was anti-coagulated with 2% sodium EDTA under addition of 10 mg acetylsalicylic acid/ml processed and centrifuged at 4°C. Plasma was removed and stored in liquid nitrogen. This blood withdrawal took place in the morning in the respective school after an at least 12 hours overnight fasting for determination of plasma 8-epi-PGF$_{2\alpha}$, creatinine, blood lipids and lipoproteins. Urine was collected over a period of 24 hours. All the children were healthy and not taking any drug since at least 4 weeks. Children with abnormal lipid-/lipoprotein profile were excluded. It was assured that they were non-smokers and that no other person regularly living in the household was a smoker. Parents were giving their written informed consent for the screening.

Table 1. Children´s Characteristics

Group	Cigarettes / Day	Boys		Girls	
		Number of Children (n)	Age, years (mean (range))	Number of Children (n)	Age, years (mean (range))
	0	14	6.2 (5-11)	17	6.8 (4-9)
A	<20	6	7.5 (5-13)	8	7.3 (4-14)
	≤40	5	7.1 (4-8)	8	6.5 (3-11)
	> 40	5	7.1 (3-14)	4	6.9 (4-13)
B	<20	5	7.8 (3-12)	11	6.2 (4-9)
	≤40	4	6.8 (3-10)	9	7.3 (4-12)
	> 40	7	7.3 (5-12)	6	7.1 (5-10)
C	<20	10	5.9 (5-8)	7	7.1 (4-11)
	≤40	7	6.9 (4-14)	7	7.0 (3-11)
	> 40	8	6.9 (4-11)	10	7.0 (5-14)

Group A = only Father smoking, Group B = only Mother smoking, Group C = Both parents smoking.

Children were divided into 4 groups if mother (group B), father (group A) or both (group C) smoked < 20 cigarettes/day (group 1; n=47; 21 boys, 26 girls; 3-14 years), < 40 cigarettes/day (group 2; n=40; 16 boys. 24 girls; 3-14 years) or > 40 cigarettes (group 3; n=40; 20 boys, 20 girls; 3-14 years) or controls of non-smoking parents (group 4; n=31; 14 boys, 17 girls, 4-11 years) (Table 1).

The number of cigarettes was defined as the total number parents together were smoking at home daily estimated for the last 8 weeks preceding the blood withdrawal.

8-Epi-PGF$_{2\alpha}$ Determination

Samples were extracted and purified and determined using a specific immunoassay as described previously [25, 27]. The cross reactivity with other prostaglandins amounted < 2.5%.

Day to day variability was $3.4 \pm 1.9\%$ in healthy adults (19-24 years n=19) determined for 5 days parallel to the screening investigation. Interassay variability was $6.7 \pm 3.1\%$ (plasma) and $5.9 \pm 2.4\%$ (urine); intraassay variability $3.8 \pm 1.9\%$ (plasma) and $3.5 \pm 1.6\%$ (urine).

Statistical Analysis

Variables were reported as means ☐ SD for continuous variables. Unpaired t-test and One-Way ANOVA with Tukey's Multiple Comparison Test were used to compare continuous variables. A value of $p<0.05$ was considered significant. All calculations were performed with the GraphPad Prism for Windows (Version 5, GraphPad Software, Inc., San Diego, CA, USA).

Results

Even if exposed to ETS of less than 20 cigarettes a day by a smoking parent, 8-epi-PGF$_{2\alpha}$ was elevated in plasma by about 35-55%, in urine by 20-30%. If parents smoke 20 to 40 cigarettes a day by a smoking parent, 8-epi-PGF$_{2\alpha}$ was elevated in plasma by about 65-75%, in urine by 30%. If both parents were smoking together more than 40 cigarettes/day plasma 8-epi-PGF$_{2\alpha}$ increased up to about 130% vs. the respective control groups, urinary 8-epi-PGF$_{2\alpha}$ up to about 65% vs. control group (Figure 1). This elevation apparently depends on the number of cigarettes the children are exposed to per day, on the other hand, whether mother or father was the only smoking parent.

Smoking behavior of the mother showed a trend wise greater influence on the increase of isoprostane levels as compared to the fathers except in the group of > 40 cigarettes at home (Figure 2). As shown in Figure 3 and Figure 4 8-epi-PGF$_{2\alpha}$ levels were higher when both parents were smokers as compared to a single smoking parent. (Figure 3)

The response of girls vs. boys to ETS in the various groups showed no statistically significant difference (Table 2a, 2b).

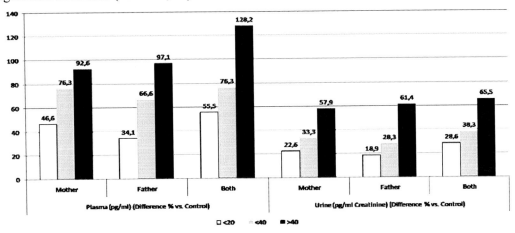

Figure 1. Plasma and Urinary 8-epi-PGF$_{2\alpha}$ levels of children with smoking parents versus children with non-smoking parents (Control). Numbers are given in percentage.

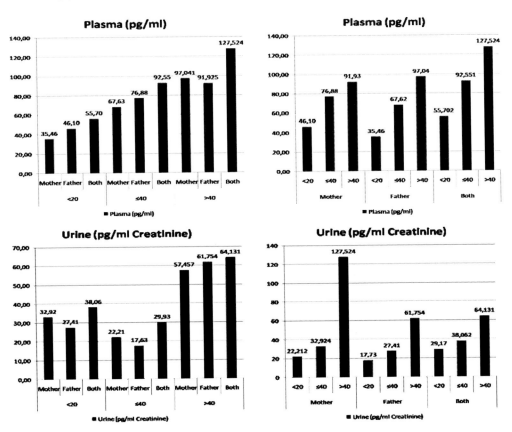

Figure 2. Comparison of male/female average plasma 8-epi-PGF$_{2\alpha}$ levels in relation to number of cigarettes smoked and the smoking parent.

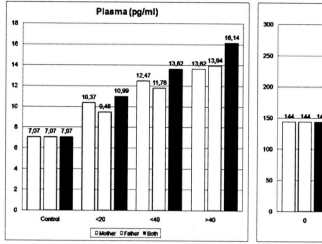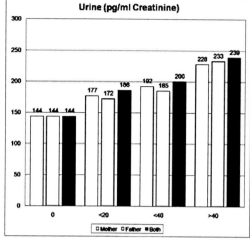

Figure 3. Children's Plasma 8-epi-PGF$_{2\alpha}$ levels (pg/ml) and Urinary 8-epi-PGF$_{2\alpha}$ levels (pg/ml Creatinine).

As we were asking total number of cigarettes smoked and how many of the cigarettes were smoked at home, a good correlation to the number of cigarettes really smoked at home was found. Attempts to calculate the total time children are spending at home vs. number of cigarettes/hour, however, as well as calculating size of the flat, did not reveal significant differences (data not shown).

Discussion

Recently not only the negative impact of active cigarette smoking [28] but also of ETS on morbidity has gained increasing interest [29], especially in children. In the United States 43% of children from 2 months to 11 years of age are exposed to ETS [30], which can cause respiratory diseases [31] and may lead to or aggravate pre-existing asthma in children [32]. Current researchers believe that the process of atherosclerosis starts in early childhood [33, 34] a potential influence of ETS on children's cardiovascular system, however, has not been addressed so far. Atherosclerotic disease has been linked to oxidation injury in previous investigations [35] and the results from our study clearly showed that there is a significant increase of oxidation injury in children exposed to ETS by their parents' smoking.

The ARIC (Atherosclerotic Risk in Communities) study [2] which investigated effects of ETS on the progression of atherosclerosis showed in 10.914 middle-aged adults an increase of the carotid intima-media thickness by 20% in patients exposed to ETS over a 3 years follow-up. Passive smoking in this trial was defined as exposure to cigarette smoke for > 1 hour a day.

There are some limitations to test and quantify ETS exposure at work [36, 37] and during social life. Exposure to ETS of (non-)smokers in a standardized room (m^3) is difficult to perform and time consuming. In addition, although well standardized, it is far from true life conditions, but allows assessing the influence of a single as well as repeated exposure to cigarette smoke.

Table 2a. Plasma 8-epi-PGF$_{2\alpha}$ levels – influence of number of cigarettes smoked, the smoking parent and gender of the child

Plasma Isoprostane Values

Cigarettes/ Day	Smoking Parents	Boys			Girls			p-Value Boys vs. Girls
		Number of children (n)	Plasma (pg/ml)	p-Value vs. Control	Number of children (n)	Plasma (pg/ml)	p-Value vs. Control	
0	-	14	7.11 ± 1.83	Control	17	7.04 ± 1.95	Control	0.9193
≤20	Mother	6	10.12 ±	0.004	8	10.55 ±	0.0003	0.6753
≤20	Father	5	9.86 ± 1.24	0.0067	11	9.31 ± 1.55	0.0032	0.4987
≤20	Both	10	10.89 ±	< 0.0001	7	11.14 ±	< 0.0001	0.7946
≤40	Mother	5	12.72 ±	< 0.0001	8	12.31 ±	< 0.0001	0.7141
≤40	Father	4	12.06 ±	0.0003	9	11.66 ±	< 0.0001	0.7254
≤40	Both	7	13.88 ± 2	< 0.0001	7	14.16 ±	< 0.0001	0.8069
>40	Mother	5	13.91 ±	< 0.0001	4	13.25 ±	< 0.0001	0.7097
>40	Father	7	13.88 ±	< 0.0001	6	14.00 ±	< 0.0001	0.9176
>40	Both	8	15.71 ±	< 0.0001	10	16.48 ±	< 0.0001	0.5539

Table 2b. Urinary 8-epi-PGF$_{2a}$ levels – influence of number of cigarettes smoked, the smoking parent and gender of child

Urine Isoprostane Values

Cigarettes / Day	Smoking Parents	Boys			Girls			p-Value Boys vs. Girls
		Number of Children (n)	Urine (pg/ml Creatinine)	p-Value vs. Control	Number of Children (n)	Urine (pg/ml Creatinine)	p-Value vs. Control	
0	-	14	147 ± 12	Control	17	142 ± 9	Control	0.1953
≤ 20	Mother	6	174 ± 17	0.0007	8	179 ± 14	<0.0001	0.5569
≤ 20	Father	5	166 ± 21	0.0232	11	174 ± 19	<0.0001	0.4616
≤ 20	Both	10	181 ± 23	0.0001	7	192 ± 15	<0.0001	0.2862
≤ 40	Mother	5	191 ± 15	<0.0001	8	193 ± 27	<0.0001	0.8833
≤ 40	Father	4	181 ± 24	0.0010	9	187 ± 26	<0.0001	0.7025
≤ 40	Both	7	203 ± 19	<0.0001	7	196 ± 21	<0.0001	0.5255
> 40	Mother	5	230 ± 22	<0.0001	4	225 ± 36	<0.0001	0.8035
> 40	Father	7	224 ± 27	<0.0001	6	243 ± 29	<0.0001	0.2469
> 40	Both	8	236 ± 30	0.000000	10	241 ± 24	0.000000	0.6992

In the course of former research, it was pointed out that a single passive exposure of smokers or non-smokers to ETS did not increase significantly oxidation susceptibility of LDL-cholesterol or isoprostane formation, the changes were only trend-wise [38], on the contrary does even a single exposure to ETS stimulate platelet activation [39].

Children living together with their (smoking) parents represent true life conditions and are thus an almost ideal group to assess potential effects of ETS. Although there are some limitations in standardizing some parameters like flat size, airing of the room, temperature, humidity, time spent at home, physical behavior, type of tobacco smoked and others.

Some years ago a series of prostaglandin (PG)-like compounds which are formed by free radical induced pe-roxidation of arachidonic acid [40] were discovered in all biological fluids and tissues in concentrations easily to proof.

Serum [41] and urinary [26] concentrations of 8-epi-$PGF_{2\alpha}$, have been extensively used as reliable markers of systemic oxidative stress [42] especially because they show neither gender differences nor circadian variations, only a trend to increase with age. Vascular 8-epi $PG_{2\alpha}$ levels are also indicating oxidative tissue stress [43] and a greater susceptibility to lipid-oxidation of atherosclerotic plaques compared with normal vascular walls [44]. Some of the biological effects of 8-epi-$PGF_{2\alpha}$ include systemic and local vasoconstriction, proliferation of vascular smooth muscle cells and enhanced platelet activation, consequently leading to CHD [45].

Enhanced isoprostane formation has been associated with increased LDL-oxidation, both in-vitro and in-vivo, and was also identified within the vascular wall. Ox-LDL exerts toxic effects on vascular cells [46], causes endothelial dysfunction [47], nitric oxide (NO) reduction [48], platelet activation and induction of a pro-coagulatory state.

To the best of our knowledge, no data on children or juveniles, ETS and iso-eicosanoid formation are currently available. Given the known effects of 8-epi-$PGF_{2\alpha}$ on hemodynamics and vessel walls homeostasis in adults, we aimed to investigate the impact of ETS on 8-epi-$PGF_{2\alpha}$ formation in children. Our data clearly indicate that in children exposed to ETS by parents smoking at home in-vivo oxidative stress increased as evidenced by an elevation of 8-epi-$PGF_{2\alpha}$ both in plasma and urine. This, in turn, may exert pro-atherogenic actions via influencing mediator release, platelet function, lipid metabolism and others. Thus ETS seems to result in a significant oxidative vascular stress already in childhood.

Feldmann J. et al. [13] has investigated the influence of ETS on lipid profile in healthy adolescents from New York by analyzing plasma cotinine levels, as marker of ETS, and lipid profiles in 444 participants. Current smoking habits of parents, siblings and friends as well as personal smoking habits and diet were evaluated by a questionnaire. ETS exposure was then compared between different groups. In participants exposed to ETS HDL-cholesterol levels were decreased by 7-9% and they had a higher ratio of total cholesterol/HDL-cholesterol as compared to controls.

Similar results in children were found by Neufeld et al. [49] who showed a reduction in HDL-cholesterol by 11.2% in children of smoking parents vs. children of non-smoking parents and in the larger Medical College of Virginia twin-study [50], where children exposed to ETS at home had significantly higher total cholesterol-, and lower HDL levels, when compared to a control group.

Our findings show for the first time a significant oxidation injury via increased levels of 8-epi-PGF$_{2\alpha}$, in plasma and urine of children exposed to ETS by smoking parents. This in combination with the above mentioned alterations in the lipid profile due to ETS, underlines the potential link of ETS to the generation of atherosclerosis in childhood. The long-term nature of this exposure underlines its relevance, the clinical value of this exposure concerning the cardiovascular risk, however, still needs to be assessed.

Limitations

Certain parameters like flat size, airing of the room, temperature, humidity, time spent at home, physical behavior of investigated children, as well as type of tobacco smoked were not standardized in this trial.

References

[1]   Streppel, M.T., et al., Mortality and life expectancy in relation to long-term cigarette, cigar and pipe smoking: the Zutphen Study. *Tob Control,* 2007. 16(2): p. 107-13.

[2]   Howard, G., et al., Cigarette smoking and progression of atherosclerosis: The Atherosclerosis Risk in Communities (ARIC) Study. *Jama,* 1998. 279(2): p. 119-24.

[3]   Enstrom, J.E. and G.C. Kabat, Environmental tobacco smoke and coronary heart disease mortality in the United States--a meta-analysis and critique. *Inhal. Toxicol,* 2006. 18(3): p. 199-210.

[4]   Glantz, S.A. and W.W. Parmley, Passive smoking and heart disease. Mechanisms and risk. *Jama,* 1995. 273(13): p. 1047-53.

[5]   Hill, S.E., et al., Mortality among lifelong nonsmokers exposed to secondhand smoke at home: cohort data and sensitivity analyses. *Am. J. Epidemiol.,* 2007. 165(5): p. 530-40.

[6]   Bartal, M., COPD and tobacco smoke. *Monaldi .Arch. Chest. Dis.,* 2005. 63(4): p. 213-25.

[7]   Hirayama, T., Non-smoking wives of heavy smokers have a higher risk of lung cancer: a study from Japan. *Br. Med. J. (Clin. Res. Ed.),* 1981. 282(6259): p. 183-5.

[8]   Klus, H. and H. Kuhn, [Chromatographic evidence for N-nitrosamines of tobacco alkaloids]. *J. Chromatogr.,* 1975. 109(2): p. 425-6.

[9]   Church, D.F. and W.A. Pryor, Free-radical chemistry of cigarette smoke and its toxicological implications. *Environ. Health Perspect,* 1985. 64: p. 111-26.

[10]   Morrow, J.D., et al., Increase in circulating products of lipid peroxidation (F2-isoprostanes) in smokers. Smoking as a cause of oxidative damage. *N. Engl. J. Med.,* 1995. 332(18): p. 1198-203.

[11]   Obot, C., et al., Characterization of mainstream cigarette smoke-induced biomarker responses in ICR and C57Bl/6 mice. *Inhal. Toxicol.,* 2004. 16(10): p. 701-19.

[12] Kato, T., et al., Short-term passive smoking causes endothelial dysfunction via oxidative stress in nonsmokers. *Can. J. Physiol. Pharmacol.*, 2006. 84(5): p. 523-9.

[13] Feldman, J., et al., Passive smoking alters lipid profiles in adolescents. *Pediatrics,* 1991. 88(2): p. 259-64.

[14] Iso, H., et al., Passive smoking and plasma fibrinogen concentrations. *Am. J. Epidemiol.,* 1996. 144(12): p. 1151-4.

[15] Lubawy, W.C. and M.A. Valentovic, Chronic exposure to high levels of sidestream smoke adversely alters 14C-arachidonic acid metabolism in rat platelets and aortas. *Prostaglandins Leukot. Med.,* 1985. 19(2): p. 131-2.

[16] Keith, R.L., et al., Pulmonary prostacyclin synthase overexpression chemoprevents tobacco smoke lung carcinogenesis in mice. *Cancer Res.,* 2004. 64(16): p. 5897-904.

[17] Davis, J.W., et al., Passive smoking affects endothelium and platelets. *Arch. Intern. Med.,* 1989. 149(2): p. 386-9.

[18] Berliner, J.A. and J.W. Heinecke, The role of oxidized lipoproteins in atherogenesis. *Free Radic. Biol. Med.,* 1996. 20(5): p. 707-27.

[19] Zhang, H., Y. Yang, and U.P. Steinbrecher, Structural requirements for the binding of modified proteins to the scavenger receptor of macrophages. *J. Biol. Chem.,* 1993. 268(8): p. 5535-42.

[20] Scheffler, E., et al., Smoking influences the atherogenic potential of low-density lipoprotein. *Clin. Investig.,* 1992. 70(3-4): p. 263-8.

[21] He, J., et al. Passive smoking and the risk of coronary heart disease--a meta-analysis of epidemiologic studies. *N. Engl. J. Med.* 1999 Mar 25 [cited 340 12]; 920-6].

[22] Kawachi, I., et al., A prospective study of passive smoking and coronary heart disease. *Circulation,* 1997. 95(10): p. 2374-9.

[23] Zhu, B.Q., et al., Passive smoking increases experimental atherosclerosis in cholesterol-fed rabbits. *J. Am. Coll .Cardiol.,* 1993. 21(1): p. 225-32.

[24] Burghuber, O.C., et al., Platelet sensitivity to prostacyclin in smokers and non-smokers. *Chest,* 1986. 90(1): p. 34-8.

[25] Morrow, J.D., et al., A series of prostaglandin F2-like compounds are produced in vivo in humans by a non-cyclooxygenase, free radical-catalyzed mechanism. *Proc. Natl. Acad. Sci. U S A,* 1990. 87(23): p. 9383-7.

[26] Wang, Z., et al., Immunological characterization of urinary 8-epi-prostaglandin F2 alpha excretion in man. *J. Pharmacol. Exp. Ther.,* 1995. 275(1): p. 94-100.

[27] Oguogho, A., et al., 6-oxo-PGF(1 alpha)and 8-epi-PGF(2 alpha)in the arterial wall layers of various species: a comparison between intact and atherosclerotic areas. *Prostaglandins Leukot. Essent. Fatty Acids,* 2001. 64(3): p. 167-71.

[28] Doll, R., et al., Mortality in relation to smoking: 40 years' observations on male British doctors. *Bmj,* 1994. 309(6959): p. 901-11.

[29] Dwyer, J.H., Exposure to environmental tobacco smoke and coronary risk. Circulation, 1997. 96(5): p. 1367-9.

[30] Pirkle, J.L., et al., Exposure of the US population to environmental tobacco smoke: the Third National Health and Nutrition Examination Survey, 1988 to 1991. *Jama,* 1996. 275(16): p. 1233-40.

[31] Rona, R.J. and S. Chinn, Lung function, respiratory illness, and passive smoking in British primary school children. *Thorax,* 1993. 48(1): p. 21-5.

[32] Magnussen, H., et al., Effects of acute passive smoking on exercise-induced bronchoconstriction in asthmatic children. *J. Appl. Physiol.,* 1993. 75(2): p. 553-8.

[33] Beauloye, V., et al., Determinants of Early Atherosclerosis in Obese Children and Adolescents. *J. Clin. Endocrinol. Metab.,* 2007. 92(8): p. 3025-3032.

[34] Misra, A., Risk factors for atherosclerosis in young individuals. *J. Cardiovasc. Risk,* 2000. 7(3): p. 215-29.

[35] Dhalla, N.S., R.M. Temsah, and T. Netticadan, Role of oxidative stress in cardiovascular diseases. *J. Hypertens.,* 2000. 18(6): p. 655-73.

[36] Kristensen, T.S., Cardiovascular diseases and the work environment. A critical review of the epidemiologic literature on chemical factors. *Scand J. Work Environ. Health,* 1989. 15(4): p. 245-64.

[37] Siegel, M., Involuntary smoking in the restaurant workplace. A review of employee exposure and health effects. *Jama,* 1993. 270(4): p. 490-3.

[38] Oguogho, A., H. Kritz, and H. Sinzinger, [Single passive smoking exposure induces no measurable oxidation of low density lipoproteins]. *Wien Klin Wochenschr,* 1996. 108(18): p. 589-92.

[39] Kritz, H. and H. Sinzinger, Passive smoking, platelet function and atherosclerosis. *Wien Klin Wochenschr,* 1996. 108(18): p. 582-8.

[40] Rokach, J., et al., The isoprostanes: a perspective. Prostaglandins, 1997. 54(6): p. 823-51.

[41] Morrow, J.D., et al., Evidence that the F2-isoprostane, 8-epi-prostaglandin F2 alpha, is formed in vivo. *Biochim. Biophys. Acta,* 1994. 1210(2): p. 244-8.

[42] Bachi, A., et al., Measurement of urinary 8-Epi-prostaglandin F2alpha, a novel index of lipid peroxidation in vivo, by immunoaffinity extraction/gas chromatography-mass spectrometry. Basal levels in smokers and nonsmokers. *Free. Radic. Biol. Med.,* 1996. 20(4): p. 619-24.

[43] Pratico, D., et al., Localization of distinct F2-isoprostanes in human atherosclerotic lesions. *J. Clin. Invest.,* 1997. 100(8): p. 2028-34.

[44] Reilly, M.P., et al., Increased formation of distinct F2 isoprostanes in hypercholesterolemia. *Circulation,* 1998. 98(25): p. 2822-8.

[45] Fukunaga, M., T. Yura, and K.F. Badr, Stimulatory effect of 8-Epi-PGF2 alpha, an F2-isoprostane, on endothelin-1 release. *J. Cardiovasc. Pharmacol.,* 1995. 26 Suppl 3: p. S51-2.

[46] Morel, D.W., J.R. Hessler, and G.M. Chisolm, Low density lipoprotein cytotoxicity induced by free radical peroxidation of lipid. *J. Lipid. Res.,* 1983. 24(8): p. 1070-6.

[47] Kugiyama, K., et al., Impairment of endothelium-dependent arterial relaxation by lysolecithin in modified low-density lipoproteins. *Nature,* 1990. 344(6262): p. 160-2.

[48] Chin, J.H., S. Azhar, and B.B. Hoffman, Inactivation of endothelial derived relaxing factor by oxidized lipoproteins. *J. Clin. Invest.,* 1992. 89(1): p. 10-8.

[49] Neufeld, E.J., et al., Passive cigarette smoking and reduced HDL cholesterol levels in children with high-risk lipid profiles. *Circulation,* 1997. 96(5): p. 1403-7.

[50] Moskowitz, W.B., et al., Lipoprotein and oxygen transport alterations in passive smoking preadolescent children. The MCV Twin Study. *Circulation,* 1990. 81(2): p. 586-92.

Index

B

D

I

J

K

L

N

S

T

X

Y

Z